# Subcortical Neurosurgery

Gabriel Zada • Gustavo Pradilla • J. D. Day
Editors

# Subcortical Neurosurgery

## Open and Parafascicular Channel-Based Approaches for Subcortical and Intraventricular Lesions

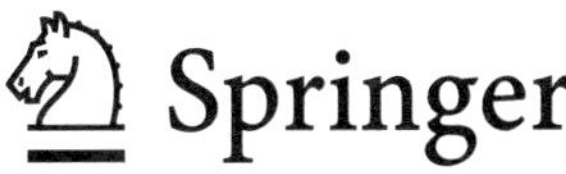 Springer

*Editors*
Gabriel Zada
Department of Neurosurgery
University of Southern California
LOS ANGELES, CA
USA

Gustavo Pradilla
School of Medicine
Emory University
Atlanta, GA
USA

J. D. Day
Department of Neurosurgery
University of Arkansas for
Medical Sciences
Little Rock, AR
USA

ISBN 978-3-030-95155-9      ISBN 978-3-030-95153-5   (eBook)
https://doi.org/10.1007/978-3-030-95153-5



This Springer imprint is published by the registered company Springer Nature Switzerland AG
The registered company address is: Gewerbestrasse 11, 6330 Cham, Switzerland

# Preface

Access to subcortical lesions has been the topic of numerous surgical and technical innovations since the beginning of neurosurgery. The concept for this textbook evolved as a result of rapid innovation within the field of subcortical surgery, and the integrated efforts of numerous scientists, biomedical engineers, neurosurgeons, and industry partners who collectively defined the subcortical space as the "final frontier" of neurological surgery in need for more accurate, precise, and effective surgical innovation.

The wide assortment of techniques developed to navigate the inherent challenges presented by the multitude of etiologies encountered in the subcortical space and the idiosyncrasies related to their location within the parenchymal substance and ventricular system traditionally failed to recognize the immense complexity of the subcortical space, which has only been elucidated recently thanks to advances in neuro-imaging (particularly diffusion tensor imaging), neuro-navigation, functional neuro-anatomy, surgical instrumentation and technique, and refinement of indications and outcomes.

A more sophisticated understanding of complex subcortical structures, the intricate relationships among them, and their plasticity under pathologic conditions was finally realized through our ability to image, map, and understand their functional correlates, resulting in a collective call for surgically applicable tools for identifying and sparing this critical anatomy to maximally preserve neurological function.

This paradigm shift in subcortical surgery **views all brain tissue as eloquent tissue**, and maintains the uncompromised principle of only traversing brain tissue on the way to a neurosurgical target with minimal collateral damage. The judicious application of this principle translated into novel approaches for a variety of subcortical and intraventricular lesions, ranging from intracerebral hemorrhages (ICH) to subcortical tumors and intraventricular colloid cysts, among many others. The concept for this textbook emerged from collaborations within the *Subcortical Surgery Group* and cooperation with key industry partners in an effort to expeditiously push this cutting edge forward.

We, the editors, would like to thank the many contributing authors of this textbook, who are each and all world experts on the front lines of the rapidly advancing field of subcortical surgery. This compendium of high-yield knowledge and surgical pearls has been selectively curated by the editorial team to provide the reader with a comprehensive understanding pertaining to the anatomy, neuro-imaging, existing technology, and surgical techniques and outcomes associated with subcortical neurosurgery. The chapters provide focused explanations of open and minimally invasive, port-based approaches to the subcortical and intraventricular spaces, case examples, and strategies to deal with selected pathology and intraoperative complications.

It is our collective hope that this textbook will provide readers with a comprehensive and one-stop reference for subcortical anatomy and surgery. It is also our hope that this book will be made obsolete soon, in the sense that this will only reflect the unprecedented pace at which the field and technology within subcortical surgery is evolving. We hope that readers derive significant benefit from the unparalleled work provided by the authorship of this book.

Los Angeles, CA, USA                                               Gabriel Zada
Atlanta, GA, USA                                               Gustavo Pradilla
Little Rock, AR, USA                                                   J. D. Day

# Contents

# Contributors

**Kumar Abhinav, FRCS (SN)** Stanford Neurosurgical Training and Innovation Center, Stanford University, Stanford, CA, USA

Department of Neurosurgery, Bristol Institute of Clinical Neuroscience, Center for Skull Base and Pituitary Neurosurgery, Southmead Hospital, Bristol, UK

Department of Neurosurgery, Stanford University School of Medicine, Stanford, CA, USA

**Juan Altafulla, MD** Jose Domingo de Obaldia Hospital, Department of Surgery, Panama, Panama

**Julian Bailes, MD** NorthShore University Health Systems, Department of Neurosurgery, Evanston, IL, USA

**Mark D. Bain, MD** Department of Neurosurgery, Cleveland Clinic Foundation, Cleveland, OH, USA

**Joshua Bakhsheshian, MD** University of Southern California, Department of Neurosurgery, Los Angeles, CA, USA

**Evan D. Bander, MD** NewYork-Presbyterian Hospital, Weill Cornell Medicine, Department of Neurosurgery, New York, NY, USA

**J. Manuel Revuelta Barbero, MD, PhD** Department of Neurosurgery, Emory University, Atlanta, GA, USA

**David Bray, MD** Department of Neurosurgery, Emory University School of Medicine, Atlanta, GA, USA

**Claudio Cavallo, MD** Vanderbilt University Medical Center, Department of Neurosurgery, Nashville, TN, USA

**Kaisorn L. Chaichana, MD, FAACS, FAANS** Department of Neurosurgery, Mayo Clinic Florida, Jacksonville, FL, USA

**Aaron Cohen-Gadol, MD** *The Neurosurgical Atlas*, Carmel, IN, USA
Department of Neurological Surgery, Indiana University, Indianapolis, IN, USA

**J. D. Day, MD** Department of Neurosurgery, University of Arkansas for Medical Sciences, Little Rock, AR, USA

**Nicholas B. Dadario, BS** Robert Wood Johnson Medical School, Rutgers University, New Brunswick, NJ, USA

**Courtney Duong, BS** David Geffen School of Medicine, Department of Neurosurgery, Los Angeles, CA, USA

**Thiago Albonette Felicio, MD** The Ohio State University Wexner Medical Center, Department of Neurological Surgery, Columbus, OH, USA

**Juan Fernandez-Miranda, MD** Stanford Neurosurgical Training and Innovation Center, Stanford University, Stanford, CA, USA
Department of Neurosurgery, Stanford University School of Medicine, Stanford, CA, USA

**Sirin Gandhi, MD** St. Joseph's Hospital and Medical Center, Department of Surgery, Phoenix, AZ, USA

**Cristian Gragnaniello, MD, PhD** Department of Neurosurgery, UT Health San Antonio, San Antonio, TX, USA

**Paul E. Kim, MD** Division of Neuroradiology, Department of Radiology, University of Southern California Keck School of Medicine, Los Angeles, CA, USA

**Won Kim, MD** Ronald Reagan UCLA Medical Center, Department of Neurosurgery, Los Angeles, CA, USA

**Aditya Kondajji, BS** Ronald Reagan UCLA Medical Center, Department of Neurosurgery, Los Angeles, CA, USA

**Charles Kulwin, MD** Goodman Campbell Brain and Spine, Carmel, IN, USA

**Mohamed A. Labib, MD** Department of Neurosurgery, University of Maryland Medical Center, Baltimore, MD, USA

**Zachary N. Litvack, MD, MCR** Neuroscience Institute, Swedish Medical Center, Seattle, WA, USA

**Lina Marenco-Hillembrand, MD** Department of Neurosurgery, Mayo Clinic Florida, Jacksonville, FL, USA

**Sandip S. Panesar** Stanford Neurosurgical Training and Innovation Center, Stanford University, Stanford, CA, USA

**Sean P. Polster, MD** University of Chicago, Department of Neurosurgery, Chicago, IL, USA

**Gustavo Pradilla, MD, FAANS** Neurological Surgery, Emory University School of Medicine, Atlanta, GA, USA

**Daniel M. Prevedello, MD** The Ohio State University Wexner Medical Center, Department of Neurological Surgery, Columbus, OH, USA

**Joshua Prickett, DO** Aiken Regional Medical Centers, Department of Surgery, Aiken, SC, USA

**Rohan Ramakrishna, MD** NewYork-Presbyterian Hospital, Weill Cornell Medicine, Department of Neurological Surgery, New York, NY, USA

**Rima Sestokas Rindler, MD** The Mayo Clinic, Department of Neurosurgery, Rochester, MN, USA

**Prasanth Romiyo, BS** Tina & Fred Segal Brain Tumor and Skull Base Research Fellow, Ronald Reagan UCLA Medical Center, Department of Neurosurgery, Los Angeles, CA, USA

**David Satzer, MD** University of Chicago, Department of Neurosurgery, Chicago, IL, USA

**Robert A. Scranton, MD** Department of Neurosurgery, Indiana University School of Medicine, Indianapolis, USA

**Mitesh V. Shah, MD** Department of Neurosurgery, Indiana University School of Medicine, Indianapolis, USA

**Mohamed A. R. Soliman, MD, MSc, PhD** Faculty of Medicine, Department of Neurosurgery, Cairo University, Cairo, Egypt

Department of Neurosurgery, Jacobs School of Medicine and Biomedical Science, University at Buffalo, New York, NY, USA

**Ben Allen Strickland, MD** Los Angeles County General Hospital, Department of Neurosurgery, Los Angeles, CA, USA

**Michael E. Sughrue, MD** Department of Neurosurgery, Prince of Wales Hospital, Sydney, NSW, Australia

**Jonathan Weyhenmeyer, MD** Department of Neurosurgery, Indiana University School of Medicine, Indianapolis, IN, USA

**Benjamin B. Whiting, MD** Department of Neurosurgery, Cleveland Clinic Foundation, Cleveland, OH, USA

**Yuanzhi Xu, MD** Stanford Neurosurgical Training and Innovation Center, Stanford University, Stanford, CA, USA

Department of Neurosurgery, Huashan Hospital, Shanghai Medical College, Fudan University, Shanghai, China

**Isaac Yang, MD** Ronald Reagan UCLA Medical Center, Department of Neurosurgery, Los Angeles, CA, USA

**Gabriel Zada, MD, MS** Keck Hospital, Neurological Surgery, Los Angeles, CA, USA

**Xiaochun Zhao, MD** OU Health, Department of Neurosurgery, Oklahoma City, OK, USA

**Peizhi Zhou, MD** Department of Neurosurgery, West China Hospital of Sichuan University, Chengdu, City, China

# Chapter 1
# The Subcortical Space: Anatomy of Subcortical White Matter

Sandip S. Panesar, Kumar Abhinav, Peizhi Zhou, Yuanzhi Xu, and Juan Fernandez-Miranda

## Introduction

A thorough understanding of subcortical white matter anatomy is critical for the neurosurgeon. Subcortical white matter consists of myelinated axon fibers arranged in anatomically relevant discrete bundles or fascicles. The subcortical white matter

S. S. Panesar
Stanford Neurosurgical Training and Innovation Center, Stanford University, Stanford, CA, USA

K. Abhinav
Stanford Neurosurgical Training and Innovation Center, Stanford University, Stanford, CA, USA

Department of Neurosurgery, Bristol Institute of Clinical Neuroscience, Center for Skull Base and Pituitary Neurosurgery, Southmead Hospital, Bristol, UK

Department of Neurosurgery, Stanford University School of Medicine, Stanford, CA, USA
e-mail: kumar.abhinav@doctors.org.uk

P. Zhou
Department of Neurosurgery, West China Hospital of Sichuan University, Chengdu City, China

Y. Xu
Stanford Neurosurgical Training and Innovation Center, Stanford University, Stanford, CA, USA

Department of Neurosurgery, Huashan Hospital, Shanghai Medical College, Fudan University, Shanghai, China

J. Fernandez-Miranda (✉)
Stanford Neurosurgical Training and Innovation Center, Stanford University, Stanford, CA, USA

Department of Neurosurgery, Stanford University School of Medicine, Stanford, CA, USA
e-mail: drjfm@stanford.edu

© Springer Nature Switzerland AG 2022
G. Zada et al. (eds.), *Subcortical Neurosurgery*,
https://doi.org/10.1007/978-3-030-95153-5_1

fasciculi are anatomo-functionally categorized into projection, association, limbic, commissural, or U-fiber systems. Aside from the U-fiber system, which, by definition, consists of short cortico-cortical fibers between adjacent gyri, the other systems consist of both long- and short-range fasciculi assuming either intra- or interlobar (or interhemispheric, if commissural) courses [1].

Traditionally, anatomical descriptions of human subcortical white matter anatomy came from postmortem dissection techniques. These descriptions persisted until the latter twentieth century until the introduction of diffusion magnetic resonance imaging (MRI) tractography. Though historically important as a foundation for anatomical understanding, postmortem dissection suffers from several key limitations including substantial time taken to acquire, prepare, and dissect specimens, permitting few subjects per study; a loss of anatomical integrity due to preparation; destruction of specimens due to a lateral-medial dissection approach; and the inability to accurately determine cortical connectivity. Radioisotope tracer injection in nonhuman primates is considered the "gold standard" approach for studying white matter cortical connectivity. Nevertheless, as these require sacrifice of the study subject, they cannot be utilized in humans. Moreover, translating simian neuroanatomical findings to humans is problematic, however, due to the evolutionary divergence between species.

MRI tractography is a technique of measuring the diffusion properties of water confined within myelinated axons noninvasively and, most importantly, in vivo [2]. The introduction of tractography toward the 1990s permitted study of white matter in large numbers of healthy and diseased subjects. Most importantly for the neurosurgeon, tractography permits the study of white matter architecture affected by the presence of space-occupying lesions [3, 4]. By visualizing white matter tract displacement, disruption, or infiltration by tumors or other pathologies, the neurosurgeon may tailor their approach to the lesion so as to cause minimal damage to the perilesional white matter while safely maximizing the extent of resection. The trade-off between the extent of resection and functional outcome may therefore be optimized, especially when preoperative tractography is utilized in conjunction with other functional adjuncts such as functional imaging or use of awake craniotomy. Intraoperative electrical stimulation (IES), in this respect, is considered a gold standard and also affords a unique opportunity to further study and understand the function of different white matter tracts.

## Projection System

The projection fasciculi subserve core sensorimotor functionality. These include the ascending sensory pathways, the descending motor pathways, and the audiovisual afferents (Fig. 1.1a).

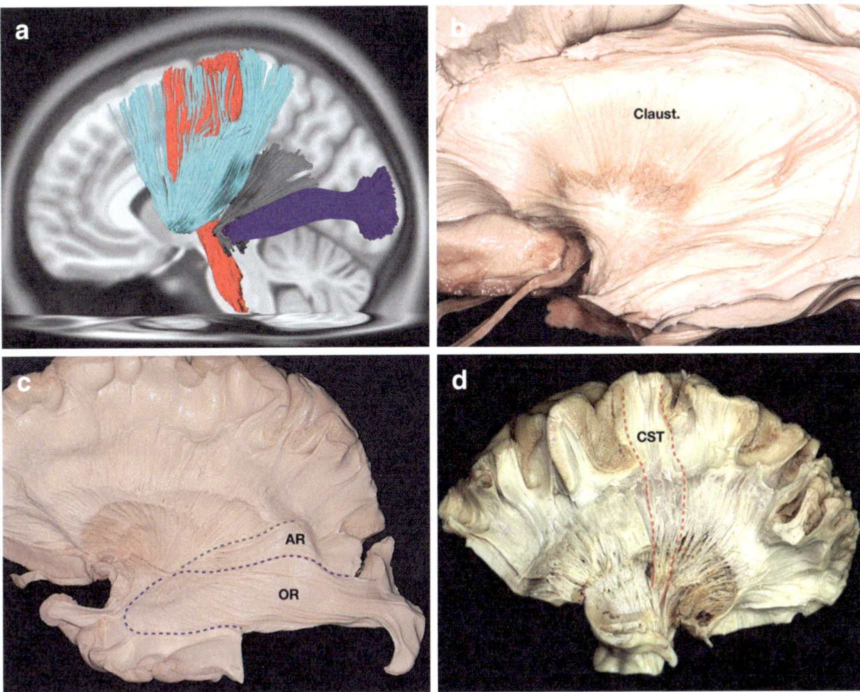

**Fig. 1.1** (**a**) Tractography of the projection white matter tracts. Left sagittal view. The claustro-cortical system (light blue) lies superficial to the cortical terminations of the corticospinal tracts (red). Rostrally-caudally are the acoustic radiations (gray) and optic radiations (purple). (**b**) Dissection of a postmortem specimen. View of the left hemisphere following removal of the gray matter, U-fibers, and superficial association system to reveal the claustrum (Claust.) lying within the extreme capsular structures. (**c**) Another view of the left hemisphere from a postmortem specimen. More white matter has been removed from the extreme and external capsules to reveal the underlying optic radiations (OR) and acoustic radiations (AR). (**d**) In this view of a postmortem left-hemisphere, the corticospinal tracts (CST) have been exposed

## *Claustro-Cortical Fibers*

The claustrum is a collection of peri-insular gray matter lying in between the extreme and external capsules. Projection fibers fan out in a sheetlike arrangement from the claustrum and travel to the superior frontal, precentral, postcentral, and posterior parietal cortices. The claustro-cortical fiber system lies dorsal to the inferior fronto-occipital and uncinate fasciculi within the external capsule (Fig. 1.1b).

## *Optic Radiations*

The optic radiations are the final portion of the visual pathways. They begin at the lateral geniculate nucleus of the thalamus before radiating anterolaterally into the substance of the temporal lobe. As they travel anteriorly, they are medial to the medial wall of the temporal horn of the lateral ventricle. The optic radiations then turn sharply, continuing to fan out while passing over the roof of the anterior temporal horn before assuming a position lateral to the lateral wall of the temporal horn and continuing posteriorly. The optic radiations remain lateral to the lateral wall of the temporal horn, traversing most medially within the sagittal stratum into the occipital lobe, where they terminate on either side of the calcarine sulcus. Like all white matter, the optic radiations are anatomo-functionally organized, with the upper division (Baum's loop) carrying sensory information from the inferior visual quadrants and the lower division (Meyer's loop) carrying sensory information from the superior visual quadrants. Lesions to the optic radiations produce characteristic visual field deficits depending upon the location of the lesion (Fig. 1.1c).

## Acoustic Radiations

The acoustic radiations originate from the medial geniculate nucleus of the thalamus. They assume a tortuous S shape and pass medially-laterally as they travel into the dorsal temporal lobe. From the medial geniculate nucleus, the acoustic radiations first pass underneath the optic radiations. They pass upward via internal capsule and backward along the inferior sulcus of the insula, into the temporal lobe, where they pass perpendicular to the fibers of the temporal stem (inferior fronto-occipital, inferior longitudinal, and uncinate fasciculi). They terminate at Heschl's gyrus of the temporal lobe, which lies on its dorsal surface, within the Sylvian fissure (Fig. 1.1c).

## Geniculate Motor Fibers

The geniculate tracts transmit motor information to the peripheral nervous system. They consist of two functionally distinct fiber populations: corticospinal (controlling limb movements) and corticobulbar (controlling cranial motor function) projections. The geniculate fibers all originate in layer V pyramidal neurons of the premotor, motor, and supplementary motor cortices. At their origin, they are fanned out radially, along the motor strip, which is bounded dorsally and medially by the sagittal sulcus, and ventrally and laterally by the Sylvian fissure. The dorsomedially originating fibers travel caudally, while the ventrolaterally originating fibers travel medially and over the dorsomedial fibers as they converge at the corona radiata. The geniculate tracts therefore assume a "twisted" arrangement. After passing through the genu of the internal capsule, the bundle travels into the brainstem via the crus cerebri. The corticospinal projections lie anterior to the corticobulbar projections. In the brainstem, corticospinal fibers pass into the medulla via the pons, prior to decussating at the pyramids and continuing as the lateral corticospinal tract. At the level of the brainstem, the corticobulbar fibers synapse upon the appropriate cranial nerve nuclei (Fig. 1.1d).

## Corticocerebellar Fibers

The corticocerebellar fibers transmit information to and from the cerebellum and its nuclei. They originate from all cortical areas and can be classified according to their site of origin from the hemispheric lobes. These fibers generally include the pontine nuclei as a waypoint between the cerebral cortices and the cerebellum and are also known as the corticopontocerebellar fibers. From their cortical origins, they all travel caudally via the internal capsule and crus cerebri in an organized fashion. For example, fibers originating from the prefrontal and frontal cortices travel most anteriorly within the internal capsule, whereas fibers originating from the occipital cortex travel most posteriorly. Corticopontocerebellar fibers from all lobes converge within the posterior limb of the internal capsule before passing via the crus cerebri to the pons where they decussate. The corticopontocerebellar fibers henceforth travel via the middle cerebellar peduncle to their cerebellar terminations.

## Sensory Projection Fibers

The dorsal columns of the spinal cord carrying vibration, proprioception, fine touch, and discriminative sensory information ascend the spinal cord, synapsing upon the gracile (below T6 level) and cuneate (above T6 level) nuclei within the medulla. From these medullary nuclei, the medial lemniscus pathway decussates and ascends via the mesencephalon to the thalamus, synapsing upon the ventral posterior nucleus of the thalamus. The anterolateral system carries sensations of crude touch and pressure (anterior spinothalamic tract) and pain and temperature (lateral spinothalamic tract). These enter the spinal cord and ascend briefly (1–2 levels) before decussating and travelling to the various thalamic nuclei. The lateral spinothalamic tract travels through the brainstem via the spinal lemniscus and synapses at the ventroposterolateral thalamic nucleus. The anterior spinothalamic tract joins the medial lemniscus to travel to the ventral posterior thalamic nucleus. From the thalamus, the sensory projections travel to the postcentral gyrus of the parietal lobe via the thalamocortical radiations, which pass through the internal capsule. Some thalamocortical projections travel to the limbic system via the cingulum.

## Projection System: Surgical Considerations

Damage to motor pathways may result in partial or complete hemiparesis. Likewise, damage to the optic radiations (e.g., during temporal lobe resections) can produce visual field deficits. Several methods exist to delineate their course both preoperatively and intraoperatively. Preoperatively, functional methods such as functional MRI (fMRI) or magnetoencephalography (MEG) may be used. These techniques permit localization of functional cortex specific to particular tasks. Nevertheless, they cannot reliably demonstrate the subcortical course of white matter tracts. Tractography is able to reliably demonstrate corticospinal projections from their cortical origin to the medullary level (or below) and has thus become commonplace for preoperative localization [3]. It can also demonstrate the optic radiations; however, some algorithms have difficulty reproducing the full extent of Meyer's loop due to its sharp turn over the anterior horn. Efforts have been made to integrate both fMRI and MEG with tractography, with the functional techniques utilized to create regions of interest from which fiber tracking algorithms may be launched [5, 6]. This is particularly useful when considering that lesions may grow within or in close proximity to eloquent white matter. In these instances, delineation of white matter anatomy is critical for presurgical planning. Intraoperative electrical stimulation (IES) is also a valuable tool [7] as it permits direct intraoperative functional localization, which may ultimately determine resection extent. The complementary use of all aforementioned techniques may ultimately enhance both preoperative and intraoperative anatomo-functional localization.

## Limbic System

The limbic system subserves emotional and memory functionality. It consists of both large and small white matter fasciculi which interconnect subcortical gray matter nuclei and the parahippocampal regions. The primary limbic white matter components are the cingulum and fornix; however, many smaller tracts also interconnect the telencephalon with the diencephalon and mesencephalon (Fig. 1.2a).

### *Cingulum*

The cingulum is the long white matter tract travelling parasagittally on either side of the central sulcus. It originates in the orbitofrontal regions, ventral to the rostrum of the corpus callosum, travelling first anteriorly, and then curving around the genu, to eventually lie dorsal to the corpus callosum along its anteroposterior course. At the posterior sagittal limit of the corpus callosum, the cingulum curves around the splenium, travelling caudally and laterally to terminate in the parahippocampal regions. The para-splenial curving cingulate fibers are also known as the isthmus. The cingulate course is contained within the cingulate gyrus, which lies atop the corpus callosum. The cingulum is unique in that it is comprised of both long and short fibers, giving off connections at all points along its longitudinal course (Fig. 1.2b).

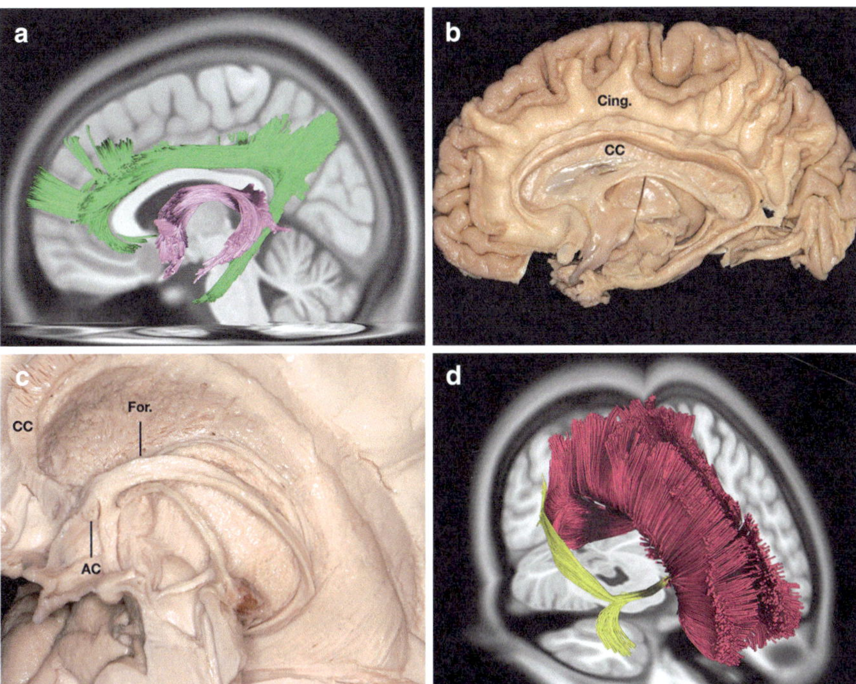

**Fig. 1.2** (**a**) Tractography of the limbic white matter tracts. Visible in this left sagittal view are the cingulum (bright green) and fornix (pink). (**b**) A medial view of the right hemisphere in a postmortem specimen. The specimen has been transected at the corpus callosum (CC). The cingulum (Cing.) has been exposed. (**c**) Further dissection of the medial aspect of the hemisphere reveals the fornix (For.) and the anterior commissure (AC) . (**d**) An oblique anterior tractographic view depicting the corpus callosum (dark purple), lying dorsal to the anterior commissure (dark yellow). The anterior and posterior fibers of the anterior commissure and its distinct handlebar shape are visible from this view

## *Fornix and Mammillothalamic Tracts*

The fornix is the main efferent limbic pathway. Within the temporal lobe, the fornix originates from the subiculum and entorhinal cortex as the fimbria travelling posterolaterally as the forniceal crus within each hemisphere. Each crus curves rostrally around its respective thalamic pulvinar to lie on top of the thalamus, where they join to form the forniceal body in the midline. The commissural fibers interconnecting each crus within the body region are known as the psalterium or the hippocampal commissure. The body continues anteriorly, to the anterior longitudinal extremity of the thalamus, where it subsequently separates again. Each hemispheric fornix subsequently divides again into anterior and posterior columns, bisected by the anterior commissure. Anterior fibers primarily terminate within the septal area, the lateral preoptic area, and the hypothalamus. The posterior columns primarily terminate within the mamillary bodies. The mammillothalamic tracts are short fibers ascending from the mamillary bodies, terminating within the anterior nucleus of the thalamus (Fig. 1.2c).

## *Limbic System: Surgical Considerations*

Lesions arising at the medial hemispheric surfaces may affect limbic structures. Dorsally, tumors may grow at any point along the cingulate gyrus: the medial surfaces of the frontal, parietal, or occipital lobes, which can impinge upon the cingulum [8]. Likewise, tumors may arise at the medial surface of the temporal lobe, which may affect the temporal components of the cingulum and fornix. Tumors may also arise within the diencephalic structures (thalamus, hypothalamus, and ventricles) and the corpus callosum. Due to the abstract functionality of the limbic structures, lesions growing within or near to limbic white matter may remain largely asymptomatic and cause relatively little distortion to surrounding white matter structures until large in size. Approaches to these lesions may include anterior, middle, or posterior interhemispheric and supracerebellar-transtentorial corridors [9]. These approaches are preferable to transcortical approaches where a certain extent of cortical transgression and disruption of the white matter is required to reach the lesion. Interhemispheric approaches, however, come with a potential risk of injuring the draining parasagittal cortical draining veins which should be studied carefully preoperatively using a MR venogram. For approaches to medial temporal structures, such as during amygdalohippocampectomy, a trans-Sylvian approach minimizes the risk of injury to the optic radiations in the roof of the temporal horn [10].

## Commissural System

### *Anterior Commissure*

The anterior commissure connects the hemispheres across the midline. It is frequently described as having a "handlebar" arrangement. The body of the anterior commissure runs transversely in the coronal plane, to cross the midline, ventral to the supraoptic recess of the third ventricle. At its lateral extents, it bifurcates into both anterior and posterior divisions. The anterior divisions run forward within the canal of Gratiolet, parallel to the temporal stem fascicles (uncinate and inferior fronto-occipital). These terminate within the anterior olfactory nucleus bilaterally. The posterior fibers travel posteriorly within the temporal lobe, deep to the lentiform nucleus, terminating within the middle temporal gyrus. Some fibers blend with the sagittal stratum of the external capsule (Fig. 1.2d).

## *Corpus Callosum*

The corpus callosum is the predominant interhemispheric conduit. It is a thick collection of transversely travelling fibers joining the two hemispheres together across the sagittal midline. When transected and viewed from a sagittal perspective, it resembles a helmet, with the third ventricle underneath and the cingulate gyri on top. The corpus callosum is routinely divided along its sagittal length, with the genu as its most rostral segment. The rostrum curves dorsally and continues posteriorly as the genu. The middle portion is known as the body, followed by the isthmus. The splenium is the posteriormost extent of the corpus callosum (Fig. 1.2c, d).

## *Commissural System: Surgical Considerations*

The corpus callosum is typically accessed using parasagittal craniotomy and dissection of the interhemispheric fissure while paying close attention to the anterior cerebral arteries. In an effort to prevent the spread of epileptiform activity across the hemispheres, partial or total division of the corpus callosum is a well-recognized surgical treatment modality [11]. Division of callosal fibers may cause disconnection syndromes depending upon the region at which they are transected: Transection of the corpus callosum at the splenium at the parieto-occipital section may produce nondominant hand agraphia and alexia without agraphia. Splitting the corpus callosum at the area of the postcentral gyrus may result in hemispatial neglect and tactile dysnomia, whereas lesions of the precentral corpus callosum may produce alien hand syndrome [12]. Typically, the risk of disconnection syndrome increases with a more posterior disruption or disconnection of the callosal fibers.

## Association System

The association system comprises the majority of subcortical white matter. Unlike the projection and limbic pathways, however, the anatomy and roles of particular association fasciculi are open to considerable debate. Traditionally, association fasciculi were grouped with adjacent association tracts and thought to be anatomo-functionally related. With the introduction of tractography, new insights into association fascicle anatomy have been gained, particularly regarding connective, volumetric, and morphological hemispheric asymmetry (Figs. 1.3 and 1.4).

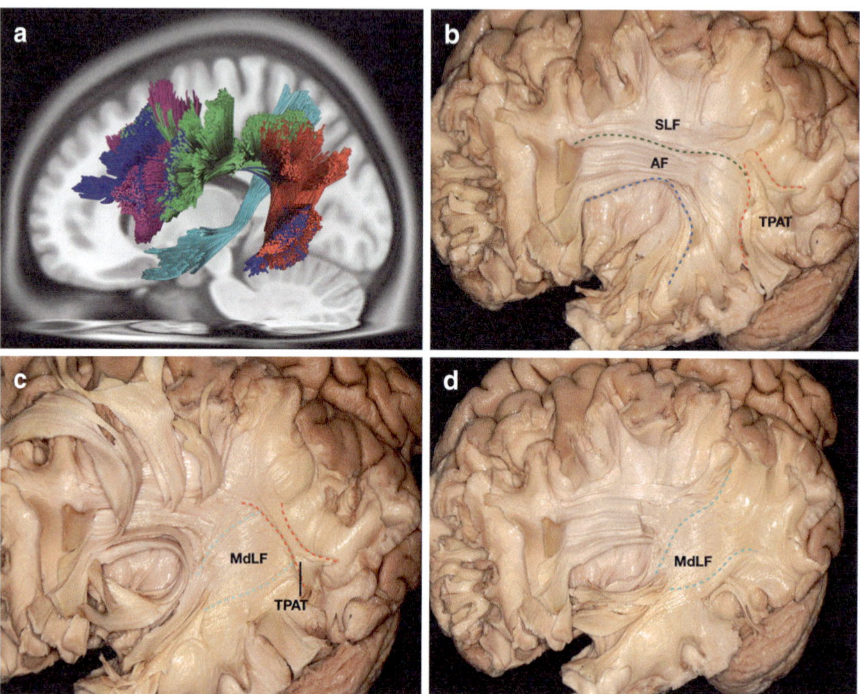



**Fig. 1.3** (**a**) Tractography of the dorsal association matter tracts. Visible in this left sagittal view are the temporoparietal aslant tract (red), superior longitudinal fasciculus (green), arcuate fasciculus (dark blue), frontal aslant tract (dark purple), and middle longitudinal fasciculus (light blue). (**b**) Dissection of a postmortem specimen. View of the left hemisphere. The cortical gray matter and underlying U-fibers have been removed to reveal the superior longitudinal fasciculus (SLF), arcuate fasciculus (AF), and temporoparietal aslant tract (TPAT). (**c**) Upon further dissection of the same specimen in 3B, the AF and SLF have been peeled away to reveal the middle longitudinal fasciculus (MdLF), leaving only the most posterior fibers of the TPAT. (**d**) Upon further dissection of the same specimen in 3A, and 3B, the TPAT has been peeled away to reveal the MdLF

## Dorsal Association Fasciculi (Superficial Deep)

### *Arcuate Fasciculus*

The arcuate fasciculus (AF) lies immediately underneath the TPAT. It is a long, leftward-lateralized fiber tract that connects the temporal and frontal lobes. The name derives from its arc-like course as it travels around the Sylvian fissure. Older descriptions of the AF described a three-part arrangement consisting of two superficial (anterior and posterior/horizontal and vertical) and a single deep "arcuate" component. With introduction of high spatial resolution tractography, this

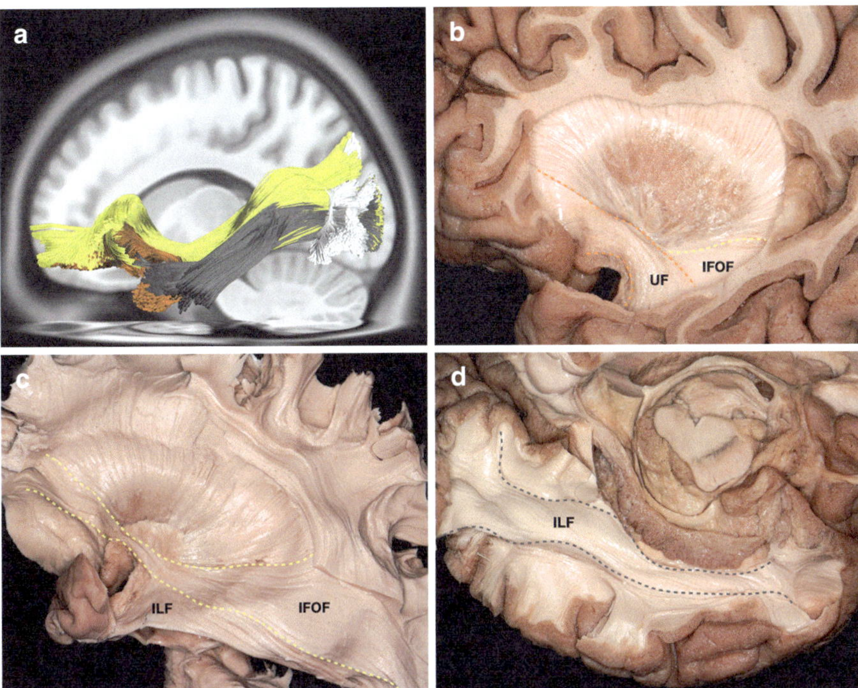

**Fig. 1.4** (**a**) Tractography of the ventral association matter tracts. Visible in this left sagittal view are the inferior longitudinal fasciculus (gray), uncinate fasciculus (orange), inferior fronto-occipital fasciculus (yellow), and vertical occipital fasciculus (white). (**b**) Dissection of a postmortem specimen. View of the left hemisphere. The cortical gray matter and underlying U-fibers have been removed to reveal the uncinate fasciculus (UF) and inferior fronto-occipital fasciculus (IFOF). (**c**) Upon further dissection, the UF has been removed to reveal the extent of IFOF in the external capsule. (**d**) An alternative inferior view of the left temporal lobe demonstrating the extent of the inferior longitudinal fasciculus (ILF)

description has been challenged: The posterior or vertical AF component is in fact the TPAT, an anatomically distinct fiber tract. The anterior or horizontal AF component belongs to the superior longitudinal fasciculus system. The AF instead has been shown to consist of dorsal and shorter ventral components [13]. The larger dorsal component connects the ventral precentral and caudal middle frontal gyri with the middle and inferior temporal gyri. The smaller ventral component connects the pars opercularis with the superficial temporal gyrus. Due to this distinct morphology, and the fact that the AF is leftward-lateralized in both morphology and volume, it should be also considered as anatomically distinct from the superior longitudinal fasciculus, which demonstrates rightward connective and volumetric lateralization patterns (Fig. 1.3b).

## *Superior Longitudinal Fasciculus*

The superior longitudinal fasciculus (SLF) lies within the same anatomical plane, yet dorsal to the AF. It connects the parietal lobe with the frontal lobe. Traditionally, the AF was considered as part of a larger SLF network due to the close proximity of the two fasciculi. Nevertheless, as previously discussed, novel investigative techniques have refuted this concept. The SLF is in fact a rightward-lateralized two-part system, also consisting of dorsal and ventral components [14]. Additionally, previous descriptions of the SLF include an extreme dorsal component (SLF-I) lying medial to the corticospinal tracts, which was later shown to be part of the cingulum [14]. The dorsal SLF (SLF-II according to old nomenclature) connects the angular gyrus to the caudal middle frontal gyrus. The ventral SLF (SLF-III according to old nomenclature) connects the supramarginal gyrus to the ventral precentral gyrus. The rightward-lateralization of SLF connectivity and volumetry serves to provide further evidence to refute the notion of its anatomical association with the AF (Fig. 1.3b).

## *Middle Longitudinal Fasciculus*

The middle longitudinal fasciculus (MdLF) is situated immediately underneath the AF's peri-Sylvian arc portion. Despite being called a "longitudinal" fasciculus, it is in fact an obliquely travelling tract connecting the temporal with caudal parietal and occipital lobes. The MdLF was initially found in the macaque monkey and subsequently found in the human brain using tractography techniques. The MdLF originates from the superior temporal gyrus, travelling dorsally and posteriorly to connect with the angular gyrus, superior parietal lobule, and superior occipital lobe [15] (Fig. 1.3c, d).

## *Temporoparietal Aslant Tract*

The temporoparietal aslant tract (TPAT) is a short, vertical tract connecting the temporal and parietal lobes. It is the most lateral association fasciculus [16]. Previously, this tract was thought to be a component of the "indirect" arcuate fasciculus. In the era of advanced tractography, this notion has been refuted however. The TPAT is anatomically distinct from both the arcuate and superior longitudinal fasciculi and can be further subdivided into dorsal and ventral components. The ventral TPAT connects the supramarginal gyrus to the middle temporal gyrus. The dorsal TPAT component primarily connects the angular gyrus with both the middle and inferior temporal gyri (Fig. 1.3c).

## *Frontal Aslant Tract*

The frontal aslant tract (FAT) is a recently described association fasciculus. Unlike other association fasciculi, it does not travel between lobes, instead interconnecting dorsomedial frontal areas with ventrolateral frontal areas in an oblique arrangement. It is a short collection of fibers originating from the superior frontal gyrus (notably the pre-supplementary motor area and the supplementary motor area), travelling ventrally and laterally in an oblique trajectory to the pars opercularis and triangularis. The FAT passes underneath and perpendicularly to the posteroanteriorly travelling portions of the AF and SLF.

## Ventral Association Fasciculi (Superficial Deep)

## *Uncinate Fasciculus*

The uncinate fasciculus (UF) is a hook-shaped ventral association tract connecting the orbitofrontal lobe with the anterior temporal lobe. Together with the inferior fronto-occipital fasciculus, it exits the frontal lobe via the temporal stem of the ventral external capsule. At its frontal extremity, it bifurcates to connect with the orbitofrontal cortex, rectus, and ventrolateral frontal gyri. Temporally, it connects with the temporal pole, uncus, and parahippocampal gyrus. There is some controversy regarding the UF's connectivity with the amygdala. The UF possesses a leftward-dominant connective and volumetric structure [17] (Fig. 1.4a, b).

## *Inferior Fronto-Occipital Fasciculus*

The inferior fronto-occipital fasciculus (IFOF) is the longest association fasciculus, travelling in a ventral longitudinal course between the frontal lobe and occipital lobe via the external capsule. In the frontal lobe, it assumes a trifurcated connectivity profile, with dorsomedial, ventromedial, and ventrolateral divisions connecting to the middle frontal gyri, frontal polar, and ventrolateral frontal gyri, respectively. Fibers from all divisions converge into a compact stem, travelling via the ventral external capsule together with the UF. Within the external capsule, the IFOF continues posteriorly to the occipital lobe via the sagittal stratum, with the ILF lying ventrally and laterally and the optic radiations situated medially. Here, it begins to fan out again, to connect with rostral parietal and occipital gyri. Traditional descriptions also describe connectivity to the basal temporal regions, namely, the fusiform gyrus; however, novel tractographic studies have disputed this finding [17]. Unlike the UF, the IFOF is not lateralized to either hemisphere in terms of connectivity or volume (Fig. 1.4c).

## Inferior Longitudinal Fasciculus

The inferior longitudinal fasciculus (ILF) is the most ventral human association fasciculus. It originates within the anterolateral temporal lobe, connecting it to caudal occipital and basal temporal lobes. Its existence became disputed during the 1980s due to simian radioisotope findings which proposed the ILF to be composed of a series of U-fibers rather as opposed to a robust fasciculus. Nevertheless, several tractography studies have proved the existence of the ILF as a distinct ventrally travelling fasciculus. Anteriorly, it originates from the lateral three temporal gyri, travelling posteriorly in a bundle to terminate within the lingual, fusiform, superior, and middle occipital gyri. The ILF is both connectively and volumetrically leftward-lateralized [18] (Fig. 1.4d).

## Vertical Occipital Fasciculus

Though anatomical descriptions of the VOF date back to early postmortem dissection studies, they disappeared from the literature throughout much of the twentieth century, prior to being rediscovered during the tractography era. It connects the basal occipitotemporal regions with the lateral occipital cortex. Some have described the VOF as being anatomically continuous with the TPAT as they lie in the same approximate plane. The VOF lies superficial and perpendicular to the occipital courses of the inferior fronto-occipital and inferior longitudinal fasciculi [16].

## Association Tracts: Surgical Considerations

Intraparenchymal tumors may arise anywhere within the hemisphere, potentially affecting multiple association tracts simultaneously. As association white matter is abundant throughout the hemispheres, it may be at risk of damage during common operative approaches. Most transcortical approaches involve passing through hemispheric association fasciculi; thus, an understanding of its lateral-medial white matter architecture and relations as outlined here is beneficial for the neurosurgeon.

Unlike the projection tracts which subserve readily assessable neurological functionality (i.e., vision, motor function, touch, etc.), function of the association tracts is subject to considerable debate. The use of IES may be beneficial in delineating the function of association fascicles in addition to guiding resection depth. As a result, many of the prevailing opinions regarding the functionality of association fascicles are derived from IES observations. Preoperative tractography may complement the use of IES by providing the surgeon with an understanding of pertinent white matter architecture in a three-dimensional fashion. A combined approach of preoperative tractography with IES may therefore optimize surgical outcomes.

## *Tractography: Technical Aspects*

Generally, tractography techniques measure diffusion characteristics of water molecules confined within myelinated axons, a property known as anisotropy. Common methods to reconstruct the acquired diffusion data are either tensor based or non-tensor based. Diffusion tensor imaging (DTI) was the first tractography method, introduced during the late 1990s. DTI algorithms utilize a Gaussian approach to reconstructing diffusion MRI data, and produce a single diffusion tensor per voxel, corresponding to principal fiber orientation contained within. The tensors' overall directionality is an averaged measurement of all constituent diffusion sampling measurements taken. The major drawback for tensor-based approaches however arises due to the fact that only a single tensor can exist per voxel. The real underlying white matter anatomy contains numerous twisting, bending, crossing, or obliquely oriented white matter fibers, which cannot be adequately represented at sub-voxel resolution using the tensor-based approach alone.

To address the angular resolution problems inherent to DTI, several other tractography methods have been devised. These include Q-ball imaging, high-angular resolution diffusion imaging (HARDI) [19], diffusion spectrum imaging (DSI) [20], and generalized Q-sampling imaging (GQI) [21]. All of these utilize different mathematical models to reconstruct diffusion data and have been utilized to differing extents by clinicians and researchers. Nevertheless, aside from GQI, few have been reliably validated for neurosurgical purposes [3, 4, 22]. Moreover, as most device manufacturers include built-in DTI acquisition sequences with MRI hardware, DTI remains the prevalent tractography technique used by neurosurgeons worldwide.

All non-tensor modalities utilize alternative intra-voxel directionality metrics which have the advantage of being able to represent greater-than-one principal fiber orientation at sub-voxel resolutions. GQI tractography, for example, utilizes a non-Gaussian method to calculate a spin distribution function (SDF) from diffusion data, which can represent crossing fiber orientations at sub-voxel resolutions. This is advantageous to neurosurgeons when considering that white matter architecture is often displaced, disrupted, or infiltrated by lesions or may be affected by edema. As peri-tumoral edema consists primarily of water, it may adversely affect diffusion signals of white matter tracts passing through the peri-tumoral areas. As a result, tracts may be falsely terminated (disrupted) within peri-tumoral vicinities. In fact, both HARDI and GQI methods have been shown to demonstrate intact white matter tracts passing through edematous peri-tumoral regions more reliably compared to DTI. This is a particularly important caveat for the neurosurgeon who may tailor their operative approach to a lesion based upon perceived white matter involvement [4, 22].

Depending upon its aggressiveness, a tumor may simply push tracts out of the way (displacement) or may invade and destroy them (infiltration). Moreover, when viewed tractographically, tumor-adjacent tracts may display a phenomenon called disruption, which is their abrupt termination in close proximity to the lesion. This is produced by compression or excess water, affecting the anisotropic diffusion signal of the peri-tumoral fiber tracts. Non-tensor fiber tracking algorithms such as generalized Q-sampling imaging (GQI) or high angular resolution diffusion imaging (HARDI) are more readily able to trace peri-tumoral white matter due to their ability to resolve multiple fiber orientations within the voxel [4] and may be more beneficial for presurgical white matter visualization.

## Conclusions

The complex arrangement of subcortical white matter represents a learning curve for the neurosurgeon. Understanding of the lateral-to-medial arrangement of white matter tracts and their interaction with parenchymal lesions may help to guide surgical approach.

## References


1. Fernández-Miranda JC, Rhoton AL, Alvarez-Linera J, Kakizawa Y, Choi C, de Oliveira EP. Three-dimensional microsurgical and tractographic anatomy of the white matter of the human brain. Neurosurgery. 2008;62(6 Suppl 3):989–1026.; discussion 1026–8. https://doi.org/10.1227/01.neu.0000333767.05328.49.
2. Basser PJ, Mattiello J, LeBihan D. MR diffusion tensor spectroscopy and imaging. Biophys J. 1994;66(1):259–67.
3. Fernandez-Miranda JC, Pathak S, Engh J, et al. High-definition fiber tractography of the human brain: neuroanatomical validation and neurosurgical applications. Neurosurgery. 2012;71(2):430–53. https://doi.org/10.1227/NEU.0b013e3182592faa.
4. Panesar SS, Abhinav K, Yeh F-C, Jacquesson T, Collins M, Fernandez-Miranda J. Tractography for surgical neuro-oncology planning: towards a gold standard. Neurother J Am Soc Exp Neurother. 2019;16(1):36–51. https://doi.org/10.1007/s13311-018-00697-x.
5. Romano A, D'Andrea G, Minniti G, et al. Pre-surgical planning and MR-tractography utility in brain tumour resection. Eur Radiol. 2009;19(12):2798. https://doi.org/10.1007/s00330-009-1483-6.
6. Kamada K, Todo T, Masutani Y, et al. Visualization of the frontotemporal language fibers by tractography combined with functional magnetic resonance imaging and magnetoencephalography. J Neurosurg. 2007;106(1):90–8. https://doi.org/10.3171/jns.2007.106.1.90.
7. Duffau H, Capelle L, Denvil D, et al. Usefulness of intraoperative electrical subcortical mapping during surgery for low-grade gliomas located within eloquent brain regions: functional results in a consecutive series of 103 patients. J Neurosurg. 2003;98(4):764–78. https://doi.org/10.3171/jns.2003.98.4.0764.
8. Shah A, Jhawar SS, Goel A. Analysis of the anatomy of the Papez circuit and adjoining limbic system by fiber dissection techniques. J Clin Neurosci. 2012;19(2):289–98. https://doi.org/10.1016/j.jocn.2011.04.039.
9. Weil AG, Middleton AL, Niazi TN, Ragheb J, Bhatia S. The supracerebellar-transtentorial approach to posteromedial temporal lesions in children with refractory epilepsy. J Neurosurg Pediatr. 2015;15(1):45–54. https://doi.org/10.3171/2014.10.PEDS14162.
10. Yaşargil MG, Krayenbühl N, Roth P, Hsu SPC, Yaşargil DCH. The selective amygdalohippocampectomy for intractable temporal limbic seizures: historical vignette. J Neurosurg. 2010;112(1):168–85. https://doi.org/10.3171/2008.12.JNS081112.

11. Asadi-Pooya AA, Sharan A, Nei M, Sperling MR. Corpus callosotomy. Epilepsy Behav. 2008;13(2):271–8. https://doi.org/10.1016/j.yebeh.2008.04.020.
12. Jea A, Vachhrajani S, Widjaja E, et al. Corpus callosotomy in children and the disconnection syndromes: a review. Childs Nerv Syst. 2008;24(6):685–92. https://doi.org/10.1007/s00381-008-0626-4.
13. Fernández-Miranda JC, Wang Y, Pathak S, Stefaneau L, Verstynen T, Yeh F-C. Asymmetry, connectivity, and segmentation of the arcuate fascicle in the human brain. Brain Struct Funct. 2015;220(3):1665–80. https://doi.org/10.1007/s00429-014-0751-7.
14. Wang X, Pathak S, Stefaneanu L, Yeh F-C, Li S, Fernandez-Miranda JC. Subcomponents and connectivity of the superior longitudinal fasciculus in the human brain. Brain Struct Funct. 2016;221(4):2075–92. https://doi.org/10.1007/s00429-015-1028-5.
15. Wang Y, Fernández-Miranda JC, Verstynen T, Pathak S, Schneider W, Yeh F-C. Rethinking the role of the middle longitudinal fascicle in language and auditory pathways. Cereb Cortex N Y N 1991. 2013;23(10):2347–56. https://doi.org/10.1093/cercor/bhs225.
16. Panesar SS, Belo JTA, Yeh F-C, Fernandez-Miranda JC. Structure, asymmetry, and connectivity of the human temporo-parietal aslant and vertical occipital fasciculi. Brain Struct Funct. 2018; https://doi.org/10.1007/s00429-018-1812-0.
17. Panesar SS, Yeh F-C, Deibert CP, et al. A diffusion spectrum imaging-based tractographic study into the anatomical subdivision and cortical connectivity of the ventral external capsule: uncinate and inferior fronto-occipital fascicles. Neuroradiology. 2017;59(10):971–87. https://doi.org/10.1007/s00234-017-1874-3.
18. Panesar SS, Yeh F-C, Jacquesson T, Hula W, Fernandez-Miranda JC. A quantitative Tractography study into the connectivity, segmentation and laterality of the human inferior longitudinal fasciculus. Front Neuroanat. 2018;12 https://doi.org/10.3389/fnana.2018.00047.
19. Tuch DS, Reese TG, Wiegell MR, Makris N, Belliveau JW, Wedeen VJ. High angular resolution diffusion imaging reveals intravoxel white matter fiber heterogeneity. Magn Reson Med. 2002;48(4):577–82. https://doi.org/10.1002/mrm.10268.
20. Wedeen VJ, Wang RP, Schmahmann JD, et al. Diffusion spectrum magnetic resonance imaging (DSI) tractography of crossing fibers. NeuroImage. 2008;41(4):1267–77.
21. Yeh F-C, Wedeen VJ, Tseng W-YI. Generalized q-sampling imaging. IEEE Trans Med Imaging. 2010;29(9):1626–35. https://doi.org/10.1109/TMI.2010.2045126.
22. Abhinav K, Yeh F-C, Mansouri A, Zadeh G, Fernandez-Miranda JC. High-definition fiber tractography for the evaluation of perilesional white matter tracts in high-grade glioma surgery. Neuro Oncol. 2015;17(9):1199–209. https://doi.org/10.1093/neuonc/nov113.

# Chapter 2
# The Ventricular System: Anatomy and Common Lesions

Robert A. Scranton and Aaron Cohen-Gadol

## Abbreviations

CT    computed tomography
MRI   magnetic resonance imaging
PICA  posterior inferior cerebellar artery

## Ventricular Anatomy

Operative anatomy of the cerebral ventricular system can conceptually be divided into three distinct parts: the lateral ventricles, the third ventricle, and the fourth ventricle. These major divisions have important implications for both the types of pathology found and the most appropriate operative approach to them.

R. A. Scranton
Department of Neurosurgery, Indiana University School of Medicine, Indianapolis, USA
e-mail: mshah2@iu.edu

A. Cohen-Gadol (✉)
*The Neurosurgical Atlas*, Carmel, IN, USA

Department of Neurological Surgery, Indiana University, Indianapolis, IN, USA
e-mail: cohen@nsatlas.com

© Springer Nature Switzerland AG 2022
G. Zada et al. (eds.), *Subcortical Neurosurgery*,
https://doi.org/10.1007/978-3-030-95153-5_2

## *Lateral Ventricle Anatomy*

The lateral ventricles are a paired C-shaped structure, as seen in the sagittal plane, that encompass the thalamus and diencephalon. Anatomically, each lateral ventricle can be divided into the following five parts: frontal horn (anterior), body, atrium (trigone), temporal horn, and occipital horn (Fig. 2.1) [1]. The lateral ventricle, from the frontal horn through the atrium, is covered on its roof by the corpus callosum, and it is covered laterally by the thalamus, except in the most posterior part, where it is replaced by the caudate. It is important to note that the genu of the internal capsule contacts the ventricular surface lateral to the foramen of Monro, separating the thalamus anteriorly and the caudate posteriorly. The posterior portion of the lateral ventricle, the occipital horn, is covered by the optic radiations, and the temporal horn is covered by the caudate.

The lateral and third ventricles communicate via the foramen of Monro. A critical structure of concern when approaching the lateral ventricle is the fornix, which begins in the alveus, connects to the fimbria, and then advances adjacent to the temporal horn. The pathway contains projection fibers that connect the hippocampus and hypothalamus. Injury in this area can result in profound memory deficits classically manifested as an anterograde deficit. Surgical approaches should be tailored around preserving this structure. The foramen of Monro is formed by the forniceal bodies on the anterior and superior borders; caution must be taken when approaching the foramen of Monro through an endoscopic approach to the third ventricle or through an anterior interhemispheric transcallosal interforniceal approach because damage can result in transient or permanent cognitive impairment.

Projecting posteriorly from the foramen of Monro is the choroidal fissure, which extends posteriorly along the lateral ventricle, atrium, and temporal horn. It

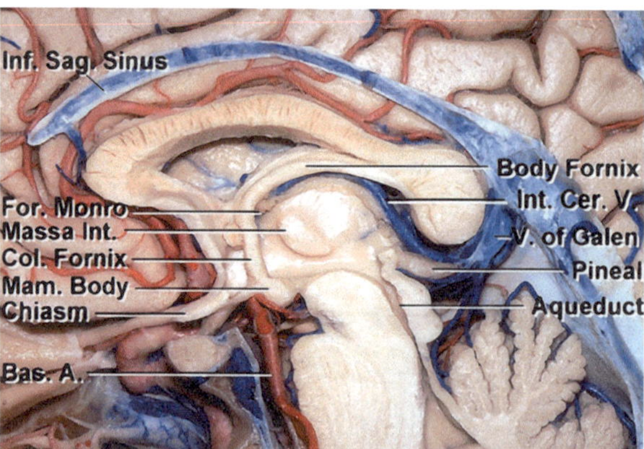


**Fig. 2.1** Anatomical sagittal section showing the corpus callosum and surrounding structures bordering the ventricular system. The corpus callosum is the largest anatomic interface with the lateral ventricle. This structure is divided into four segments. From anterior to posterior, these segments are the rostrum, the genu, the body, and the splenium. (Image courtesy of A. L. Rhoton, Jr.) (With permission from *The Neurosurgical Atlas* by Aaron Cohen-Gadol, MD)

represents the separation between the thalamus and fornix and is covered by choroid plexus. The choroid plexus and its vessels play an important role in providing a vascular supply to tumors encountered in this location through the anterior and posterior choroidal arteries. Early ligation of these connections between the choroid plexus and tumor, when possible, is advised.

The venous anatomy within the lateral ventricular system is intricate, and a good working knowledge of it is required to perform surgery in the area. Important vessels include the anterior septal veins, superior choroidal vein, medial and lateral atrial veins, thalamostriate vein, inferior ventricular vein, and the inferior choroidal vein. The major outflow goes through the internal cerebral veins and the basal veins of Rosenthal. The thalamostriate vein projects from lateral to medial toward the choroidal fissure, where it joins the anterior septal vein and the superior choroidal vein. Transection of the septal vein just before its junction with the thalamostriate, the venous angle, is considered safe and enables the surgeon to use an expanded transforaminal route to the third ventricle. Retraction injury still remains a concern. The thalamostriate vein serves as an important landmark for identifying which lateral ventricle has been entered during surgery, and it should be preserved.

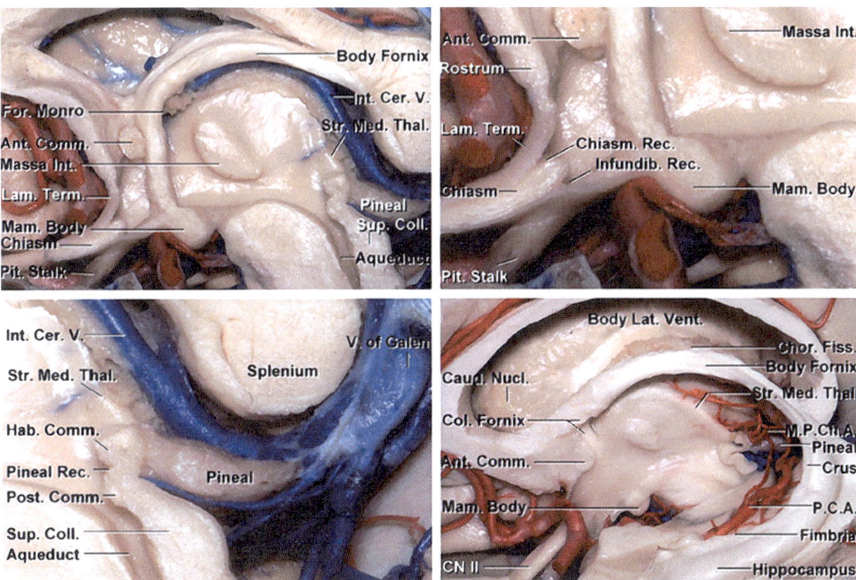


**Fig. 2.2** Midsagittal anatomical picture showing the relevant anatomy surrounding the area of the third ventricle. The anterior border of the third ventricle is composed of the region between the optic chiasm and the foramen of Monro. The structures in this region include the optic chiasm, lamina terminalis, anterior commissure, and columns of the fornix. The posterior border of the third ventricle is composed of the region between the aqueduct of Sylvius and the suprapineal recess. The structures composing this region include the posterior commissure, pineal body, and habenular commissure. (Images courtesy of A. L. Rhoton, Jr.) (With permission from *The Neurosurgical Atlas* by Aaron Cohen-Gadol, MD)

## Third Ventricle Anatomy

The third ventricle connects the lateral ventricles via the foramen of Monro to the fourth ventricle via the aqueduct of Sylvius (cerebral aqueduct). Relevant terms to use when describing the anatomy of the third ventricle include the anterior, posterior, lateral, cranial (roof), and caudal (floor) borders (Fig. 2.2).

The anterior border extends from the optic chiasm to the foramen of Monro and is formed by the anterior commissure, lamina terminalis, optic chiasm, and columns of the fornix. The posterior border is roughly the region between the aqueduct of Sylvius and the suprapineal recess, and it includes the posterior commissure, pineal body, and habenular commissure.

The lateral walls are formed by the thalamus and hypothalamus, and the massa intermedia, an interconnection between the adjacent walls of the third ventricle, might be found here. Caudally, the floor is formed by the posterior perforated substance, mamillary bodies, tuber cinereum, and infundibulum.

The roof of the third ventricle is a complex structure composed of five distinct layers. From deep to superficial, they include the choroid plexus, the inferior layer of tela choroidea, the vascular layer (velum interpositum), the superior layer of tela choroidea, and, last, a forniceal layer. The vascular layer contains the medial posterior choroidal arteries and internal cerebral veins. Given the vital structures that border the third ventricle, especially the floor and walls, surgical transgression can be devastating.

## Fourth Ventricle Anatomy

The borders of the fourth ventricle, cranially to caudally, are as follows:

- Anterior (floor)—midbrain, pons, and medulla.
- Lateral—superior, middle, and inferior cerebellar peduncles.
- Posterior (roof)—superior medullary velum, cerebellar lingula, and fastigium.
- Inferior—choroid plexus, tela choroidea, inferior medullar velum, cerebellar uvula, and nodulus.

When viewing the floor of the fourth ventricle from a telovelar approach, a midline raphe can be seen; the medial sulcus with the facial colliculi lateral to this raphe are at the level of the middle cerebellar peduncle, which is then bordered laterally by the sulcus limitans (Fig. 2.3). Caudal to the facial colliculus, the striae medullaris will be evident coming laterally around the inferior cerebellar peduncle to terminate in the medial sulcus and is followed more caudally by the hypoglossal and then vagal triangles.

Understanding the vascular anatomy of the posterior inferior cerebellar artery (PICA) and the regions it supplies is critical to this approach. There are five

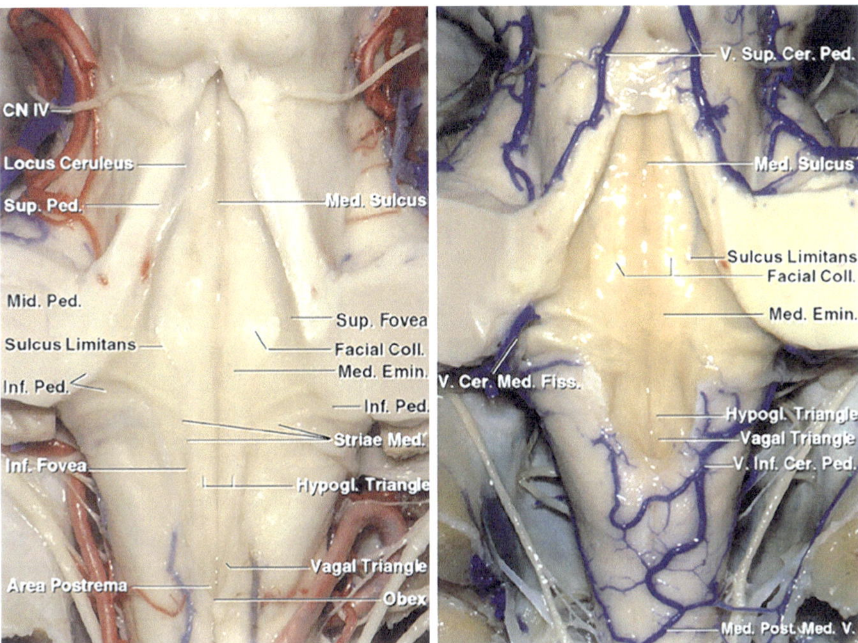


**Fig. 2.3** Anatomical dissection showing the posterior view of the floor of the fourth ventricle. The topography of the eloquent fourth ventricular floor is mapped. The locations of the facial colliculus and the hypoglossal and vagal triangles are evident. Stimulation mapping can effectively guide the surgeon to avoid these critical structures during surgery of the floor. (Images courtesy of A. L. Rhoton, Jr.) (With permission from *The Neurosurgical Atlas* by Aaron Cohen-Gadol, MD)

anatomical divisions of the PICA, including the anterior medullary, lateral medullary, tonsillomedullary, telovelotonsillar, and cortical segments (Fig. 2.4). The surgeon must understand that the first three segments give rise to brainstem perforators and must be preserved.

## Ventricular Pathology

Ventricular tumors account for 0.8% to 1.6% of intracranial masses and present a technical challenge because of their deep location and surrounding structures [2, 3]. Primary tumors that can involve the ventricular system include colloid cysts, cavernomas, craniopharyngiomas, astrocytomas, choroid plexus papillomas, ependymomas, subependymomas, lymphoma, germ cell tumors, astrocytomas, and epidermoid and dermoid cysts. Secondary tumors include meningiomas, gliomas, pituitary adenomas, metastasis to the choroid plexus, and arachnoid cysts [2, 4, 5]. These tumors usually follow a very slow, benign course and present in patients as a result

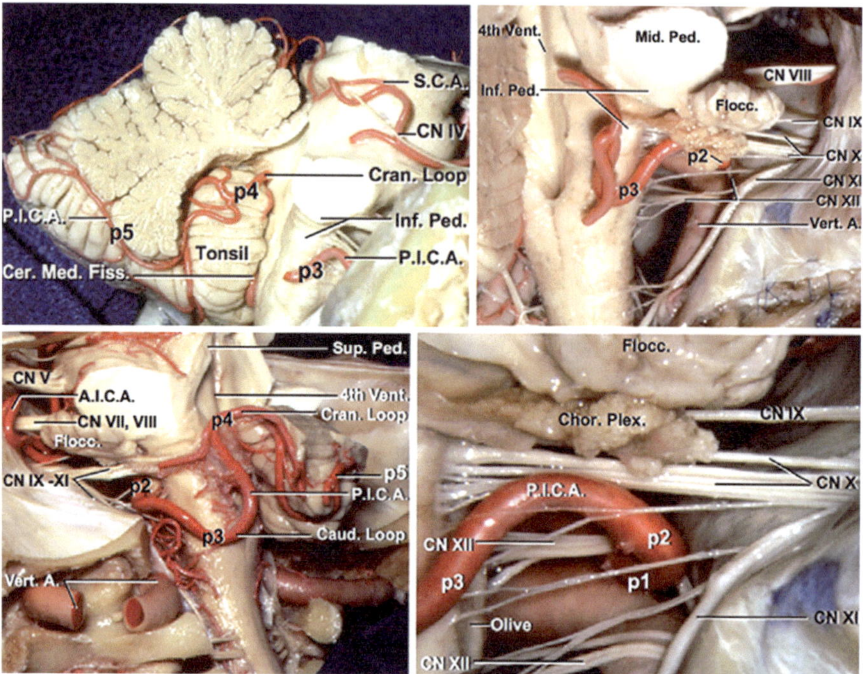



**Fig. 2.4** Morphology of the left PICA from a posterior view. The first three major PICA segments, namely, the anterior medullary, lateral medullary, and tonsillomedullary segments, also provide the major arterial supply to the brainstem. Any segment of the PICA in close proximity of the brainstem can provide vascular support to the brainstem and should be preserved. (Images courtesy of A. L. Rhoton, Jr.) (With permission from *The Neurosurgical Atlas* by Aaron Cohen-Gadol, MD)

of a headache workup, as obstructive hydrocephalus, or from mass effect and compression.

Presenting complaints typically involve headache, imbalance, cognitive dysfunction, and personality changes or motor weakness from masses that arise in the lateral or third ventricle [6–8]. Masses in the pineal region can cause compression of the tectal plate, which leads to dorsal midbrain (or Parinaud) syndrome. This syndrome is characterized by upward gaze palsy, light-near dissociation, and a convergence retraction nystagmus and is a result of compression of the rostral interstitial nucleus of the medial longitudinal fasciculus [9, 10]. Tumors of the fourth ventricle often present with ataxia from compression of the cerebellar tracts.

The preoperative differential diagnosis has implications for the surgical plan and approach chosen. This diagnosis is normally based on patient presentation and key imaging characteristics on magnetic resonance imaging (MRI) and computed tomography (CT) (Table 2.1). Ventricular pathology should, at a minimum, be evaluated before surgery using MRI with contrast; CT also can be helpful for narrowing the differential diagnosis. Vascular imaging can also be invaluable for studying both the anatomical relationship between the pathology and the normal arteries and

**Table 2.1** Tumor-specific CT and MRI findings for ventricular tumors

| Tumor type | Key findings | |
| --- | --- | --- |
| | MRI | CT |
| Colloid cyst | T1-weighted homogeneous hyperintensity; T2-weighted homogeneous hypointensity with hyperintense circumferential rim | Homogeneously isodense to mildly hyperdense lesion; commonly observed in foramen of Monro; rare calcifications |
| Craniopharyngioma | Heterogeneous cystic and solid features; heterogeneous intensity within solid tumor; T1-weighted hyperintensity within cystic components; intense contrast enhancement | Heterogeneously cystic and solid components with calcification; contrast enhancement in solid tumor |
| Low-grade astrocytoma | T1-weighted hypointensity; T2-weighted hyperintensity; minimal or absent contrast enhancement | Hypodensity; calcifications (15%); minimal or absent contrast enhancement |
| Cavernous malformation | Mixed intensity; minimal or absent contrast enhancement; microhemorrhages appear as hemosiderin rims | Hyperdensity; well-delineated round to ovoid mass; do not demonstrate intralesional hemorrhage or mass effect |
| Glioblastoma | T1-weighted heterogeneous hypointensity; T2-weighted hyperintensity; ring contrast enhancement surrounding necrotic core | Peripheral heterogeneous contrast enhancement; intralesional hypodensity |
| Subependymoma | Lobulated appearance; T1-weighted hypointense to isointense lesion; T2-weighted hyperintense lesion; minimal or absent contrast enhancement | Well-delineated isodense to hyperdense lesion; minimal or no contrast enhancement |
| Meningioma | T1-weighted isointensity; homogeneous contrast enhancement | Well-delineated hyperdensity |
| Central neurocytoma | Heterogeneous hyperintensity from cysts, calcifications, and core necrosis; moderate contrast enhancement | Hyperdense; calcifications |
| Pineocytoma | T1-weighted hypointensity; T2-weighted hyperintensity; homogeneous contrast enhancement | Well-delineated hypodense to hyperdense lesion; homogeneous contrast enhancement; calcifications |
| Anaplastic astrocytoma | T1-weighted hypointensity; T2-weighted hyperintensity; heterogeneous contrast enhancement | Heterogeneous contrast enhancement; rare calcifications |
| Ependymoma | Heterogeneously hypointense to isointense lesion on T1 and T2; cystic features; intralesional necrosis, hemorrhage, vascularity, and hemosiderin deposition | Homogeneous contrast enhancement; cystic features; calcifications (50%) |

(continued)

**Table 2.1** (continued)

| Tumor type | Key findings | |
| --- | --- | --- |
| | MRI | CT |
| Pineoblastoma | T1-weighted hypointense to isointense; T2-weighted hyperintensity; signs of parenchyma invasion | Not well delineated from surrounding tissue; heterogeneous contrast enhancement; calcifications |
| Choroid plexus papilloma | T1-weighted isointense; T2-weighted isointense; homogeneous contrast enhancement; MRI insufficient to differentiate choroid plexus papillomas from carcinomas | Majority demonstrate delineated isodense to hyperdense lesion; contrast enhancement; intralesional hemorrhage; calcifications are common |

veins. Early identification and ligation of a tumor's vascular supply is a standard tenet of tumor surgery and is especially important in difficult areas such as the ventricular system. Tumors associated with the ventricular system, especially in the lateral ventricles, most often derive their blood supply from branches of the choroidal vessels. They typically are not seen until late in the operation, which can create an additional challenge. Any approach that enables early visualization would offer an advantage.

When a surgeon is operating in the lateral ventricles, special care should be taken to respect the venous anatomy; damage to the thalamostriate and/or internal cerebral veins can be devastating. Many of the tumors encountered in this area, such as colloid cysts and subependymomas, have a relatively benign course, and subtotal resection should be considered in situations in which neurological deficit as a consequence of its removal is likely.

Surgical manipulation of tumors in the third and fourth ventricles with intact walls is associated with significant morbidity. Subtotal resection should be strongly considered, especially for an infiltrating tumor.

Tumors in the fourth ventricle usually originate in the floor from the choroid plexus or tela choroidea. The majority of lesions arise outside the ventricle and extend into it, including medullary, tectal, and cerebellar hemispheric masses, which means that the telovelar approach should be strongly considered.

# References


1. Yasargil MG, Abdulrauf SI. Surgery of intraventricular tumors. Neurosurgery. 2008;62(6 Suppl 3):1029–40. discussion 1040–1021.
2. Agarwal A, Kanekar S. Intraventricular Tumors. Semin Ultrasound CT MR. 2016;37(2):150–8.
3. Lapras C, Deruty R, Bret P. Tumors of the lateral ventricles. Adv Tech Stand Neurosurg. 1984;11:103–67.
4. Delfini R, Acqui M, Oppido PA, Capone R, Santoro A, Ferrante L. Tumors of the lateral ventricles. Neurosurg Rev. 1991;14(2):127–33.

5. Koeller KK, Sandberg GD. From the archives of the AFIP. Cerebral intraventricular neoplasms: radiologic-pathologic correlation. Radiographics. 2002;22(6):1473–505.
6. Gokalp HZ, Yuceer N, Arasil E, et al. Tumours of the lateral ventricle. A retrospective review of 112 cases operated upon 1970-1997. Neurosurg Rev. 1998;21(2–3):126–37.
7. Ellenbogen RG. Transcortical surgery for lateral ventricular tumors. Neurosurg Focus. 2001;10(6):E2.
8. Piepmeier JM. Tumors and approaches to the lateral ventricles. Introduction and overview. J Neuro-Oncol. 1996;30(3):267–74.
9. Strupp M, Kremmyda O, Adamczyk C, et al. Central ocular motor disorders, including gaze palsy and nystagmus. J Neurol. 2014;261(Suppl 2):S542–58.
10. Pearce JM. Parinaud's syndrome. J Neurol Neurosurg Psychiatry. 2005;76(1):99.

# Chapter 3
# Advanced Neuroimaging of the Subcortical Space: Connectomics in Brain Surgery

Nicholas B. Dadario and Michael E. Sughrue

## An Introduction to Connectomic Neuroimaging

Connectomics borrows the "-omics" suffix from genomics as it is a big data approach to analyzing the massive datasets produced by functional and structural brain imaging. More specifically, the "connectome" refers to the entire set of axonal connections in the brain [1]. Obviously, this is a question of frame of reference as no existing technique currently shows all of the connections, but more accurately, the present use of the term connectome for neurosurgery focuses on the large-scale connections between sections of cortex and many underlying subcortical structures.

The ability to show ourselves the functional organization of the cortex before cutting into the brain has obvious and profound potential toward reducing morbidity [2]. A lack of proper understanding of how the brain works is at the heart of most of our failures with glioma surgery [3, 4], as we often are left scratching our head about what is going on exactly. Despite this, logistics have kept these imaging platforms limited to the most ivory of towers, namely, centers with in-house experts to navigate the complexities of image acquisition and processing, and the numerous steps necessary to implement these in a surgical workflow. Additionally, relative lack of knowledge by neurosurgeons about these evolving techniques has led to many misconceptions among neurosurgeons about how these techniques work and what they tell us [5, 6].

N. B. Dadario
Robert Wood Johnson Medical School, Rutgers University, New Brunswick, NJ, USA

M. E. Sughrue (✉)
Department of Neurosurgery, Prince of Wales Hospital, Sydney, NSW, Australia

© Springer Nature Switzerland AG 2022
G. Zada et al. (eds.), *Subcortical Neurosurgery*,
https://doi.org/10.1007/978-3-030-95153-5_3

## Diffusion Tractography

Diffusion tractography refers to the utilization of diffusion-weighted MRI, long used in diagnostic imaging for cerebral ischemia, to model the direction of white matter fibers in the brain [7]. This is accomplished by performing diffusion imaging at different gradient strengths (a.k.a. the B-values) and in numerous different directions (a.k.a. the B-vectors). Increasing the number of directions diffusion imaging is acquired or acquiring multiple nonzero B-values are the principal differences between the quality of different diffusion imaging protocols. Diffusion directions for protocols can vary from 20 directions to as many as 200 in different imaging protocols with the principal trade-off being imaging time, which is not an insignificant issue in busy centers [8].

Following acquisition, two typical corrections for known distortions are eddy current correction and distortion correction, in addition to standard head motion correction [9]. After this, the path from raw data to diffusion tensor can best be explained to nonexperts as a three-step process: first, calculating the fractional anisotropy (FA) map; second, modeling the diffusion tensors; and third, performing tractography using the diffusion tensors. A schematic demonstrating these steps in a simplified format is seen in Fig. 3.1.

Fractional anisotropy refers to the observation that Brownian motion in pure water moves equally in all directions (isotropically) but, when restricted in some form, moves more one way than others (anisotropically). In the brain, the most notable cause of anisotropic diffusion is axons, which cause anisotropy in the direction of their fibers [10]. Collecting and modeling these structures as ellipsoids at every voxel is the process of creating an FA map, or a map of anisotropy. In reality, this map is represented by a matrix of FA measured in the various sampled directions, and all further steps are linear algebra transformations on this matrix.

Because the end goal is to line up a set of vectors to estimate the direction and course of white matter bundles, the estimation of the FA in each voxel as a vector is the key step in the creation of diffusion-based tractography. In fact, the difference in how this is modeled is the main difference in most of the current variations on the original paradigm of diffusion tensor imaging (DTI). DTI analyzes the FA in a voxel and assigns the vector for that voxel as the dominant eigenvector for that voxel. In other words, it is a winner-take-all strategy. This has the limitation of not being able to resolve crossing fibers well, and this makes it less effective at resolving the anatomy of smaller tracts or ones which run orthogonal to larger bundles [11]. Notably, roughly 70% of voxels have crossing fibers, so this is not a trivial concern [12]. Dense data seeding with interpolation can deal with some of these problems, but this is always a limit of the imaging.

Newer ways to model the vectors have been devised, and it is presently an area of active research. For example, diffusion spectrum imaging (DSI) models the data by collecting many more directions and modeling several eigenvectors per voxel [13]. Similar variations include HARDI-Q-ball imaging and several other variations on this theme, which are beyond the scope of this book. DSI is great as a research tool but practically difficult to implement in clinical practice with imaging times well over an hour. Constrained spherical deconvolution (CSD) fits the data using prestructured models of the anisotropic ellipsoid [14]. These have promise but presently are not incorporated into clinical image guidance pipelines very often.

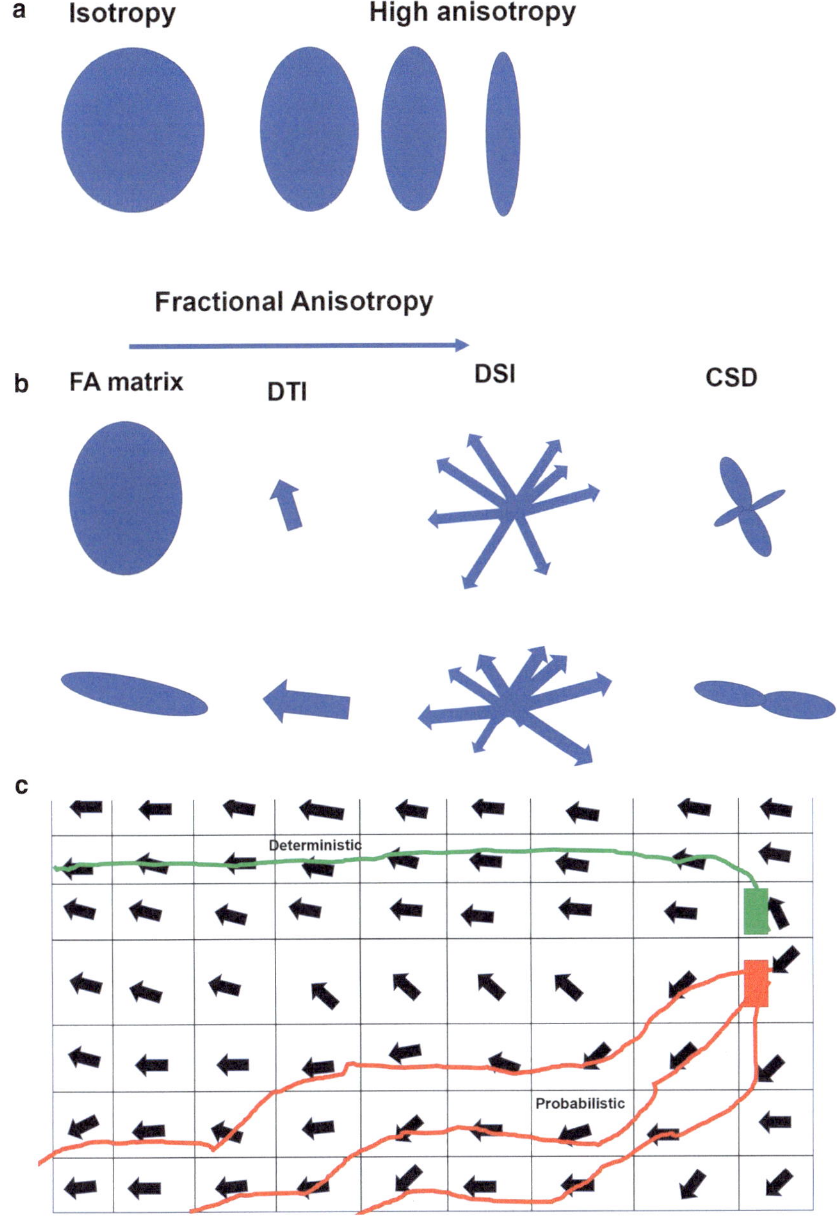



**Fig. 3.1** This schematic demonstrates a conceptualization of the steps of creating a diffusion tensor imaging (DTI) tractographic image. (**a**) This image demonstrates the basic concept behind anisotropy as a matrix describing basic shape of anisotropy. In reality, this is a high-dimensional vector set. (**b**) This image demonstrates the different methods of modeling a set of vectors from the FA matrix. Note that while DTI models this as the dominant eigenvector, diffusion spectrum imaging (DSI) models multiple vectors, and constrained spherical deconvolution (CSD) uses a collection of predetermined ellipsoids to model the vector set. (**c**) Finally, the vector map is translated to tractography by laying seeds and tracing the vectors using a set of conditions. Deterministic tractography maps one tract set per seed and works by sequentially laying more seeds in turn. Probabilistic maps all possible vector alignments in a seed and calculates the set of probable pathways based on a collection of tracts. Most surgical diffusion imaging is deterministic

Once the vectors are modeled, tractography is the process of lining up vectors into tracts. The two main processes for doing so include probabilistic, which models all possible streamlines from a seed and weights them based on the probability of their existence, and deterministic, which lays a seed and sequentially aligns a single set of vectors from that seed until a preset termination threshold has been reached, either by the vector taking a sharper angle than the chosen threshold or by the magnitude changing more than a threshold [15]. Presently, all clinical grade tractography is deterministic to our knowledge.

Understanding this process, the potential limitations are more easily understood. For example, vasogenic edema interferes with the process and makes the absence of tracts less reliable. Also, the process of aligning vectors can lead to missed tracts or false tracts due to the algorithm following a false path [16]. It should also be clear that small and crossing fibers are a big deal. Thus, tractography is not a foolproof technique.

## Functional MRI

Functional MRI (fMRI) is a well-known technique to neurosurgeons, but in our experience many of them generally misunderstand what it really says and what it does not. The technique often utilizes the blood oxygen level-dependent (BOLD) signal changes which occur when a brain region is activated, and it in turn causes a vasodilation that causes the hemoglobin oxygen level to change which can be detected and back calculated from a sequential acquisition of an echo planar image (EPI) [17].

The processing of an EPI image into a useable fMRI map involves the following steps: (1) head motion, even minor, needs to be corrected and realigned or the voxels cannot be made into a time course, (2) corrects for cardiac and respiratory signals and their effect on BOLD need to be made to delete these signals, and (3) artifacts from MRI field inhomogeneities, CSF, and large vessel pulsations need to be corrected or deleted. The skull and meninges need to be stripped.

fMRI can be acquired in two principal paradigms: task-based fMRI and resting state fMRI (rfMRI) [18]. Task-based fMRI involves comparing a baseline condition to the BOLD signal during a task of some form. While this has the benefit of having a clear idea of the context of what was activating the area of interest, it is not trivial to obtain as it requires an MRI paradigm and a trained person administering the task. This is not usually feasible at most places doing neurosurgery.

rfMRI relies on the fact that large-scale brain networks constantly co-activate each other even when at rest. While resting state images do not provide certainty of task context, when combined with our prior knowledge of the anatomy of large-scale brain networks, rfMRI provides the ability to map all of the brain networks at once, with an 8- to 10-minute image, with no expert in the room [19]. The advantage of this too busy neurosurgery imaging pipelines is obvious.

rfMRI can be processed a number of ways [20]. One is a seed-based correlation, which identifies areas which have signal time courses which correlate with that seen in the selected region of interest. This is simple to understand but can be time-consuming and prone to human bias. A more interesting paradigm is independent component analysis (ICA) [21]. The cocktail party analogy often used to describe ICA is outlined in Fig. 3.2. In more formal terms, it involves taking the

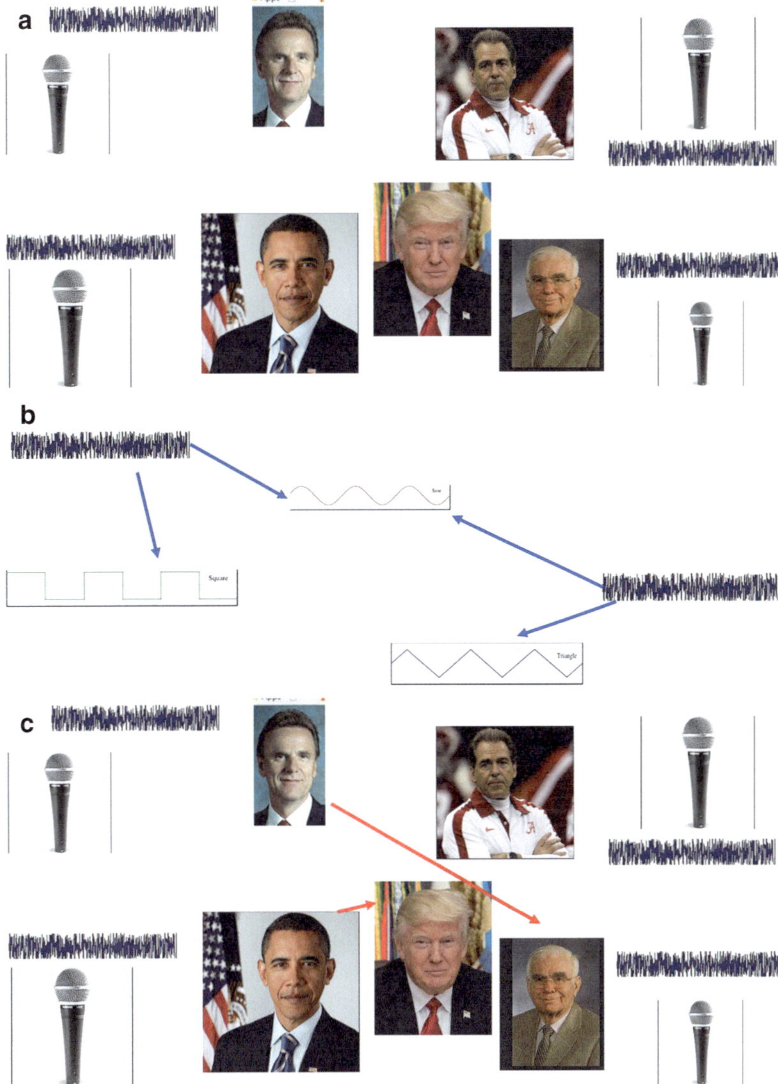


**Fig. 3.2** A conceptual description of analyzing functional brain imaging using ICA analysis. (**a**) The idea is that there are multiple locations receiving a mixture of periodic signal (in this analogy, it is a mixture of sounds from conversation). (**b**) Our goal is to separate out the conversations into independent sets of waves which explain the variance. This is achieved by a series of matrix transformations which decompose the signal into components which explain the variance and are statistically independent of each other. (**c**) ICA analysis can show us who is mostly talking to who. In the brain, these are wide-scale brain networks which fire on similar time courses. It is important to note that ICA does not exclude that areas sometimes talk to other areas and is simply finding the dominant components of the variance

cross talk between areas and finding the cross talk which behaves independently of other areas and which explains the largest fraction of the variance.

While ICA components (or ICA networks) can contain noise or cardiorespiratory artifacts, and even tumor blush, and thus helps clean the signal, a number of common components are usually seen in most ICA analyses. Such components are sometimes called the canonical ICA networks and have been robustly identified and studied extensively. The anatomy of these networks can be outlined with a combination of diffusion tractography and ICA to provide excellent views of the network brain anatomy for intraoperative navigation. These are described below.

## Anatomy of the Human Brain Networks

The Human Connectome Project (HCP) recently published their scheme for parcellating the human neocortex based on functional connectivity and physical characteristics [22]. Figure 3.2 provides an example of the scheme, which we have heavily utilized to describe brain connectivity in ways which can be compared, reproduced, and utilized by surgeons. What follows are our mapping of the anatomy of the large-scale functional networks in HCP parcellation format with diffusion spectrum tractography to provide the best possible anatomic model for these networks given existing technology [19, 23]. Interindividual variability in the human cortex is extreme, and gliomas can cause functional reorganization, so these models are merely the starting point in the discussion, but a key starting point compared to a previous lack of knowledge of these areas.

## The Motor System

Most neurosurgeons have long viewed the motor system as basically being the motor strip and perhaps the SMA. However, as Fig. 3.3 demonstrates, it is a more complex system of at least four components, including the sensorimotor strips, the supplementary motor area (SMA) [24], and the dorsal and ventral premotor areas [25], as well as their thalamic and basal ganglia connections. These usually form a single bilateral ICA network. Figure 3.3 highlights the "bouquet of flowers" arrangement of the system which in this diagram is demonstrated using the dorsal premotor system and sensory and motor strips.

## Networks inside of the SLF System

### Semantic Language

This left-sided network involves many of the familiar players, areas 44 and 45, the posterior MTG and superior temporal sulcus, and the arcuate connecting them (Fig. 3.4) [26, 27]. New to this model is area 55b, which is connected to the semantic

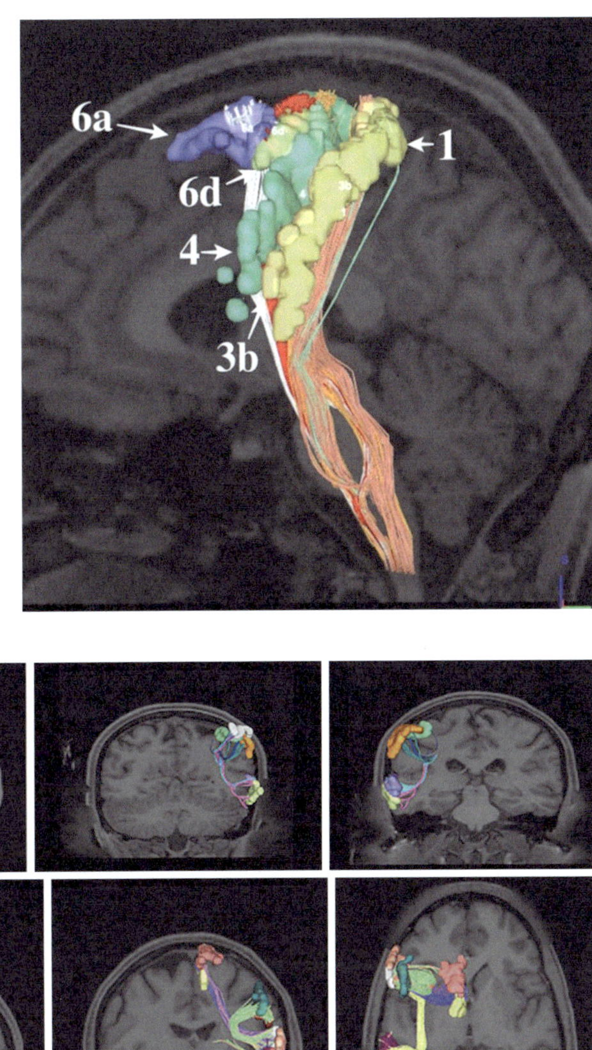

**Fig. 3.3** Network map of the dorsal premotor system



**Fig. 3.4** Network map of the language networks

language areas by SLF-2, as well as parietal contributions. SMA contributions to area 44 and neighboring areas like area 8C come from the frontal aslant tract (FAT).

## Auditory Network

Connectomics has shown us that the auditory areas are highly complex with several subregions in the Heschl's gyrus and superior temporal gyrus (Fig. 3.5) [28]. These

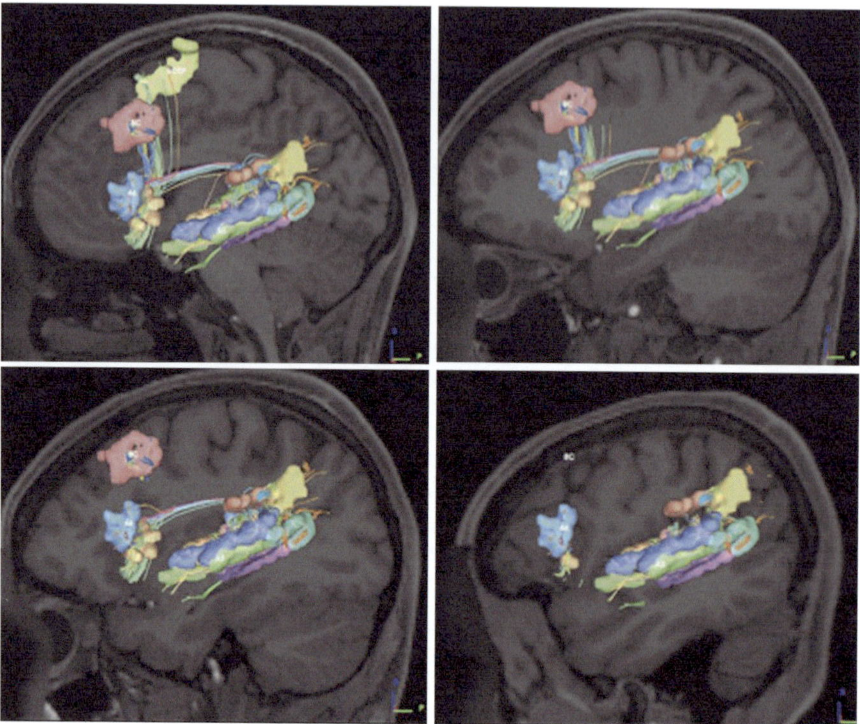

**Fig. 3.5** Network map of the auditory network

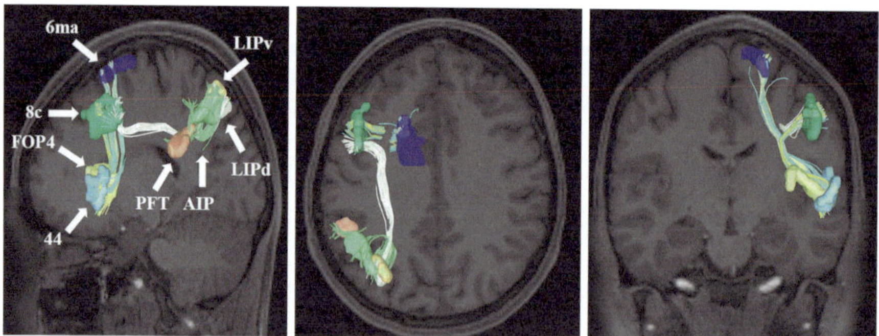


**Fig. 3.6** Network map of the praxis system

bilateral networks have their own connections via the arcuate to area 44, which is also part of this network, as is 8C and the SMA.

## Praxis Network

Tool use is a left SLF network, though interestingly it also involves area 44 and other frontal regions involved in speech (Fig. 3.6). This highlights the fact that Broca's area is more complex than we have given it credit for.

## Neglect

Our studies confirm other works that neglect results from damage to the right SLF (Fig. 3.7) [29]. The network model is interesting, and despite our initial thought that this would result from the dorsal or ventral attention networks, the data support a more complex model linking parts of the olfactory, auditory, somatosensory, executive, and dorsal attention networks as well as an analog of the semantic network on the right at the superior temporal sulcus. Our best hypothesis is that the true network is not the cortical areas but the fibers which connect them in the SLF. This is consistent with the binding problem neglect has thought to represent, namely, creating a coherent view of the world from mixed sensory modalities.

## Dorsal Attention Network

This network (Fig. 3.8) is bilateral and is inside the SLF that involved the frontal eye fields, the intraparietal sulcus, and the lateral visual areas [30]. Interestingly, this network has shown up in many of our studies of higher cognitive abilities, such as math, and we currently think it is part of allocating cognitive resources to higher tasks along with the top-down processing of stimuli.

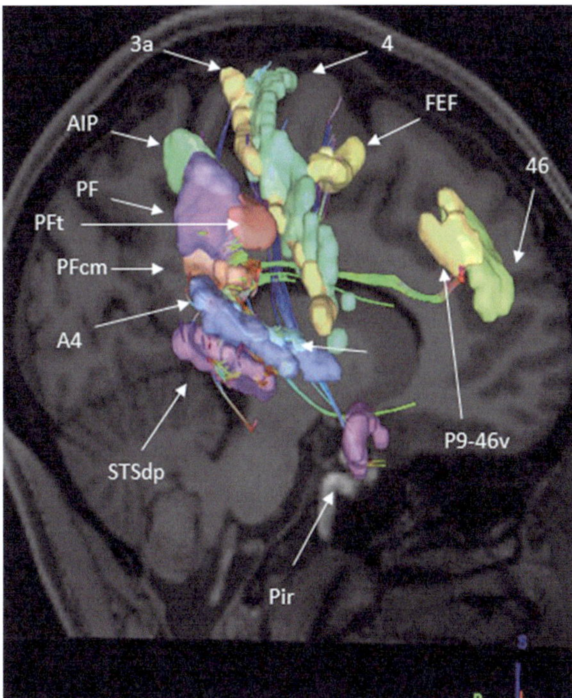


**Fig. 3.7** Network map of the neglect system

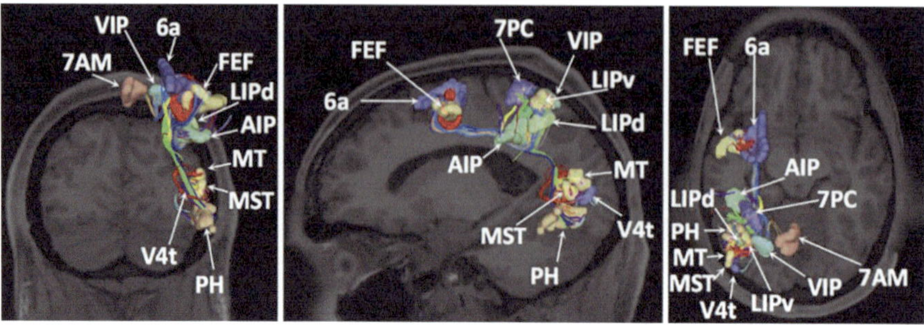

**Fig. 3.8** Network map of the dorsal attention network

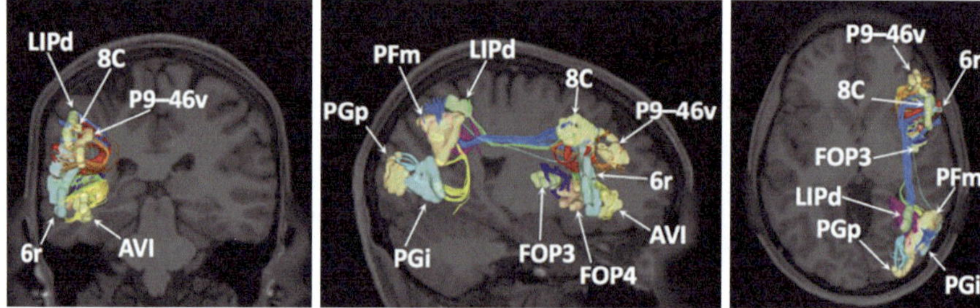

**Fig. 3.9** Network map of the ventral attention network

## Ventral Attention Network

This is a right-sided network which also is an SLF network (Fig. 3.9) [31]. Its function in the greater context of human cognition is not entirely clear to us, but compared to the DAN, the VAN reorients attention more specifically to behaviorally relevant stimuli.

## Central Executive Network

This is one of the dominant networks of the human cerebrum and is involved in organizing goal-directed behaviors [32]. It is discussed further with the control networks, such as DMN and salience networks.

## *Inferior Fronto-Occipital Fasciculus*

The IFOF is a large tract; however, it has a specific clinically important aspect of its anatomy (Fig. 3.10). It runs from anterior to posterior connecting the inferior occipital and frontal lobes. While the tract fans out anteriorly in the frontal lobe and

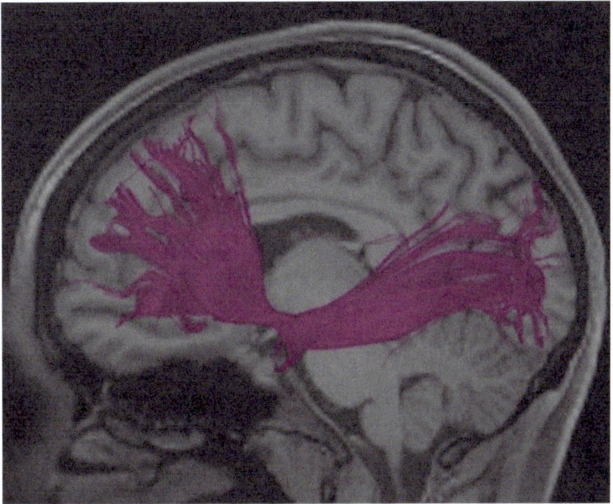

**Fig. 3.10** Image of the inferior frontal occipital fasciculus (IFOF)

posteriorly in the occipital lobe, it is a tight bundle in the insula and limen insula. This means that if you are in IFOF fibers in the frontal or occipital regions, then you are working on fibers relevant to the area you have cut into, but in the insula, you can destroy a lot of the tract all at once.

The occipital origins of this tract are principally in the lingual gyrus and cuneus and after hooking superiorly around the preoccipital notch before diverging from the ILF and crossing at the TPO junction as a largely compact bundle. After bending anterosuperiorly at the limen insula, the fibers fan out. The bulk of these fibers head to the SFG where they interact with a large length of the gyrus. There are also communications with the IFG and a lesser communication with the MFG.

## *Inferior Longitudinal Fasciculus (ILF)*

The ILF is an anterior to posterior tract running from the occipital pole to the temporal pole running just deep to the fusiform gyrus on the inferior temporal/occipital surface. This tract does not typically block a lateral approach to a deeper target in the way other lateral tracts do; however, it is a common path for spread of gliomas.

It primarily connects the inferior temporal gyrus to the lingual gyrus though some fibers extend superiorly into the temporal pole.

## *Uncinate Fasciculus*

Most of us are aware that this tract is running in the limen insula and connects the frontal and occipital lobes. Specifically, it connects the inferior frontal gyrus and pars triangularis to the anterior temporal lobe.

## *IFOF/ILF/Uncinate and the Role of the Temporal Pole in Language*

There are ample data supporting the role of the left temporal pole in language [26]. This has been termed semantic language; however, this is an unfortunate term as the semantic areas (those which activate during tasks of semantic language) do not have substantial connections via the IFOF or ILF to the temporal pole. Various two pathway models have been proposed about how these language problems occur. One model involves visual information flowing to area 45 via the IFOF. The problem we have found with this model is that none of the visual areas we have found connected to IFOF are high-level visual areas involved in object recognition; they are mostly connected to V1–4 and the dorsal visual stream ("where" pathway), neither of which seems to directly provide information needed to make visual matches by itself. Another involves the ILF carrying visual information to the temporal pole via ILF, which then communicates with area 45 via the uncinate. This is possible but the meaning of words is strongly localized to the back of the left temporal lobe in most people, and it's hard to fit the ILF into that model. The most plausible model we are aware of (Fig. 3.11) involves a band of U-fibers in the middle temporal gyrus which directly links the semantic areas to the temporal pole [26]. The functional

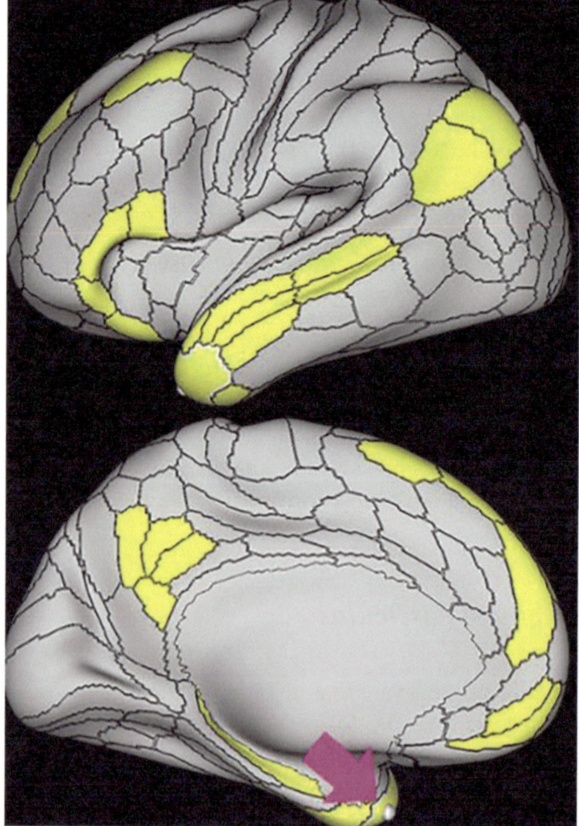

**Fig. 3.11** Functional connectivity of the area TGd which is the temporal polar region. It shows connectivity with the language area in a band of connected areas as well as with the DMN

connectivity map strongly suggests this is the connection. This does not preclude a role for ILF or IFOF in the cognitive aspects of speech as the visual system requires a large amount of top-down regulation to determine its processing scheme, and ILF and IFOF are well connected to do this. It is just hard for us to believe that by themselves, they can help match visual images to words given their connection patterns.

## The Visual System

It is an understatement to say that the human visual system is highly complex despite being localized to the occipital lobe (Fig. 3.12) [33]. A substantial percentage of the white matter in the brain aims to link the visual system to the rest of the brain.

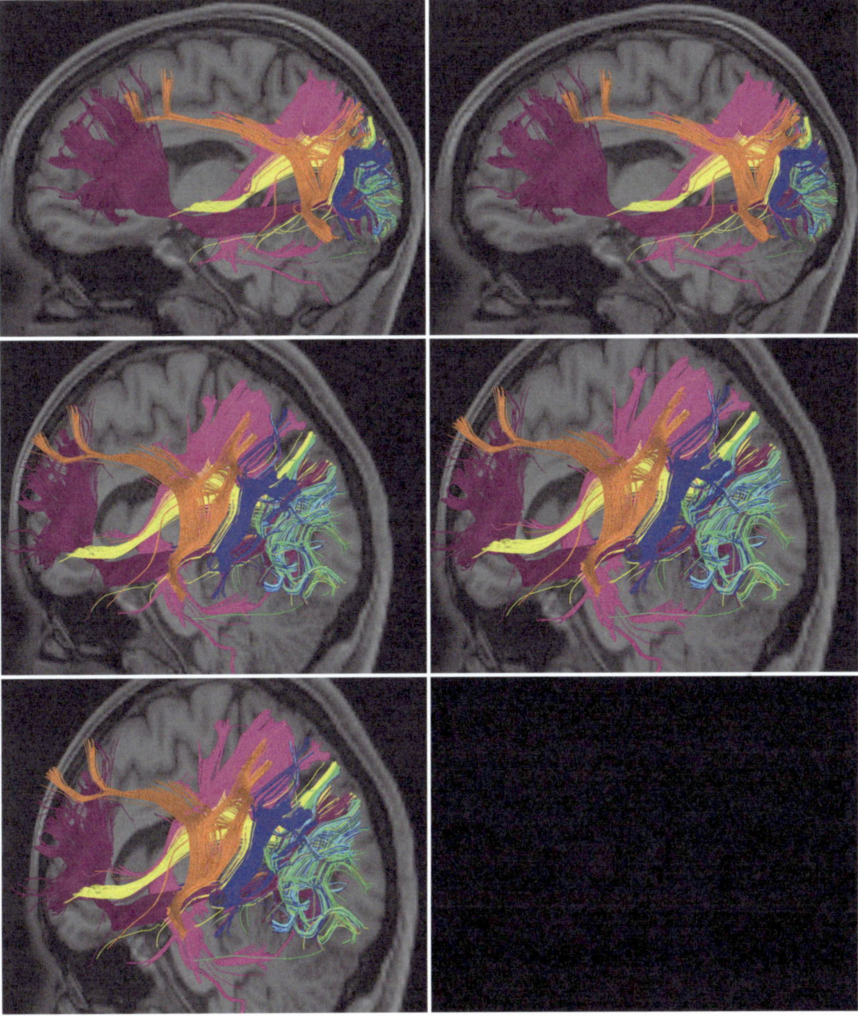

**Fig. 3.12** Network map of the visual system

## *Optic Radiations*

It is also of relevance to note that the visual system probably works in large part by communications with the pulvinar which are critical in serial visual processing. These fibers generally run in the same bundle as the optic radiations.

## *Middle Longitudinal Fasciculus (MdLF)*

It principally connects the upper cuneus to the superior temporal gyrus. The most logical explanation is this is a mechanism of linking the dorsal visual pathway (which has later level processing cortices in these regions) with the semantic areas.

## *Vertical Occipital Fasciculus (VOF)*

While there has long been a goal to segregate the visual processing into the ventral ("what" pathway) and dorsal ("where" pathway) streams, the VOF is a vertical pathway which directly connects these two areas.

## *Occipitotemporal System (OTS)*

The OTS is the system of the lateral occipital lobe and is comprised of a dense collection of large and small U-fibers which connect the lateral occipital lobe. It is most likely involved in reading.

## The Prefrontal Cognitive Initiation Axis

The initiation axis is a string of prefrontal, higher-order networks involving the default mode network, the central executive network, and the salience network [34, 35].

The default mode network (DMN) is anatomically included in the anteromedial frontal lobe, the posterior cingulate cortex (PCC), and the lateral parietal lobe that are activated only in the task negative state. The DMN is probably the most consistently identifiable network in the brain and is involved in numerous complex cognitive abilities, such as speech, theory of mind, and memory, among others [36]. It is functionally opposite of the central executive network, suggesting the contrast between our internal (DMN) and external (CEN) minds.

The salience network is a third network which appears to be key in this transition [37]. Failure to alternate these networks has been found in minimally conscious and vegetative patients and has been shown to be impaired in schizophrenics with severe negative symptoms and also depression [38, 39]. Thus, it seems reasonable to hypothesize that disruption of this system might impair a patient's ability to organize their thoughts, create a plan, and transition toward doing this, though obviously this is a complex process.

## *Default Mode Network*

The DMN (Fig. 3.13) is classically a three-part system with hubs anteromedial frontal lobe, PCC, and angular gyrus [40]. Careful study shows this is not entirely adequate as parts of the middle temporal gyrus, the thalamus, and the hippocampus also strongly correlate with these regions in many datasets. Figure 3.3 shows our model of the DMN. The anterior frontal regions include areas a24, s32, p32, and 10r; the PCC areas include areas 31a, 31pd, 31 pv, d23ab, v23ab, 7 m, POS1, and POS2; and the retrosplenial cortex (RSC) and the lateral parietal regions include PFm, PGs, and PGi. The anterior frontal and PCC areas are clearly joined by the cingulum [41]. There does not seem to be direct white matter connection of the lateral parietal regions and the medial regions, and this suggests that the network is functionally constructed by the thalamocortical rhythms or by interplay with other neighboring areas (see below).

## *Salience Network*

The salience network (Fig. 3.14) is a middle cingulate and anterior insula network [37]. Its middle cingulate structure includes areas a32prime, p32prime, and SCEF (supplementary and cingulate eye field), and its insular regions include AVI (anterior ventral insula), MI (middle insula), and the frontal opercular areas FOP4 and

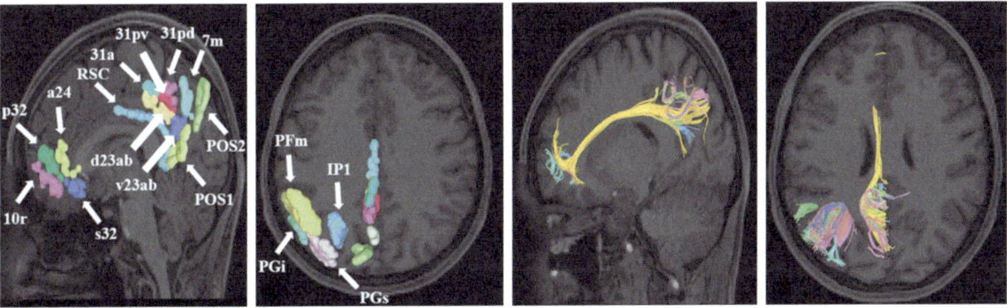


**Fig. 3.13** Network map of the default mode network

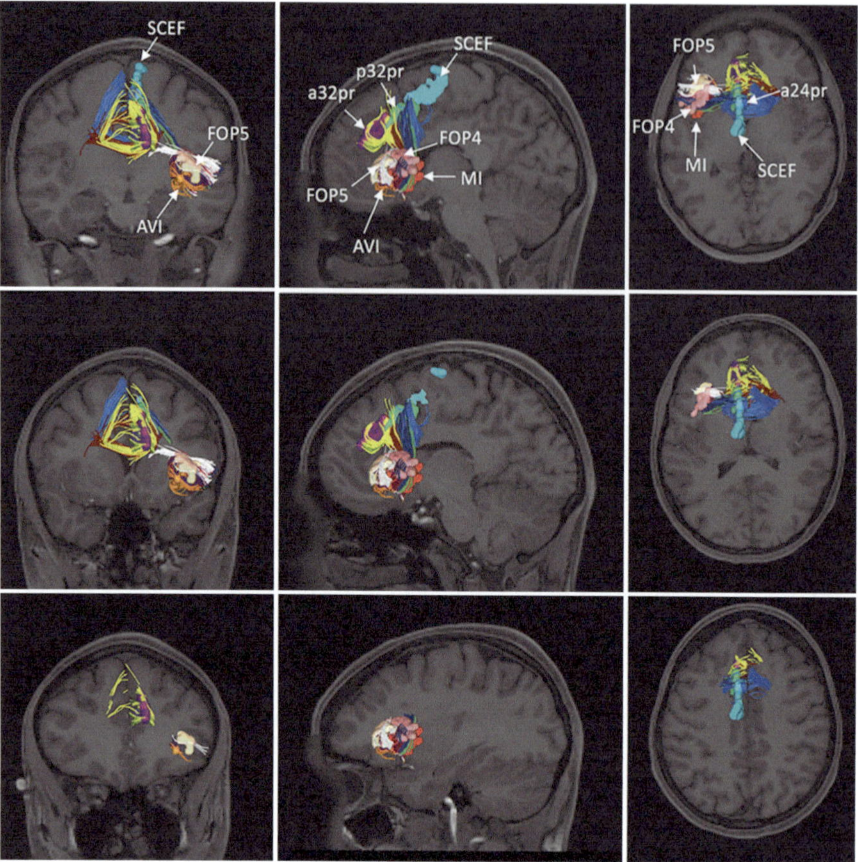


**Fig. 3.14** Network map of the salience network

FOP5. These are linked via the FAT. Most interestingly, the SCEF is also a part of the SMA complex, providing a critical link between the large-scale networks and the motor planning system.

## *Central Executive Network (CEN)*

The CEN is basically a frontopolar and parietal network (Fig. 3.15). Presently, we think this likely involves connections between HCP areas; prefrontal areas 9a, 9p, 9-46d, a9-46v, and 46; polar areas a10p and p10p; and inferior frontal sulcus areas IFSa and IFSp with the parietal areas Pft and PF, opercular area OP4, and intraparietal sulcus areas AIP, IP1, and IP2. These areas are probably linked by the superior longitudinal fasciculus [32].

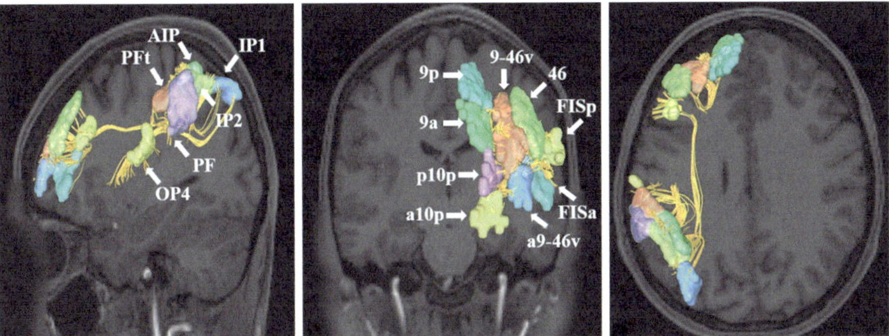


**Fig. 3.15**  Network map of the central executive network

## *Supplementary Motor Area*

These areas in the medial bank of the posterior superior frontal gyrus include areas 6ma, 6mp, and SCEF and superior frontal language area (SFL) (Fig. 3.6) [24]. In addition to its immediate neighbors, the SMA connects to the contralateral SMA via the corpus callosum; the ipsilateral premotor, opercular, and insular areas via the FAT; and the contralateral premotor areas via the crossed FAT which runs in the middle callosum, as well as contributing to fibers entering the basal ganglia and corticospinal tract. Interestingly, direct connections to the primary motor cortex are surprisingly sparse. The fact that the SMA contains a connection between the superior frontal language area and the canonical Broca's regions such as area 44 is a likely mechanism behind the mutism component of SMA syndrome [34].

## Conclusion

This chapter attempts to summarize an enormous topic and focus it toward the needs of neurosurgeons. It is important to note that we expect that a chapter like this written in 5 years from the current date will look different as this is a dynamic area which is evolving quickly. However, improved understanding of how to model and apply knowledge about the large-scale brain networks can better inform neurosurgical decision-making by better exposing the risks and benefits associated with certain tumors and related surgical decision-making.

## References


1. Bullmore E, Sporns O. The economy of brain network organization. Nat Rev Neurosci. 2012;13(5):336–49. https://doi.org/10.1038/nrn3214.
2. Dadario NB, Brahimaj B, Yeung J, Sughrue ME. Reducing the cognitive footprint of brain tumor surgery. Front Neurol. 2021;12:711646. https://doi.org/10.3389/fneur.2021.711646.

3. Dhandapani M, Gupta S, Mohanty M, Gupta SK, Dhandapani S. Trends in cognitive dysfunction following surgery for intracranial tumors. Surg Neurol Int. 2016;7(Suppl 7):S190–5. https://doi.org/10.4103/2152-7806.179229.

4. Herbet G, Moritz-Gasser S. Beyond language: mapping cognition and emotion. Neurosurg Clin N Am. 2019;30(1):75–83. https://doi.org/10.1016/j.nec.2018.08.004.

5. Schilling KG, Petit L, Rheault F, et al. Brain connections derived from diffusion MRI tractography can be highly anatomically accurate—if we know where white matter pathways start, where they end, and where they do not go. Brain Struct Funct. 2020;225(8):2387–402. https://doi.org/10.1007/s00429-020-02129-z.

6. O'Donnell LJ, Pasternak O. Does diffusion MRI tell us anything about the white matter? An overview of methods and pitfalls. Schizophr Res. 2015;161(1):133–41. https://doi.org/10.1016/j.schres.2014.09.007.

7. Stejskal EO, Tanner JE. Spin diffusion measurements: spin echoes in the presence of a time-dependent field gradient. J Chem Phys. 1965;42:288. https://doi.org/10.1063/1.1695690.

8. Setsompop K, Cohen-Adad J, Gagoski BA, et al. Improving diffusion MRI using simultaneous multi-slice echo planar imaging. NeuroImage. 2012;63(1):569–80. https://doi.org/10.1016/j.neuroimage.2012.06.033.

9. Andersson JLR, Sotiropoulos SN. An integrated approach to correction for off-resonance effects and subject movement in diffusion MR imaging. NeuroImage. 2016;125:1063–78. https://doi.org/10.1016/j.neuroimage.2015.10.019.

10. Yeh F-C, Verstynen TD, Wang Y, Fernández-Miranda JC, Tseng W-YI. Deterministic diffusion fiber tracking improved by quantitative anisotropy. PLoS One. 2013;8(11):e80713.

11. Grisot G, Haber SN, Yendiki A. Diffusion MRI and anatomic tracing in the same brain reveal common failure modes of tractography. NeuroImage. 2021;239:118300. https://doi.org/10.1016/j.neuroimage.2021.118300.

12. O'Neal CM, Ahsan SA, Dadario NB, et al. A connectivity model of the anatomic substrates underlying ideomotor apraxia: a meta-analysis of functional neuroimaging studies. Clin Neurol Neurosurg. 2021;207:106765. https://doi.org/10.1016/j.clineuro.2021.106765.

13. Wedeen VJ, Wang RP, Schmahmann JD, et al. Diffusion spectrum magnetic resonance imaging (DSI) tractography of crossing fibers. Neuroimage. 2008;41(4):1267–77. https://doi.org/10.1016/j.neuroimage.2008.03.036.

14. Morez J, Sijbers J, Vanhevel F, Jeurissen B. Constrained spherical deconvolution of nonspherically sampled diffusion MRI data. Hum Brain Mapp. 2021;42(2):521–38. https://doi.org/10.1002/hbm.25241.

15. Sarwar T, Ramamohanarao K, Zalesky A. Mapping connectomes with diffusion MRI: deterministic or probabilistic tractography? Magn Reson Med. 2019;81(2):1368–84. https://doi.org/10.1002/mrm.27471.

16. Yeh F-C, Irimia A, Bastos DCdA, Golby AJ. Tractography methods and findings in brain tumors and traumatic brain injury. NeuroImage. 2021;245:118651. https://doi.org/10.1016/j.neuroimage.2021.118651.

17. Fornito A, Bullmore ET. What can spontaneous fluctuations of the blood oxygenation-level-dependent signal tell us about psychiatric disorders? Curr Opin Psychiatry. 2010;23(3)

18. Park KY, Lee JJ, Dierker D, et al. Mapping language function with task-based vs. resting-state functional MRI. PLoS One. 2020;15(7):e0236423. https://doi.org/10.1371/journal.pone.0236423.

19. Baker CM, Burks JD, Briggs RG, et al. A connectomic atlas of the human cerebrum-chapter 1: introduction, methods, and significance. Oper Neurosurg (Hagerstown). 2018;15(suppl_1):S1–9. https://doi.org/10.1093/ons/opy253.

20. Lee MH, Smyser CD, Shimony JS. Resting-state fMRI: a review of methods and clinical applications. AJNR Am J Neuroradiol. 2013;34(10):1866–72. https://doi.org/10.3174/ajnr.A3263.

21. Beckmann CF, DeLuca M, Devlin JT, Smith SM. Investigations into resting-state connectivity using independent component analysis. Philos Trans R Soc Lond Ser B Biol Sci. 2005;360(1457):1001–13. https://doi.org/10.1098/rstb.2005.1634.

22. Glasser MF, Coalson TS, Robinson EC, et al. A multi-modal parcellation of human cerebral cortex. Nature. 2016;536(7615):171–8. https://doi.org/10.1038/nature18933.
23. Briggs RG, Conner AK, Baker CM, et al. A connectomic atlas of the human cerebrum-chapter 18: the connectional anatomy of human brain networks. Oper Neurosurg (Hagerstown). 2018;15(suppl_1):S470–s480. https://doi.org/10.1093/ons/opy272.
24. Sheets JR, Briggs RG, Young IM, et al. Parcellation-based modeling of the supplementary motor area. J Neurol Sci. 2021;421:117322. https://doi.org/10.1016/j.jns.2021.117322.
25. Sheets JR, Briggs RG, Dadario NB, et al. A cortical Parcellation based analysis of ventral premotor area connectivity. Neurol Res. 2021;43(7):595–607. https://doi.org/10.1080/0161641 2.2021.1902702.
26. Briggs RG, Tanglay O, Dadario NB, et al. The unique Fiber anatomy of middle temporal gyrus default mode connectivity. Oper Neurosurg (Hagerstown). 2021;21(1):E8–E14. https://doi.org/10.1093/ons/opab109.
27. Poologaindran A, Lowe SR, Sughrue ME. The cortical organization of language: distilling human connectome insights for supratentorial neurosurgery. J Neurosurg. 2020;134(6):1959–66. https://doi.org/10.3171/2020.5.JNS191281.
28. Kuiper JJ, Lin YH, Young IM, et al. A parcellation-based model of the auditory network. Hear Res. 2020;396:108078. https://doi.org/10.1016/j.heares.2020.108078.
29. Conner AK, Briggs RG, Rahimi M, et al. A connectomic atlas of the human cerebrum-chapter 10: tractographic description of the superior longitudinal fasciculus. Oper Neurosurg (Hagerstown). 2018;15(suppl_1):S407-s422. https://doi.org/10.1093/ons/opy264.
30. Allan PG, Briggs RG, Conner AK, et al. Parcellation-based tractographic modeling of the dorsal attention network. Brain Behav. 2019;9(10):e01365. https://doi.org/10.1002/brb3.1365.
31. Allan PG, Briggs RG, Conner AK, et al. Parcellation-based tractographic modeling of the ventral attention network. J Neurol Sci. 2020;408:116548. https://doi.org/10.1016/j.jns.2019.116548.
32. Niendam TA, Laird AR, Ray KL, Dean YM, Glahn DC, Carter CS. Meta-analytic evidence for a superordinate cognitive control network subserving diverse executive functions. Cogn Affect Behav Neurosci. 2012;12(2):241–68. https://doi.org/10.3758/s13415-011-0083-5.
33. Palejwala AH, Dadario NB, Young IM, et al. Anatomy and white matter connections of the lingual gyrus and cuneus. World Neurosurg. 2021;151:e426–37. https://doi.org/10.1016/j.wneu.2021.04.050.
34. Briggs RG, Allan PG, Poologaindran A, et al. The frontal aslant tract and supplementary motor area syndrome: moving towards a connectomic initiation axis. Cancers (Basel). 2021;13(5) https://doi.org/10.3390/cancers13051116.
35. Darby RR, Joutsa J, Burke MJ, Fox MD. Lesion network localization of free will. Proc Natl Acad Sci U S A. 2018;115(42):10792–7. https://doi.org/10.1073/pnas.1814117115.
36. Andrews-Hanna JR, Reidler JS, Sepulcre J, Poulin R, Buckner RL. Functional-anatomic fractionation of the brain's default network. Neuron. 2010;65(4):550–62. https://doi.org/10.1016/j.neuron.2010.02.005.
37. Seeley WW, Menon V, Schatzberg AF, et al. Dissociable intrinsic connectivity networks for salience processing and executive control. J Neurosci. 2007;27(9):2349–56. https://doi.org/10.1523/JNEUROSCI.5587-06.2007.
38. Menon V. Large-scale brain networks and psychopathology: a unifying triple network model. Trends Cogn Sci. 2011;15(10):483–506. https://doi.org/10.1016/j.tics.2011.08.003.
39. Kaiser RH, Andrews-Hanna JR, Wager TD, Pizzagalli DA. Large-scale network dysfunction in major depressive disorder: a meta-analysis of resting-state functional connectivity. JAMA Psychiat. 2015;72(6):603–11. https://doi.org/10.1001/jamapsychiatry.2015.0071.
40. Sandhu Z, Tanglay O, Young IM, et al. Parcellation-based anatomic modeling of the default mode network. Brain Behav. 2021;11(2):e01976. https://doi.org/10.1002/brb3.1976.
41. Burks JD, Bonney PA, Conner AK, et al. A method for safely resecting anterior butterfly gliomas: the surgical anatomy of the default mode network and the relevance of its preservation. J Neurosurg. 2017;126(6):1795–811. https://doi.org/10.3171/2016.5.JNS153006.

# Chapter 4
# Advanced Neuroimaging of the Ventricular System

Paul E. Kim

## Introduction

The spatial complexity of the ventricular system and its deep position within the brain poses a problem for conceptualizing its anatomy. An additional problem with understanding its anatomy is that the ventricles are essentially comprised of spaces rather than solid parenchymal structures. Thus, imaging has provided greater understanding of its anatomical complexity and variation than has cadaveric dissection, which is otherwise considered the gold standard for anatomic education.

The first use of X-rays for a neurological disorder by Harvey Cushing in 1896 (a gunshot wound to the neck causing a Brown-Sequard syndrome) [14] was a year after the discovery of X-rays by Wilhelm Roentgen. However, until Walter Dandy's pneumoencephalogram in 1918 [16], direct imaging of the intracranial contents in general and ventricular system in particular was limited to fortuitous instances of calcified intra- or periventricular tumors or post-inflammatory calcifications dense enough to outline portions of the ventricles on a plain X-ray [28, 29]. The development of computerized tomographic imaging and nuclear magnetic resonance imaging in 1973 [5, 37] was the paradigm shift that transitioned neuroimaging into the modern age. The consequences on neurosurgical therapeutic interventions cannot be understated. Ongoing advances in MRI techniques have further driven the understanding of ventricular physiology and CSF flow dynamics in ways not heretofore possible.

P. E. Kim (✉)
Division of Neuroradiology, Department of Radiology, University of Southern California
Keck School of Medicine, Los Angeles, CA, USA
e-mail: paul.kim@med.usc.edu

© Springer Nature Switzerland AG 2022
G. Zada et al. (eds.), *Subcortical Neurosurgery*,
https://doi.org/10.1007/978-3-030-95153-5_4

## Magnetic Resonance Imaging

Normal cerebrospinal fluid (CSF) outlines the ventricular system on MRI and follows the simple signal characteristics of water: hypointense on T1-weighted images and hyperintense on T2-weighted images. Suppression of CSF signal using inversion recovery techniques can be accomplished on both T1- and T2-weighted acquisitions recognized as FLAIR (Fluid-Attenuated Inversion Recovery) [17, 26].

High-resolution MRI techniques utilize 3D acquisitions such as 3D SPACE (Sampling Perfection with Application-optimized Contrasts using different flip angle Evolution, Siemens), and steady-state acquisitions 3D-CISS (Constructive Interference in the Steady State, Siemens), 3D-FIESTA (Fast Imaging Employing Steady-state Acquisition, GE), and 3D-FASE (Fast Advanced Spin Echo, Canon) can provide submillimeter isotropic resolution. These techniques are capable of resolving thin membranes within the subarachnoid space or ventricles such as the membrane of Liliequist, which is an important structure to recognize prior to performing endoscopic third ventriculostomy (ETV) [23] (Fig. 4.1). Because they are high-resolution 3D datasets, they can be reconstructed in multiple ways to depict information that would otherwise difficult to conceptualize. They can be of

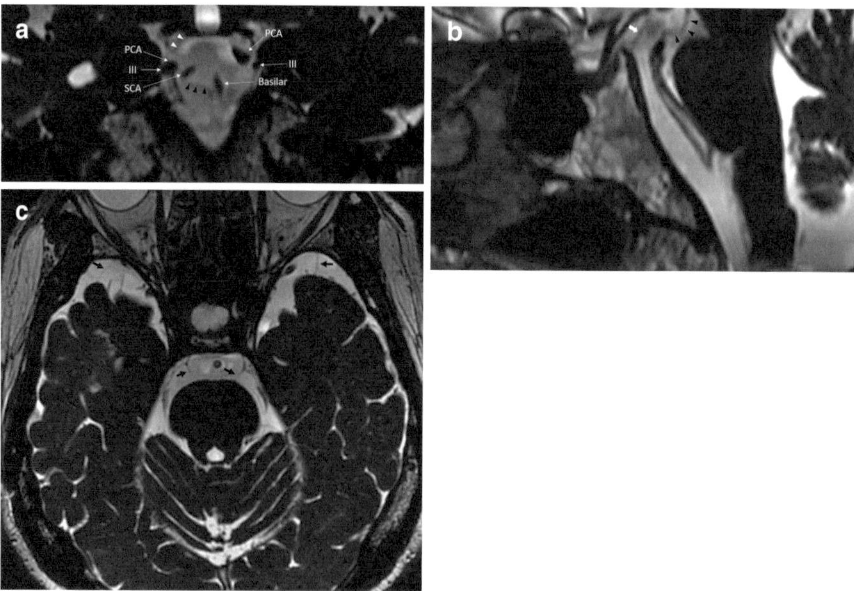


**Fig. 4.1** High-resolution 3D FIESTA demonstrating several of the arachnoid membranes in the basilar cisterns: (**a**) Coronal multiplanar reformat (MPR) of 3D FIESTA dataset can resolve the mesencephalic portion of Liliequist's membrane (black arrowheads), hypothalamic membrane (white arrowheads), posterior cerebral artery (PCA), basilar artery, and oculomotor nerve (III). (**b**) Sagittal MPR midsagittal view demonstrating the sellar segment (white arrow) and mesencephalic segment (black arrowheads) of Liliequist's membrane. (**c**) Axial view through the rostral pons demonstrating multiple subarachnoid membranes in the prepontine cistern and middle cranial fossa

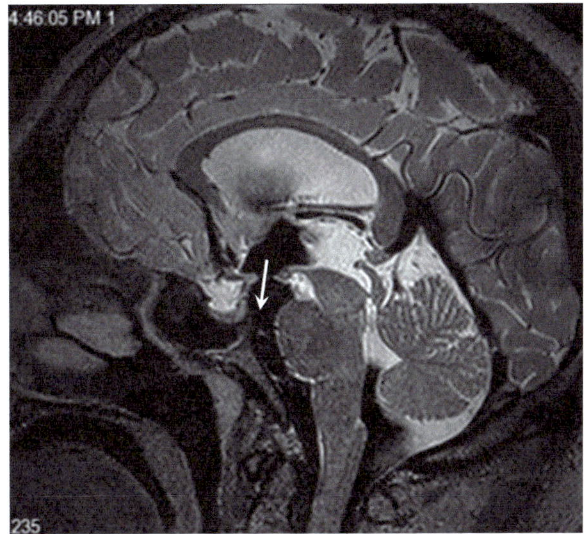

**Fig. 4.2** Endoscopic third ventriculostomy (ETV) imaging using high-resolution MRI techniques: 3D SPACE sagittal image demonstrating normal caudal antegrade CSF flow void from the third ventricle through a functioning patent ETV (arrow). (Reprinted from Kartal and Algin [32])

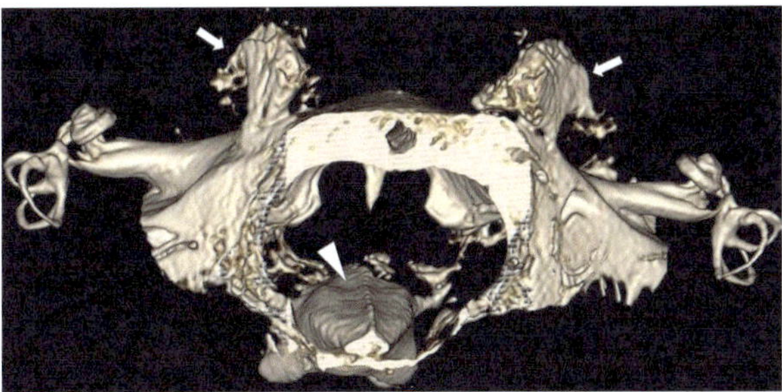

**Fig. 4.3** 3D volume rendering of posterior fossa cisterns and fourth ventricle viewed from above, obtained from 3D FIESTA dataset, applicable to creating virtual endoscopy and surgical models. Note the highly detailed "cast" of the fourth ventricle with clear 3D rendering of the facial colliculus (white arrowhead), bilateral internal auditory canals and membranous labyrinth, and bilateral Meckel's caves (white arrows)

particular value in studying the CSF pathway in hydrocephalus resulting from subarachnoid or intraventricular membranes and arachnoid cysts and after endoscopic third ventriculostomy [3, 19, 20, 23, 35, 36], [18] (Fig. 4.2). These membranes are typically not resolved at the level of spatial resolution offered in routine brain MRI sequences. The degree of anatomic precision offered by these datasets also provides the level of volume rendering detail needed for virtual endoscopy and 3D modeling [33, 58] (Fig. 4.3).

## *CSF Imaging*

The principal artifact encountered in MR imaging of the ventricles is *phase-encoding artifact* related to CSF pulsations [39, 55]. Normal CSF pulsations produce fairly characteristic, albeit variable appearances on conventional MRI sequences (Fig. 4.4). *Abnormal* CSF motion through the ventricle can sometimes be distinguished from normal artifacts on conventional MR imaging by visual inspection when CSF pulsation artifacts are excessively prominent in communicating hydrocephalus or completely absent in obstructive hydrocephalus but usually requires other flow-sensitive and/or quantitative techniques to assess adequately.

CSF flow is pulsatile, with a to-and-fro movement resulting from expansion and contraction of the intracranial vessels associated with the cardiac cycle [39]. CSF flow imaging utilizes the motion of CSF to generate images and is used to assess clinical situations such as aqueductal stenosis, normal pressure hydrocephalus (NPH), patency of third ventriculostomy, and flow at the cervicomedullary junction in Chiari 1 malformation or achondroplasia [40]. There are a variety of MRI techniques that both qualitatively and *quantitatively* assess CSF flow.

### Phase Contrast CSF Flow Imaging

The most common technique used is time-resolved 2D phase contrast MRI with velocity encoding. This technique relies upon location-specific sequential application

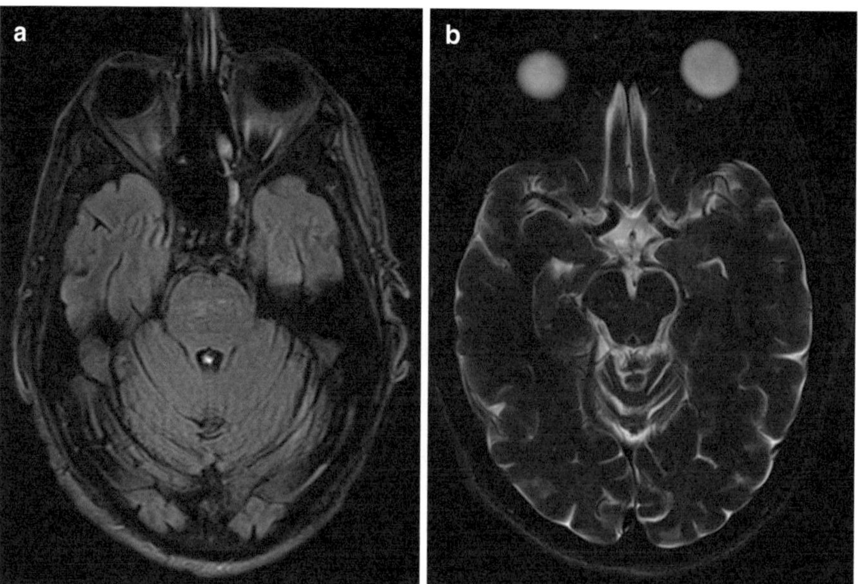


**Fig. 4.4** Typical normal CSF pulsation artifacts seen as high signal absence of CSF nulling in the fourth ventricle on T2 FLAIR (**a**) or distinct hypointense signal flow void in the aqueduct of Sylvius on T2-weighted images (**b**)

of a pair of phase-encoding pulses in opposite directions. Stationary protons will experience the same pulse at both times and therefore return no signal. Protons that are in motion will be subject to different phase-encoding pulses and will thus be visible [8, 12, 44]. With this technique, the expected velocity of CSF flow is stated as velocity encoding (VENC) and is noted in cm/sec. Typical normal CSF flow is 5–8 cm/sec. In patients with hyperdynamic circulation (e.g., NPH, communicating hydrocephalus), much higher velocities can be encountered relying on higher VENCs (up to 25 cm/s). Quantification of flow can be generated by defining a region of interest (e.g., cross-sectional area of the aqueduct of Sylvius) and charting velocity versus time, which is typically pulsatile – forward during systole and backward during diastole. The area under the curve for each cardiac phase generates values of flow forward and flow backward, notably increasing in both directions in communicating hydrocephalus and NPH [8] (Fig. 4.5).

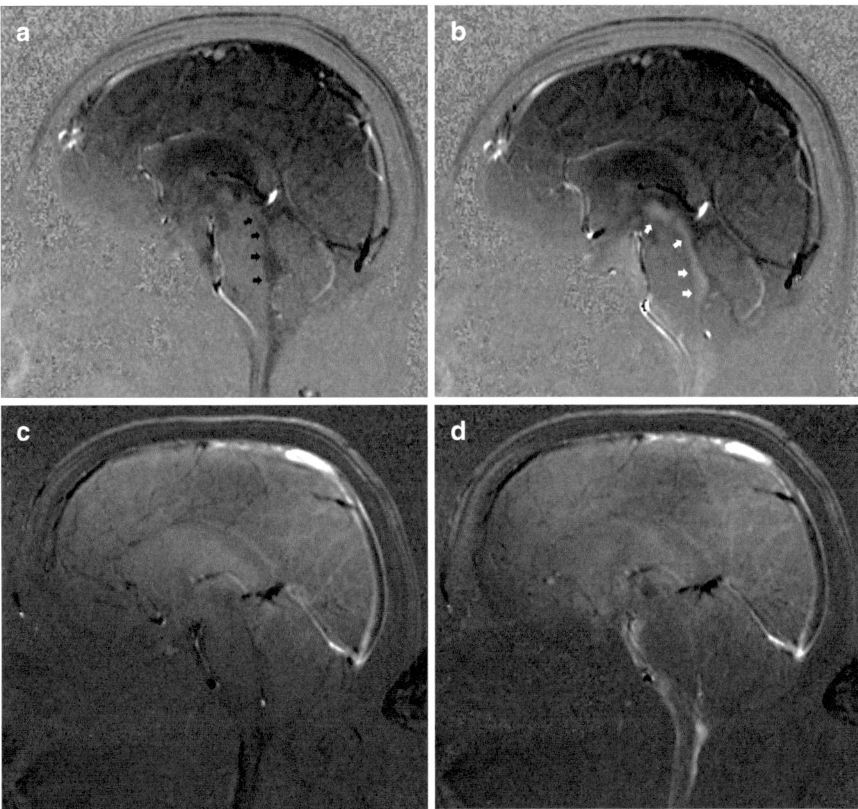

**Fig. 4.5** Phase contrast cine CSF flow study in normal pressure hydrocephalus. (**a**) Abnormally prominent antegrade flow of CSF in systole is dark signal flowing caudally through the aqueduct, fourth ventricle, and outlet foramina to the subarachnoid space of the cervicomedullary junction (black arrows). (**b**) Excessive retrograde flow in diastole is demonstrated as bright signal flowing rostrally into the third ventricle (white arrows). By comparison, normal systolic and diastolic appearances are shown in (**c**) and (**d**)

## Time-Spatial Labeling Inversion Pulse (Time-SLIP)

CSF imaging with the time-SLIP technique is based on an arterial spin-labeling technique, utilizing the "black-blood double inversion recovery" technique commonly used in cardiac imaging to create intrinsic contrast in a fluid (e.g., blood or CSF) as it flows into a specific area of interest from another area [22]. After inverting the overall signals with a nonselective inversion recovery (IR) pulse, a selective IR pulse (tag) is set for CSF in arbitrary cross sections and directions, and then movement of CSF is captured at each black-blood time-inversion pulse (BBTI). Thus, CSF within this selected area is labeled as an endogenous tracer without using a contrast medium [1] (Fig. 4.6).

## *Ventriculography*

Despite good anatomic demonstration of brain parenchyma and CSF with aforementioned conventional and advanced MRI techniques, there remain a number of instances in which CSF contrast enhancement may yield more diagnostic information, such as detailed assessment of communication between normal CSF and abnormal CSF collections, arachnoid cysts, membranes, and leakage.

Contrast ventriculography can be obtained with CT with iodinated contrast media or MRI with gadolinium-based contrast media. While it can be accomplished through cisternal puncture such as LP by allowing reflux or gravity to move contrast into the ventricles, it more typically requires direct intraventricular injection of contrast to obtain diagnostically adequate opacification [24, 42] (Fig. 4.7).

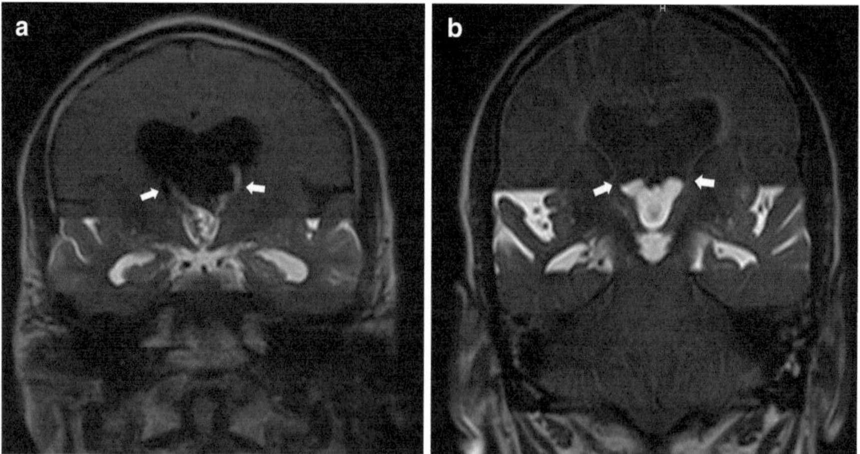

**Fig. 4.6** Time-SLIP evaluation of reflux from the third ventricle to the lateral ventricles through the foramina of Monro in normal (**a**) and normal pressure hydrocephalus (**b**). Normally, high signal-labeled CSF is seen refluxing into the lateral ventricles through the foramina of Monro (white arrows in **a**). In NPH, this normal reflux is absent (white arrows in **b**)

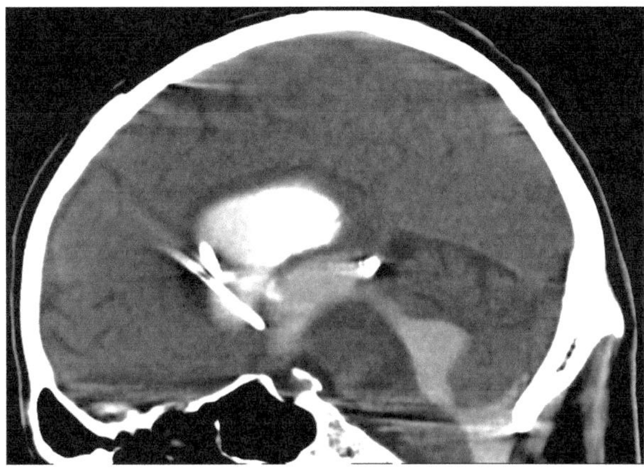

**Fig. 4.7** Contrast ventriculography performed by injection of iodinated contrast through a ventriculostomy. Despite ventricular enlargement, free flow of contrast was noted through the ventricular system into the perimedullary and upper cervical cisterns

## Imaging Ventricular Pathology

Ventricular abnormalities are, with only a few exceptions, a secondary phenomenon to pathology outside the ventricular system itself. The manifestations are rather limited: abnormal ventricular size and/or shape. Abnormal enlargement of the ventricles, *hydrocephalus*, is most commonly encountered, but abnormal diminution of ventricular size is also pathological, whether from mass effect or insufficient CSF volume. Pathological deformity of the normal ventricular contour may be the result of any space-occupying lesion inside or outside the ventricular system, as well as a sequela of inflammatory processes.

## *Hydrocephalus*

Walter Dandy first characterized the basic mechanism hydrocephalus as obstructive or nonobstructive over a century ago [15], and current classification systems still rely upon Dandy's classification scheme. Because the elements of hydrocephalus are so complex and diverse, definitions and classifications continue to be fluid within the scientific community, and there is yet to be a universally accepted definition of hydrocephalus [49]. The most commonly accepted definition is "…active distention of the ventricular system of the brain resulting from inadequate passage of CSF from its point of origin within the cerebral ventricles to its point of absorption into the systemic circulation" [50]. This definition supports a concept of hydrocephalus as an active process, produced by obstruction along the course of CSF flow or overproduction of CSF, and can be evaluated with morphologic or physiologic imaging [25]. Notably, this definition excludes the category of "*hydrocephalus ex vacuo*" resulting from loss of parenchymal volume.

## Conventional Imaging Diagnosis

The concept of enlarged ventricles appears simple, and severe abnormal ventriculomegaly with transependymal interstitial edema (Fig. 4.8) is usually easy to appreciate on imaging as active hydrocephalus. However, when hydrocephalus is early, mild or chronic, and "compensated," there can be significant ambiguity when evaluating an imaging exam isolated to a single timepoint. There have been multiple attempts at creating quantitative criteria for the diagnosis of hydrocephalus, beginning with the Evans Index in 1942 [57], with many others following, such as the bicaudate index [21], third ventricular width, fronto-occipital horn ratio [47, 48], and a number of others. Used alone, quantitative assessments – whether linear- or volume-based measurements – have ultimately fallen short, and there continues to be no entirely reliable imaging stigmata of hydrocephalus. More recent approaches using multiple criteria including linear measurements, volumetric data, and flow analysis have increased specificity [43], but despite general correlation between individual linear measurements and presence of hydrocephalus, specificity remains unreliably low in cases of mild ventricular enlargement [48]. The temporal horns have the greatest capacitance of the ventricular system, and enlargement is typically the earliest sign of hydrocephalus [51].

Noncommunicating ("obstructive") hydrocephalus is defined as obstruction at any point between the site of CSF production (choroid plexus) and the outlet foramina of the fourth ventricle. Communicating ("nonobstructive") hydrocephalus is defined as obstruction at an extraventricular level, essentially anywhere within the subarachnoid space to the site of CSF reabsorption, the arachnoid granulations. This distinction is thus artificial and made for its therapeutic implications as all hydrocephalus is pathophysiologically obstructive at some point between the ventricles and the systemic venous circulation, except for the relatively uncommon cases of

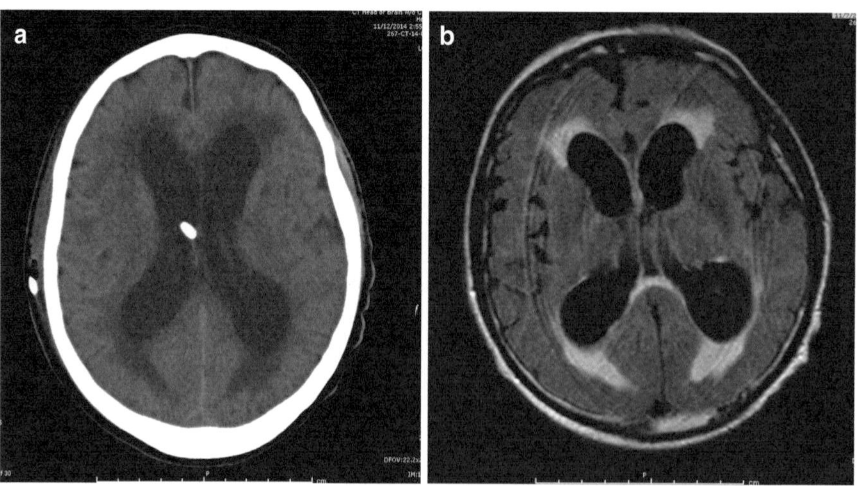

**Fig. 4.8** Typical transependymal edema seen at the external angles of the lateral ventricles on CT (**a**) and T2 FLAIR MRI (**b**)

overproduction of CSF occurring with choroid plexus tumors. Much as imaging criteria for hydrocephalus itself may be ambiguous, criterion for the imaging distinction between "noncommunicating" and "communicating" hydrocephalus is also problematic with significant overlap in the appearance of both types. For example, presence or absence of enlargement of the fourth ventricle, as well as the ratio between the third and fourth ventricular sizes, is not reliable in this distinction [34].

**Advanced Imaging Diagnosis – Assessment of CSF Flow**

Imaging techniques assessing CSF flow dynamics are the principal advanced methods for the evaluation of hydrocephalus. Noncommunicating (obstructive) hydrocephalus results in significantly diminished CSF flow rates and stroke volumes through the ventricular system, particularly the aqueduct of Sylvius, allowing for sensitive and specific identification, as well as reliable distinction from communicating hydrocephalus [54] (Fig. 4.9).

The same level of reliability in diagnosis of communicating hydrocephalus using CSF flow imaging techniques, however, remains more elusive, although these advanced methods do provide improved sensitivity and specificity compared to the static anatomic measurement methods noted previously [11]. Phase contrast techniques allow quantitative assessments of CSF flow, yielding various parameters of CSF flow, such as peak systolic velocity and stroke volume. In communicating hydrocephalus, the compliance of the entire downstream extraventricular CSF compartment results in relative hyperdynamic pulsatile flow of CSF through the aqueduct, typically manifested as an increase in peak systolic velocity and stroke volume [7, 13, 27] (Fig. 4.5). There is wide variability in reported normal peak CSF flow velocity at the cerebral aqueduct, but most reports range from approximately 2 to 5 cm/sec but can be as high as 10 cm/sec. In contrast, peak velocities in communicating NPH patients typically were greater than 6 cm/second [38, 53]. Notably then, there is significant overlap between normal volunteers and hydrocephalus patients. Increase in stroke volume has been cited as a more reliable parameter for identifying communicating hydrocephalus patients [56]. Time-SLIP has also been used to delineate normal and abnormal CSF flow dynamics. In a setting of NPH, the normal reflux of CSF from the third ventricle into the lateral ventricles through the foramina of Monro is largely absent or diminished [59] (Fig. 4.6).

Clinically, however, the NPH patient's response to shunting, not imaging metrics, is the raison d'etre of these evaluations. In this regard, these techniques unfortunately have not proven to be reliable enough to completely supplant clinical assessment measures after lumbar drain or large-volume lumbar puncture [11, 52, 56].

## *Lesions Involving the Intraventricular Space*

The intraventricular space, as has been noted, represents predominantly a fluid-filled *cavity* rather than an organic tissue structure, so with the exception of purely intraventricular lesions such as arachnoid cysts or cysticercosis, involvement in

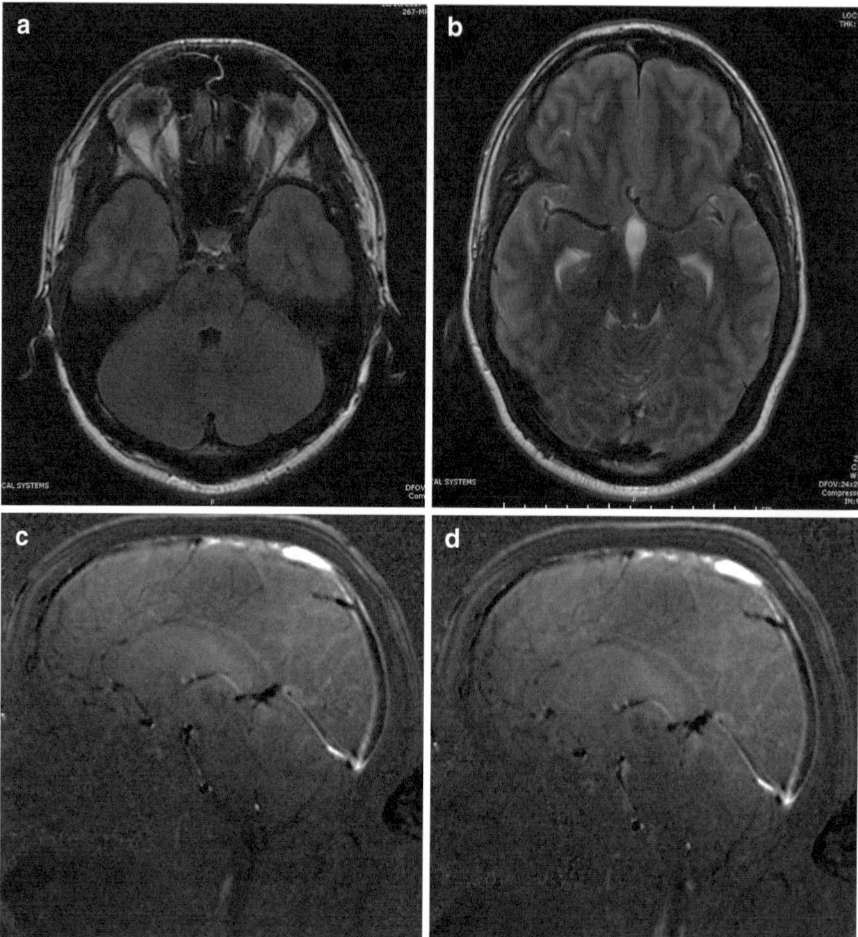

Fig. 4.9 Obstructive hydrocephalus. There is absence of normal bright signal CSF pulsation phase-encoding artifacts in the fourth ventricle on T2 FLAIR (**a**) and absence of the normal dark flow void seen in the aqueduct of Sylvius on T2-weighted images (**b**). Phase contrast cine-CSF flow study demonstrates significantly diminished dark antegrade systolic flow through the aqueduct and fourth ventricle (**c**) and bright retrograde diastolic flow (**d**). Note the contrast with normal flow and increased flow in NPH in Fig. 4.5

disease processes is actually secondary in most cases – resulting from intraventricular extension of parenchymal processes or arising from the wall of the ventricle (Table 4.1). However, there are structures which actually do lie completely within the intraventricular space, so lesions arising from these structures can be considered as truly of intraventricular origin, namely, the choroid plexus and tela choroidea. Choroid plexus cysts, papilloma, meningioma, and colloid cyst of the third ventricle are the most notable lesions arising from these structures.

**Table 4.1** Ventricular pathology by site of origin

| *Neoplasms of the ventricular wall and septum pellucidum* |
| --- |
| Ependymoma |
| Subependymoma |
| Central neurocytoma |
| Subependymal giant cell astrocytoma |
| Metastasis, lymphoma |
| *Neoplasms of the choroid plexus* |
| Choroid plexus papilloma |
| Choroid plexus carcinoma |
| Meningioma |
| Metastasis, lymphoma |
| *Parenchymal neoplasms with intraventricular extension* |
| Glioma |
| Medulloblastoma |
| Primitive neuroectodermal tumor |
| Sarcoma |
| Intraventricular teratoma |
| Metastasis, lymphoma |
| *Nonneoplastic lesions* |
| Colloid cysts |
| Neurocysticercosis |
| Intracranial hydatid cyst |
| Intracranial tuberculoma |

## Choroid Plexus Cyst (Xanthogranuloma)

Choroid plexus xanthogranulomas are common incidental lesions occurring in the glomus of the choroid plexus of the lateral ventricular atria, occurring in up to 7% of adults [31, 45]. They are nearly always incidental, with symptomatic cysts being extremely rare [30]. It is unclear in much of the literature whether they represent a distinct entity from adult choroid plexus cysts, but the distinction is irrelevant for all practical purposes – both clinically and radiographically. Signal characteristics on MRI are variable depending on the mixture of lipid, fluid, and blood products, but generally, they have an intermediate to low signal on T1 and intermediate to mildly hyperintense on T2 FLAIR, typically with a fine "foamy" internal architecture. Most distinctively, they demonstrate significant diffusion restriction on diffusion-weighted imaging (DWI) (Fig. 4.10).

## Meningioma

Meningiomas are the most common lesion arising from the choroid plexus in adults and derive from embryological invagination of arachnoid cap cells into the choroid plexus [10]. MRI features of intraventricular meningiomas do not deviate from

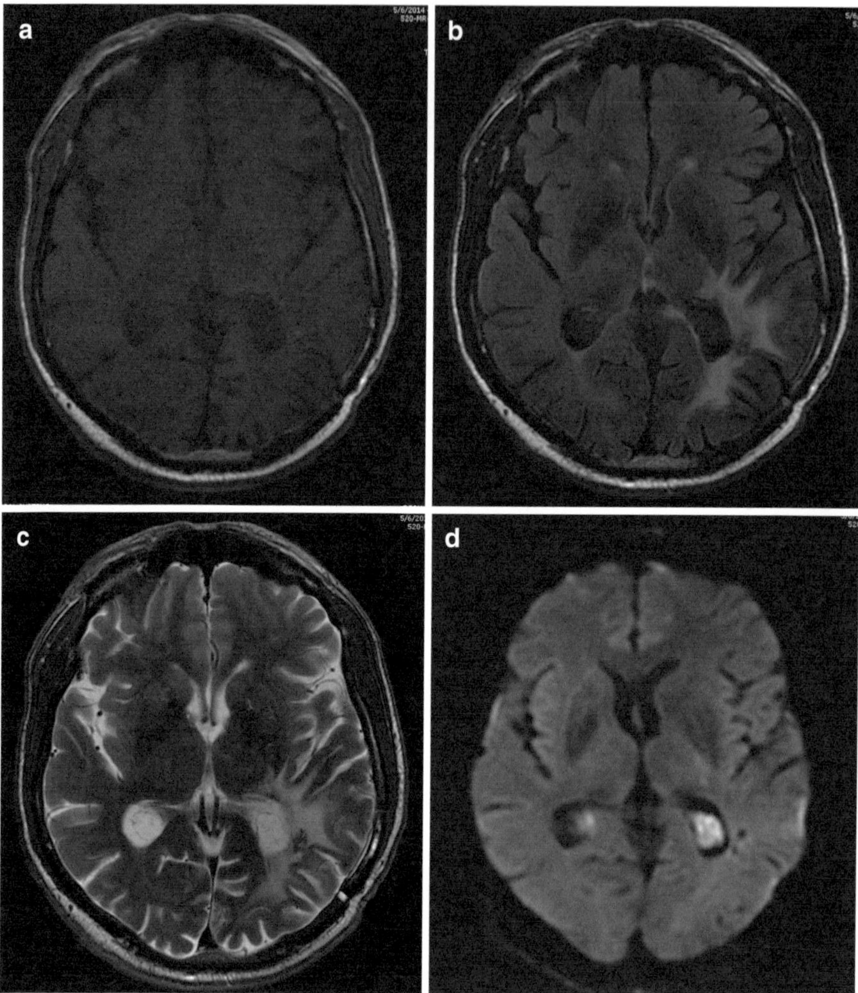

**Fig. 4.10** Xanthogranuloma of the choroid plexus. Typical appearance on MRI involving the glomus of the choroid plexus bilaterally in the atria of the lateral ventricles. These are typically mildly hypointense and homogeneous on T1 (**a**) and T2 FLAIR (**b**), while they are hyperintense on T2 (**c**) and demonstrate diffusion restriction with prominent high signal on DWI (**d**)

other meningiomas that more typically arise from the convexity or skull base, most commonly demonstrating homogeneous isointense signal on both T1- and T2-weighted images, homogeneous moderate to avid contrast enhancement, and variable calcification. They most commonly arise in the glomus of the choroid plexus in the lateral ventricle (Fig. 4.11). Although they are overall uncommon lesions, atrial intraventricular meningiomas are among the most common tumors seen in the lateral ventricle. On CT, they are sharply demarcated, lobular, and typically mildly hyperdense. On MRI, the lesion can appear as iso- to hypointense relative to gray matter on T1-weighted images and iso- to hypointense on T2-weighted images, with homogeneous moderate contrast enhancement of the mass. The

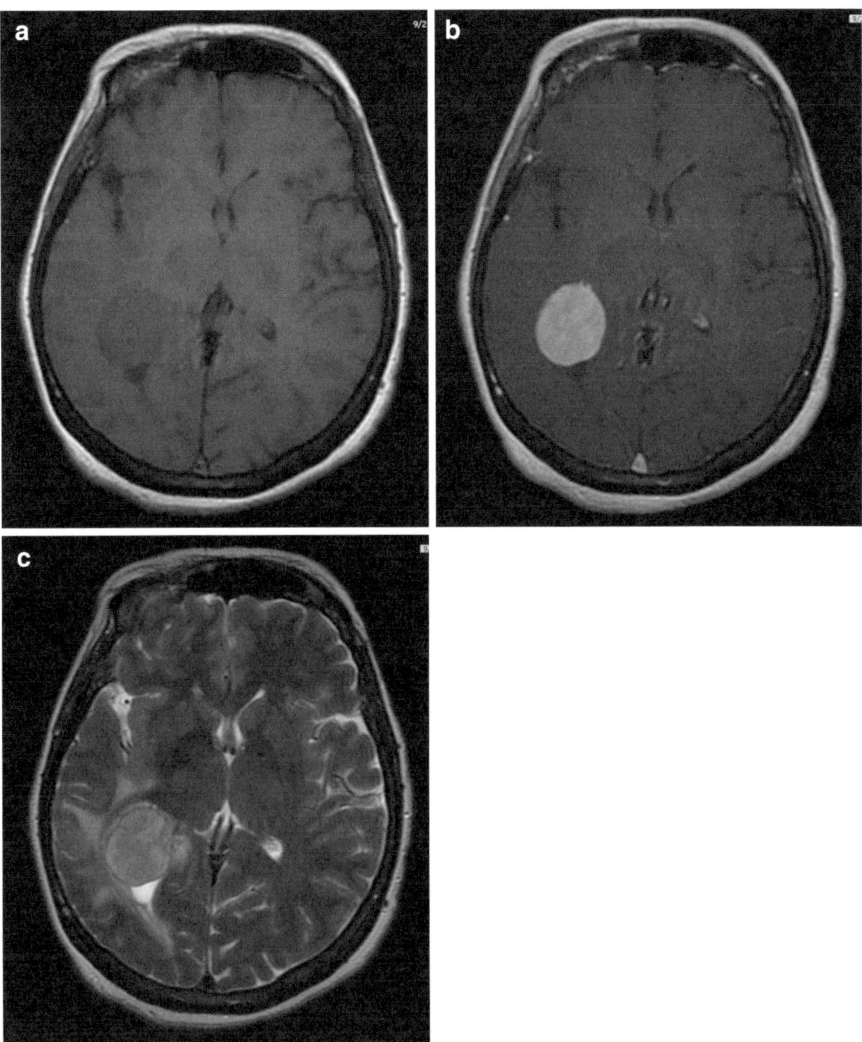

**Fig. 4.11** Intraventricular meningioma. Typically arising within the glomus of the lateral ventricles, they share virtually all features of meningiomas arising in other parts of the cranial vault: homogeneous intermediate signal on T1-weighted images (**a**), moderately avid and strikingly homogeneous contrast enhancement with gadolinium (**b**), and homogeneous mildly hypointense signal on T2-weighted images (**c**)

intermediate to low signal intensity on T2-weighted images is one of the key features of meningioma, and they typically do not show diffusion restriction on DWI.

## Choroid Plexus Tumors

Choroid plexus papilloma typically arises from the glomus of the choroid plexus, most commonly in the fourth ventricle in adults, and in the atria of the lateral ventricles in children. The tumors usually appear as a well-defined lobulated mass with identifiable fine, frond-like morphology. They are typically isointense on T1 and iso- to hyperintense on T2-weighted images with marked homogeneous gadolinium contrast enhancement. Small flow voids may sometimes be seen within the tumor on T2-weighted images reflecting their relative hypervascularity. On CT, fine speckled calcifications are seen in approximately 25% of cases [41]. Hydrocephalus resulting from tumor-associated CSF overproduction is frequently seen (Fig. 4.12). Choroid plexus carcinomas occur almost exclusively in the pediatric patient population and are difficult to distinguish from choroid plexus papillomas by imaging. Carcinomas can have more heterogeneous enhancement, and invasion of brain parenchyma may also be a clue [46].

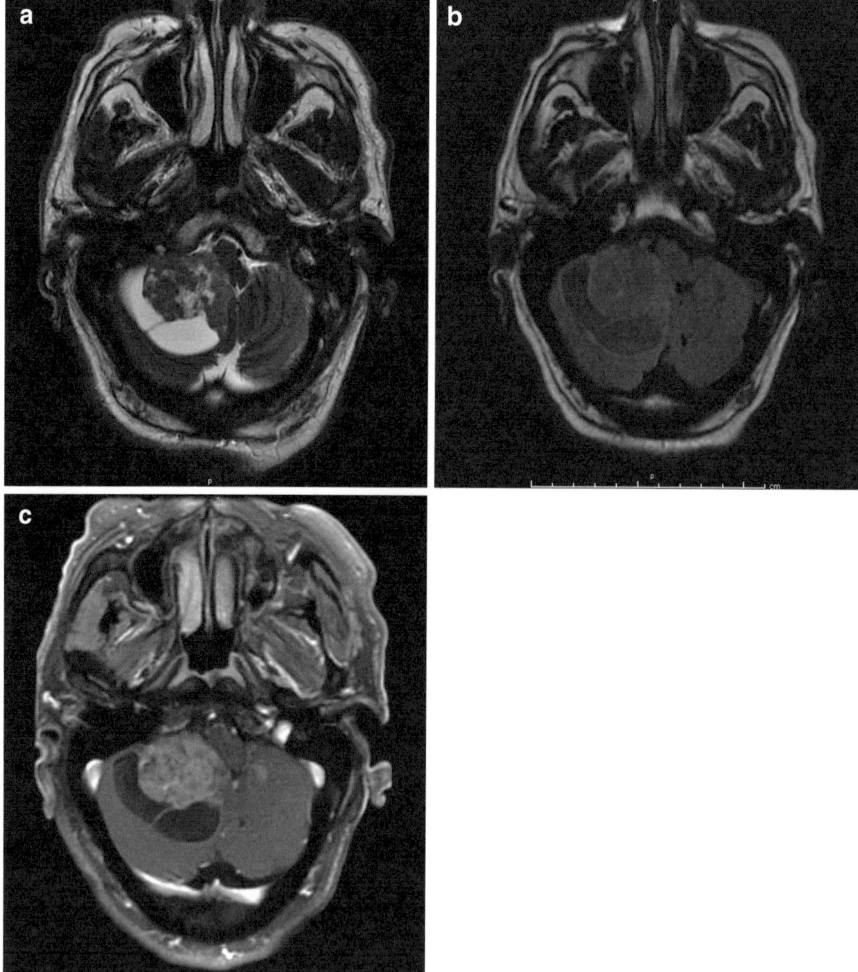

**Fig. 4.12** Choroid plexus papilloma arising from the lateral floccular portion of fourth ventricular choroid plexus. MRI appearance is characterized by solid intermediate to low signal components on T2 and T2 FLAIR (**a**, **b**) and moderately avid contrast enhancement on T1 post-contrast imaging (**c**), with characteristic "papillary" lobulated internal architecture

## Colloid Cyst of Third Ventricle

Colloid cysts are nonneoplastic lesions thought to arise from either neuroepithelial or endodermal remnants in the tela choroidea of the choroid plexus [4]. Colloid cysts have a variable appearance on MRI due to variable protein, water, cholesterol, and ionic content [6]. Most cysts are hyperintense on T1-weighted and isointense on T2-weighted imaging. T1 hyperintensity is thought to be due to the high protein content of cyst fluid [2]. When protein content is so high that water content diminishes, or if calcification is present, cyst fluid can appear hypointense on T2-weighted imaging. There is typically no diffusion restriction, and colloid cysts typically do not enhance, although thin rim enhancement of the cyst wall may rarely be seen [9] (Fig. 4.13).

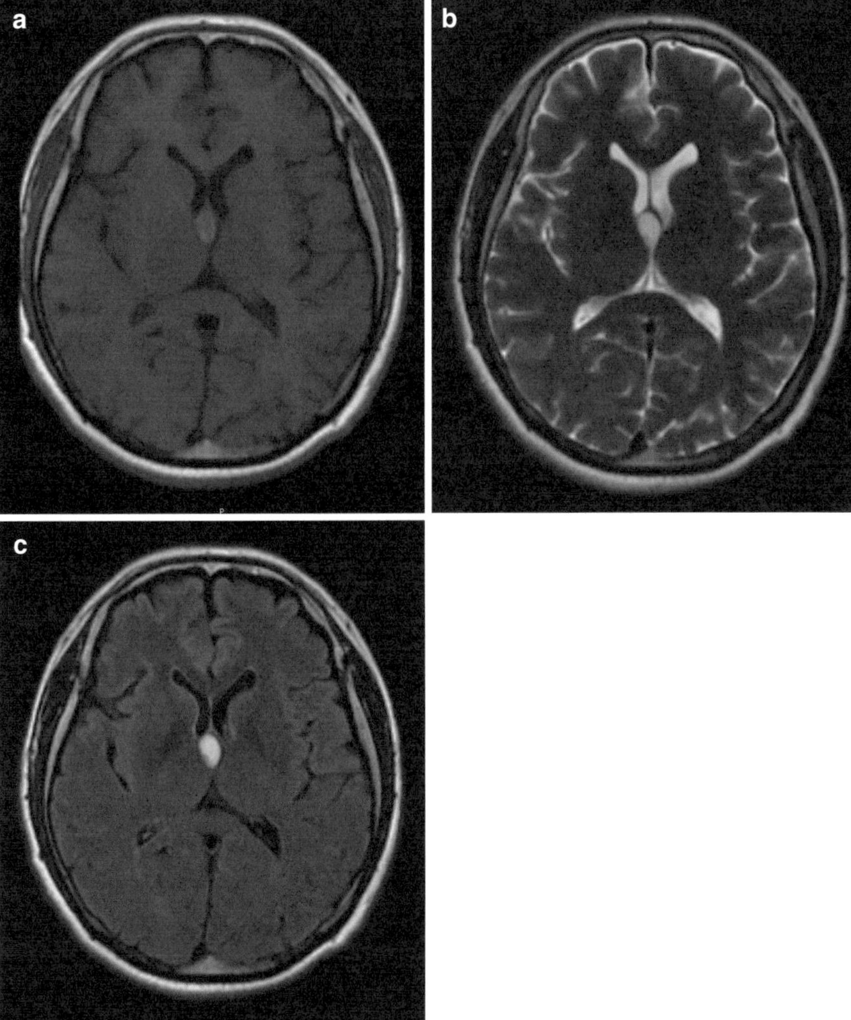

**Fig. 4.13** Colloid cyst of the third ventricle is typically sharply circumscribed in the anterior third ventricle adjacent to the foramina of Monro. Although signal intensities can vary depending on cyst contents, they are typically hyperintense on T1 (**a**), T2 (**b**), and T2 FLAIR (**c**)

# References


1. Abe K, Ono Y, Yoneyama H, Nishina Y, Aihara Y, Okada Y, Sakai S. Assessment of cerebrospinal fluid flow patterns using the time-spatial labeling inversion pulse technique with 3T MRI: early clinical experiences. Neuroradiol J. 2014;27(3):268–79.
2. Ahmadi J, Savabi F, Apuzzo ML, Segall HD, Hinton D. Magnetic resonance imaging and quantitative analysis of intracranial cystic lesions: surgical implication. Neurosurgery. 1994;35(2):199–207.
3. Aleman J, Jokura H, Higano S, et al. Value of constructive interference in steady-state three-dimensional, Fourier transformation magnetic resonance imaging for the neuroendoscopic treatment of hydrocephalus and intracranial cysts. Neurosurgery. 2001;48:1291–5.
4. Al-Sharydah AM, Al-Suhibani SS, Al-Abdulwahhab AH, Al-Aftan MS, Gashgari AF. A unique finding of cavum velum interpositum colloid-like cyst and literature review of a commonplace lesion in an uncommon place. Int J Gen Med. 2018;11:301–5.
5. Ambrose J. Computerized transverse axial scanning (tomography). 2. Clinical application. Br J Radiol. 1973;46:1023–47.
6. Armao D, Castillo M, Chen H, Kwock L. Colloid cyst of the third ventricle: imaging-pathologic correlation. AJNR Am J Neuroradiol. 2000;21(8):1470–7.
7. Baledent O, Gondry-Jouet C, Meyer M, et al. Relationship between cerebrospinal fluid and blood dynamics in healthy volunteers and patients with communicating hydrocephalus. Investig Radiol. 2004;39:45–55.
8. Battal B, Kocaoglu M, Bulakbasi N, et-al. Cerebrospinal fluid flow imaging by using phase-contrast MR technique. Br J Radiol. 2004;2011(84):758–65.
9. Bender B, Honegger JB, Beschorner R, Ernemann U, Horger M. MR imaging findings in colloid cysts of the sellar region: comparison with colloid cysts of the third ventricle and Rathke's cleft cysts. Acad Radiol. 2013;20(11):1457–65.
10. Bhatoe HS, Singh P, Dutta V. Intraventricular meningiomas: a clinicopathological study and review. Neurosurg Focus. 2006;20(3):E9.
11. Blitz AM, Shin J, Balédent O, Pagé G, Bonham LW, Herzka DA, Moghekar AR, Rigamonti D. Does phase-contrast imaging through the cerebral aqueduct predict the outcome of lumbar CSF drainage or shunt surgery in patients with suspected adult hydrocephalus? AJNR Am J Neuroradiol. 2018;39(12):2224–30.
12. Bradley WG, Scalzo D, Queralt J, et al. Normal-pressure hydrocephalus: evaluation with cerebrospinal fluid flow measurements at MR imaging. Radiology. 1996;198:523–9.
13. Chiang WW, Takoudis CG, Lee SH, Weis-McNulty A, Glick R, Alperin N. Relationship between ventricular morphology and aqueductal cerebrospinal fluid flow in healthy and communicating hydrocephalus. Investig Radiol. 2009;44(4):192–9.
14. Cushing H. Haematomyelia from gunshot wound of the cervical spine. Bull Johns Hopkins Hosp. 1897;8:195–7.
15. Dandy WE, Blackfan KD. Internal hydrocephalus: an experimental, clinical and pathological study. Am J Dis Child. 1914;8(6):406–82.
16. Dandy WE. Ventriculography following the injection of air into the cerebral ventricles. Ann Surg. 1918;68:5–11.
17. De Coene B, Hajnal JV, Gatehouse P, et al. MR of the brain using fluid-attenuated inversion recovery (FLAIR) pulse sequences. AJNR Am J Neuroradiol. 1992;13:1555–64.
18. Dias DA, Castro FL, Yared JH, Lucas Júnior A, Ferreira Filho LA, Ferreira NF. Liliequist membrane: radiological evaluation, clinical and therapeutic implications. Radiol Bras. 2014;47(3):182–5. https://doi.org/10.1590/0100-3984.2013.1809. PMID: 25741076; PMCID: PMC4337143.
19. Dinçer A, Kohan S, Ozek MM. Is all "communicating" hydrocephalus really communicating? Prospective study on the value of 3D-constructive interference in steady state sequence at 3T. AJNR Am J Neuroradiol. 2009;30(10):1898–906.
20. Doll A, Christmann D, Kehrli P, et al. Contribution of 3D CISS MRI for pre and post-therapeutic monitoring of obstructive hydrocephalus. J Neuroradiol. 2000;27:218–25.

21. Dupont S, Rabinstein AA. CT evaluation of lateral ventricular dilatation after subarachnoid hemorrhage: baseline bicaudate index values [correction of balues]. Neurol Res. 2013;35(2):103–6.
22. Edelman RR, Chien D, Kim D. Fast selective black blood MR imaging. Radiology. 1991;181:655–60.
23. Fushimi Y, Miki Y, Ueba T, Kanagaki M, Takahashi T, Yamamoto A, Haque TL, Konishi J, Takahashi JA, Hashimoto N, Konishi J. Liliequist membrane: three-dimensional constructive interference in steady state MR imaging. Radiology. 2003;229(2):360–5.
24. Gandhoke GS, Frassanito P, Chandra N, Ojha BK, Singh A. Role of magnetic resonance ventriculography in multiloculated hydrocephalus. J Neurosurg Pediatr. 2013;11(6):697–703.
25. Gibbs WN, Tanenbaum LN. Imaging of hydrocephalus. Appl Radiol. 2018;47(5):5–13.
26. Hajnal JV, Bryant DJ, Kasuboski L. Use of fluid attenuated inversion recovery (FLAIR) pulse sequences in MRI of the brain. J Comput Assist Tomogr. 1992;16:841–4.
27. Henry-Feugeas M, Idy-Peretti I, Bale'dent O, et al. Cerebrospinal fluid flow waveforms: MR analysis in chronic adult hydrocephalus. Investig Radiol. 2001;36:146–54.
28. Heuer GJ, Dandy WE. A report of seventy cases of brain tumor. Bull Johns Hopkins Hosp. 1916a;27:224–37.
29. Heuer GJ, Dandy WE. Roentgenography in the localization of brain tumor, based upon a series of one hundred consecutive cases. Bull Johns Hopkins Hosp. 1916b;27:311–22.
30. Hicks MJ, Albrecht S, Trask T, Byrne ME, Narayan RK, Goodman JC. Symptomatic choroid plexus xanthogranuloma of the lateral ventricle. Case report and brief critical review of xanthogranulomatous lesions of the brain. Clin Neuropathol. 1993;12(2):92–6.
31. Kadota T, Mihara N, Tsuji N, et al. MR of xanthogranuloma of the choroid plexus. AJNR Am J Neuroradiol. 1996;17(8):1595–7.
32. Kartal MG, Algin O. Evaluation of hydrocephalus and other cerebrospinal fluid disorders with MRI: an update. Insights Imaging. 2014;5(4):531–41.
33. Kin T, Nakatomi H, Shono N, Nomura S, Saito T, Oyama H, Saito N. Neurosurgical virtual reality simulation for brain tumor using high-definition computer graphics: a review of the literature. Neurol Med Chir (Tokyo). 2017;57(10):513–20.
34. Knol DS, van Gijn J, Kruitwagen CL, Rinkel GJ. Size of third and fourth ventricle in obstructive and communicating acute hydrocephalus after aneurysmal subarachnoid hemorrhage. J Neurol. 2011 Jan;258(1):44–9.
35. Kunz M, Schulte-Altedorneburg G, Uhl E, et al. Three-dimensional constructive interference in steady-state magnetic resonance imaging in obstructive hydrocephalus: relevance for endoscopic third ventriculostomy and clinical results. J Neurosurg. 2008;109:931–8.
36. Laitt RD, Mallucci CL, Jaspan T, et al. Constructive interference in steady-state 3D Fourier-transform MRI in the management of hydrocephalus and third ventriculostomy. Neuroradiology. 1999;41:117–23.
37. Lauterbur PC. Image formation by induced local interactions: examples employing nuclear magnetic resonance. Nature. 1973;242:190–1.
38. Lee JH, Lee HK, Kim JK, Kim HJ, Park JK, Choi CG. CSF flow quantification of the cerebral aqueduct in normal volunteers using phase contrast cine MR imaging. Korean J Radiol. 2004;5(2):81–6.
39. Lisanti C, Carlin C, Banks KP, Wang D. Normal MRI appearance and motion-related phenomena of CSF. AJR Am J Roentgenol. 2007;188(3):716–25.
40. Mbonane S, Andronikou S. Interpretation and value of MR CSF flow studies for paediatric neurosurgery. S Afr J Radiol. 2013;17(1)
41. Mishra A, Ojha BK, Chandra A, et al. Choroid plexus papilloma of posterior third ventricle: a case report and review of literature. Asian J Neurosurg. 2014;9:238.
42. Muñoz A, Hinojosa J, Esparza J. Cisternography and ventriculography gadopentate dimeglumine-enhanced MR imaging in pediatric patients: preliminary report. AJNR Am J Neuroradiol. 2007;28(5):889–94.
43. Ng SE, Low AM, Tang KK, Chan YH, Kwok RK. Value of quantitative MRI biomarkers (Evans' index, aqueductal flow rate, and apparent diffusion coefficient) in idiopathic normal pressure hydrocephalus. J Magn Reson Imaging. 2009;30(4):708–15.

44. Nitz WR, Bradley WG, Watanabe AS, et al. Flow dynamics of cerebrospinal fluid: assessment with phase-contrast velocity MR imaging performed with retrospective cardiac gating. Radiology. 1992;183:395–405.
45. Pear BL. Xanthogranuloma of the choroid plexus. AJR Am J Roentgenol. 1984;143(2):401–2.
46. Pencalet P, Sainte-Rose C, Lellouch-Tubiana A, et al. Papillomas and carcinomas of the choroid plexus in children. J Neurosurg. 1998;88:521–8.
47. Ragan DK, Cerqua J, Nash T, McKinstry RC, Shimony JS, Jones BV, Mangano FT, Holland SK, Yuan W, Limbrick DD Jr. The accuracy of linear indices of ventricular volume in pediatric hydrocephalus: technical note. J Neurosurg Pediatr. 2015;15(6):547–51.
48. Reinard K, Basheer A, Phillips S, Snyder A, Agarwal A, Jafari-Khouzani K, Soltanian-Zadeh H, Schultz L, Aho T, Schwalb JM. Simple and reproducible linear measurements to determine ventricular enlargement in adults. Surg Neurol Int. 2015;9(6):59.
49. Rekate HL. The definition and classification of hydrocephalus: a personal recommendation to stimulate debate. Cerebrospinal Fluid Res. 2008;5:2.
50. Rekate HL. A consensus on the classification of hydrocephalus: its utility in the assessment of abnormalities of cerebrospinal fluid dynamics. Childs Nerv Syst. 2011;27(10):1535–41.
51. Rekate HL, Blitz AM. Hydrocephalus in children. Handb Clin Neurol. 2016;136:1261–73.
52. Shanks J, Markenroth Bloch K, Laurell K, Cesarini KG, Fahlström M, Larsson EM, Virhammar J. Aqueductal CSF stroke volume is increased in patients with idiopathic Normal pressure hydrocephalus and decreases after shunt surgery. AJNR Am J Neuroradiol. 2019;40(3):453–9.
53. Sharma AK, Gaikwad S, Gupta V, Garg A, Mishra NK. Measurement of peak CSF flow velocity at cerebral aqueduct, before and after lumbar CSF drainage, by use of phase-contrast MRI: utility in the management of idiopathic normal pressure hydrocephalus. Clin Neurol Neurosurg. 2008;110(4):363–8.
54. Stoquart-El Sankari S, Lehmann P, Gondry-Jouet C, Fichten A, Godefroy O, Meyer ME, Baledent O. Phase-contrast MR imaging support for the diagnosis of aqueductal stenosis. AJNR Am J Neuroradiol. 2009;30(1):209–14.
55. Szeverenyi NM, Kieffer SA, Cacayorin ED. Correction of CSF motion artifact on MR images of the brain and spine by pulse sequence modification: clinical evaluation. AJNR Am J Neuroradiol. 1988;9(6):1069–74.
56. Tawfik AM, Elsorogy L, Abdelghaffar R, Naby AA, Elmenshawi I. Phase-contrast MRI CSF flow measurements for the diagnosis of Normal-pressure hydrocephalus: observer agreement of velocity versus volume parameters. AJR Am J Roentgenol. 2017;208(4):838–43.
57. Toma AK, Holl E, Kitchen ND, Watkins LD. Evans' index revisited: the need for an alternative in normal pressure hydrocephalus. Neurosurgery. 2011;68(4):939–44.
58. Weinstock P, Rehder R, Prabhu SP, Forbes PW, Roussin CJ, Cohen AR. Creation of a novel simulator for minimally invasive neurosurgery: fusion of 3D printing and special effects. J Neurosurg Pediatr. 2017;20(1):1–9.
59. Yamada S, Tsuchiya K, Bradley WG, Law M, Winkler ML, Borzage MT, Miyazaki M, Kelly EJ, McComb JG. Current and emerging MR imaging techniques for the diagnosis and management of CSF flow disorders: a review of phase-contrast and time-spatial labeling inversion pulse. AJNR Am J Neuroradiol. 2015;36(4):623–30.

# Chapter 5
# The Evolution of Trans-Sulcal Channel-Based Parafascicular Surgery

**Thiago Albonette Felicio and Daniel M. Prevedello**

## Introduction

Since the dawn of neurosurgery, attempting to achieve maximal resection of brain lesions with no or minimal collateral damage to the normal surrounding tissues has been the goal. This assertion is even more valid for deep-seated subcortical brain lesions. For most of these lesions, the shortest way to reach them is via a trans-sulcal or a transcortical approach followed by white matter dissection, thereby creating a working channel to the lesion. This corridor needs to be kept open by some sort of brain retraction as the brain tends to close that passage.

## Brain Retraction

The soft consistency of the brain itself makes it fall into the field of vision while operating into the deep subcortical region, and as an unobstructed path is required in order to allow illumination and visualization, retraction becomes essential. It could be achieved by either a tubular or flat spatula retractor.

However, one should always keep in mind that retraction has the potential to cause injury [1] since the pressure applied from the retractor is transmitted to the underlying brain. Once it deforms tissues, it can either cause direct injury or lead to partial or total occlusion of the microvasculature, impairing oxygen delivery and

**Submission Statement**

The contents of this manuscript have not been copyrighted or published previously.

T. A. Felicio · D. M. Prevedello (✉)
The Ohio State University Wexner Medical Center, Department of Neurological Surgery, Columbus, OH, USA

© Springer Nature Switzerland AG 2022
G. Zada et al. (eds.), *Subcortical Neurosurgery*,
https://doi.org/10.1007/978-3-030-95153-5_5

consequently resulting in ischemia. Its severity depends on factors such as the brain retraction pressure distribution, geometry, area of contact, vascular pressure, and the duration of retraction.

Another concern, while working on the subcortical region, is disruption of white matter tracts, which may lead to disastrous consequences, comparably to the lesions located in eloquent cortical areas, for example, the motor and visual cortex [2]. Similar to the concept of eloquent cortical areas, there are also eloquent white matter fascicles or tracts that should be taken in consideration when dealing with deep-seated brain lesions, such as the corticospinal tract, the optic radiations, the superior longitudinal fasciculus, and others. This idea is supported by imaging studies, such as resting state functional magnetic resonance imaging (RS-fMRI), magnetoencephalography (MEG), and diffusion tensor imaging (DTI) [3], and anatomical studies [4–6]. Hence, knowing the white matter tract anatomy is paramount.

## Tubular Retractors

The tubular retractors have evolved since their first report in the early 1980s, from metal-based to transparent plastic conduits, along with improvements in navigation systems and neuroimaging. Basically, the tubular retractor differs from the traditional spatula retractor in terms of relative surface area, which reflects on the amount and the distribution of pressure over the tissues. Considering the formula $P = F \div a$ (where $P$ is pressure, $F$ is force, and $a$ is surface area), it can be inferred that a lesser pressure value requires greater surface area. So it seems intuitive that the pressure exerted by the tubular retractor will be lesser when compared to the flat spatula since the former has a relative greater surface area evenly distributed. A flat spatula retractor has a very small area of tissue contact on the edges resulting in extremely elevated pressure, which could lacerate the tissue.

### *First Tubular Retractor*

Since the advent of the computed axial tomography scan (CAT scan) in 1972 [7], small subcortical lesions could be revealed radiographically and addressed. Conventional frame-based stereotactic arcs were used in such cases. Interestingly, the same basic working principle is still in use by the modern navigation systems. Briefly, the images from the CT scan are used to calculate the position of the lesion on the three orthogonal planes (sagittal, coronal, and axial), yielding three measurements: latero-lateral (x), dorsoventral (y), and rostro-caudal (z). With these measurements, the arc accurately localizes the lesion on the three-dimensional space.

Despite being ingenious, the stereotactic arc only allowed for biopsy of subcortical lesions, as oppose to the microsurgical approach, which could allow direct visualization and dissection of the lesion. However, this limitation changed with the use of the tubular retractor deployed under stereotactic arc guidance. Microsurgery through a tube precisely planned and inserted became then possible.

The first tubular retractor use was reported by Kelly et al. [8–11] in 1980, and it consisted of a hollow cylinder (2 or 3 cm in diameter) made of metal and a bullet-shape tip dilator. The bullet-shape tip allowed split of the white matter tracts, and the hollow cylinder worked as a channel for microscope visualization and for performing microsurgical resection. This set was meant to be delivered through the stereotactic arc, ensuring precision when reaching the target. Their technique is briefly described as follows: First, after proper setting of the stereotactic arc and retractor accordingly to the calculated coordinates and computer guidance to perform skin incision and craniotomy, the cortex was incised by a $CO_2$ laser beam through the tubular retractor; second, the bullet-shaped dilator was introduced within the retractor, and the set retractor-dilator was advanced through the incision made, 5–10 mm at each time; third, the dilator was removed, and the incision was deepened; again, the set was advanced, and the process was repeated until the desired target lesion was reached, always under microscope visualization; then the lesion was vaporized by the laser. Interestingly, this tubular retractor proved to have great value as the authors have used the same technique for over 30 years in brain neoplasms, showing good results in terms of extent of resection and functional outcomes [12].

Other retractors were also reported later on, similar to the one described above. These authors reported good results too, emphasizing the low rate of surgical complications [13–17].

In summary, the common characteristic for this period (1980–2000) was the use of tubular retractors coupled to the stereotactic frame-based arc, which perhaps has contributed to the limited spread of the technique. One of the reasons could be the relatively high costs associated with the equipment and the relatively less freedom of movement when operating using the arc.

## *Plastic Retractor*

Plastic retractors have made transparent wall a reality, making it possible to view the surrounding tissues through the retractor wall, which allowed improvements in hemostasis and in distinguishing the normal from the abnormal tissue.

In 2000, attempting to overcome the deleterious effects of the spontaneous intracerebral hemorrhage (ICH), Nishihara et al. [18] were the first to report the use of a plastic tubular retractor (6 mm in diameter) to treat ICH. Here, the authors did not use a navigation system. Instead, they used the preoperative image to determine the entry point and the trajectory, allowing them to puncture the hematoma, similar to a ventricular catheterization. An endoscope was held by one hand and a suction-cautery device by the other. Remarkably, the authors reported a great amount of hematoma removal, with no surgical complications and no rebleeding, a well-known complication after ICH surgery [19].

Following the path of Nishihara [18], others [20, 21] used plastic retractors to treat colloid cysts. They reported improved rates of total removal and less recurrence, which was attributed to the ability to operate in an air medium provided by the tubular retractor as opposed to the liquid medium as in traditional ventricular neuroendoscopy.

## Other Materials

Since 2005, many have reported to have adapted different available surgical materials in order to use as tubular retractors. This was the case of Harris et al. [22]. They adapted a thoracic port, which looks like a bullet-shaped tip cylinder within a plastic sheath, to operate subcortical brain neoplasms and colloid cysts. Interestingly, they used a stereotactic needle biopsy to reach the lesion. Having the needle as a guide, the port was slid over the needle, entering into the brain through twisting movements. Subsequently, an endoscope was used, held by an arm holder, to operate in 11.5 mm in diameter channel with bimanual microsurgical technique. As stated, a stereotactic arc was used, but the same group [23] published their experience 4 years later with a frameless navigation system in 21 patients harboring subcortical brain neoplasms, where they reported two minor surgical complications and no worsened neurological deficits.

Following this trail, there were many reports mentioning the use of adapted tubular retractors from several materials available in the operating room, such as polyester film [24], microdrill wrap [25, 26], nelaton tubes [27, 28], GORE-TEX sheet [29], and spinal tubular retractors [30–33]. Despite the materials being conceived for other purposes, all these authors reported safety and low complication rates.

Noteworthy, Ogura et al. [24] and Waran et al. [34] measured the intracranial pressure (ICP) while using tubular retractors. The first authors measured the ICP around the tubular retractor in two patients harboring subcortical brain neoplasms and found that the ICP was always less than 10 mmHg in all measurements. Likewise, the latter authors, operating on a patient with intracerebral hemorrhage (ICH), measured the ICP during the retractor insertion and immediately after initial ICH removal, showing a slight and brief elevation of the ICP, which lasted less than 20 seconds, followed by an enormous drop as the hematoma was evacuated. These findings corroborated the minimal effect on ICP posed by the tubular retractor.

## Technological Advancements

Since the late 2000s, in addition to conventional MRI, DTI sequences have been increasingly used in preoperative planning in order to localize important white matter tracts and also determine their relationship with the lesion, allowing the neurosurgeon to anticipate risk to these tracts and, thus, to modify the trajectory to be parallel to rather than traversing them. Also, novel and promising devices for visualization have emerged, such as the exoscope [35–38]. This device, like the endoscope, has the image projected on a high-definition screen, but contrary to the endoscope, the exoscope is positioned 50–70 cm away from the surgical field, pro-portionating more space and freedom of movements to the surgeon and assistant. The exoscope can be held by an automated robotic arm holder that follows the direction of the tube, decreasing downtime of repositioning the scope while chang-ing the angle of the retractor.

Additionally, there were technological improvements on the microscope and the endoscope as well, for example, with the emergence of the 3D endoscopes and the new powerful microscopes. Finally, there are currently two commercial, FDA-approved tubular retractor systems FDA-approved: the ViewSite Brain Access System (Vycor Medical Inc., Boca Raton, FL) [39] and the BrainPath (Nico Corp., Indianapolis, IN) [40]. Both can be used with frameless stereotac-tic navigation system and have a variety of lengths and widths available (Fig. 5.1).

## Operative Technique

The general surgical technique is described as follows. After appropriate patient selection and preoperative planning with thin-slice MRI, ideally with DTI, a non-eloquent entry point and a trajectory parallel to the important white matter tracts are selected. The entry site is marked with the guidance of a frameless stereotactic navi-gation system. The skin incision is performed according to the neurosurgeon's pref-erence, and a craniotomy with 3–4 cm in diameter is sufficient. Following this, the dura is opened in a cruciate way in a size sufficient to fit the tubular retractor. In sequence, whenever possible, a sulcus is selected and the arachnoid over the sulcus is dissected in a sharp way under microscopic visualization, sufficient to fit the retractor, preserving the adjacent vessels. Alternatively, a small corticectomy can be

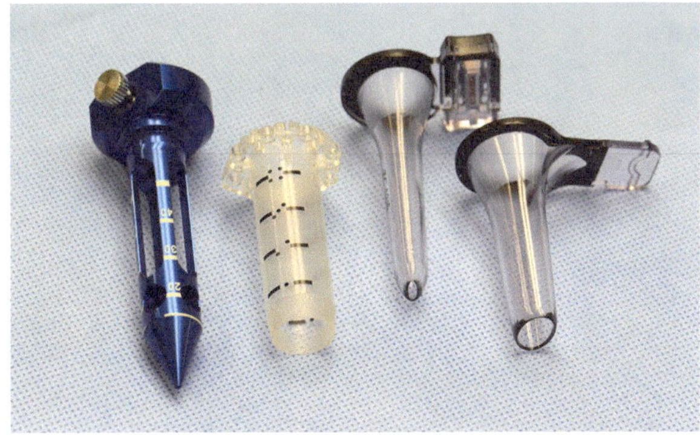

**Fig. 5.1** Commercially available tubular retractor. BrainPath on the left and ViewSite on the right

done. At this point, in our service, we introduce an 18-FR Peel-Away catheter, under imaging guidance, in order to create the first pathway to the retractor. Then, the tubular retractor, usually the smallest width possible, is advanced through the incision into the brain under real-time navigation guidance, stopping before or after the lesion, depending if the lesion is firm or soft, respectively, because this maneuver will prevent the parenchyma collapsing into the field. Next, the preferred device for visualization (microscope, endoscope, or exoscope) is brought to the field, and the lesion resection is performed using standard bimanual microsurgical technique. If required, the retractor can be changed for one with a greater width. In our service, we have been using the microscope as the main visualization tool. One of the downsides of using a microscope is the fact that its angle of visualization needs to be adjusted every time the port (retractor) is repositioned in a different angle. Furthermore, the microscope offers a low volume of focused depth of field in comparison to the exoscope. However, the microscope allows 3D visualization, whereas the current exoscopes do not provide 3D visualization. New 3D exoscopes are currently invading the market, and they likely will be replacing the microscope particularly when associated with the advantage of automatic repositioning performed by a robotic arm.

## Illustrative Case

A 49-year-old female, with a prior history of esophageal carcinoma, presented with headache, nausea, vomiting, and a slight left-sided weakness. Brain MRI showed a 3.4 x 3.2 cm right posterior frontal periventricular lesion. Surgical removal was undertaken as above described, revealing the lesion was a metastasis. There were no complications, and the patient remained neurologically stable (Figs. 5.2, 5.3, and 5.4).

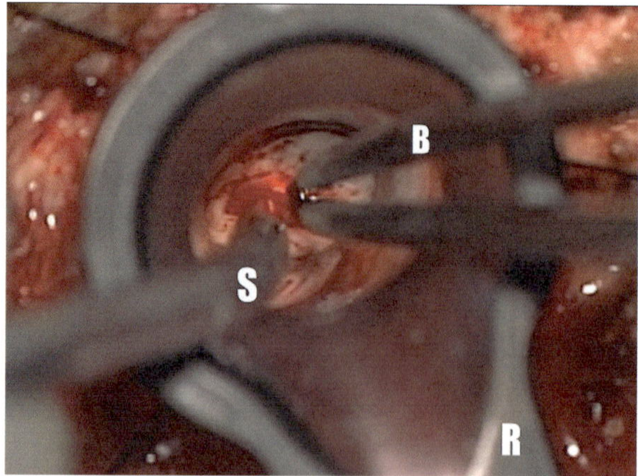


**Fig. 5.2** Microscopic intraoperative image showing suction (S) and bipolar (B) within the retractor (R)

**Fig. 5.3** Microscopic intraoperative image, high magnification, showing tumor (arrow) at the tip of the suction (S) being dissected from the white matter (*) within the retractor (R)

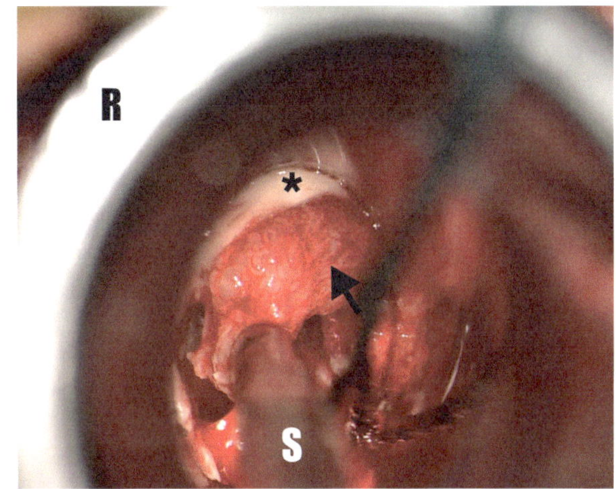

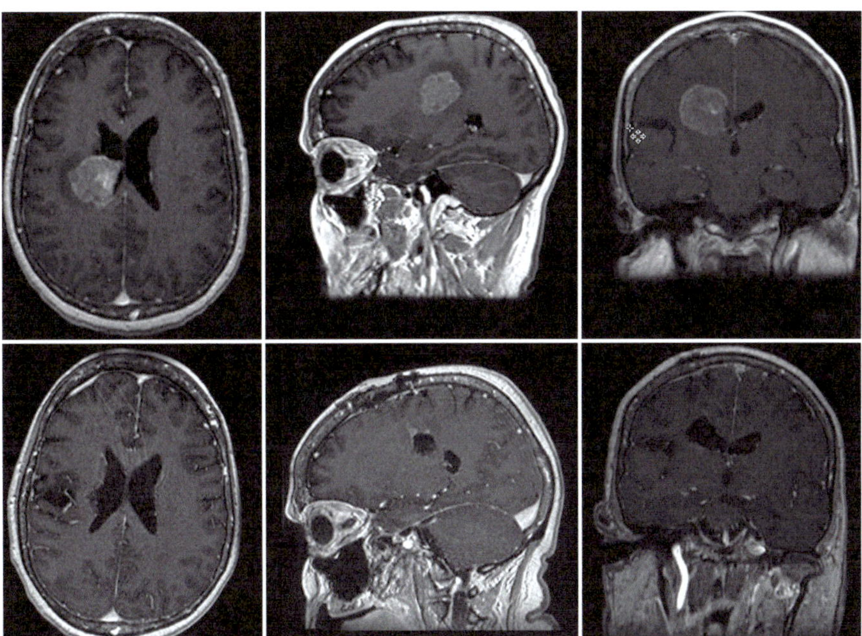

**Fig. 5.4** Axial, sagittal, and coronal T1-weighted imaging (T1WI) with gadolinium contrast MRI pre- (top) and postoperative (bottom)

## Discussion

Some nuances in the surgical technique for channel-based surgery are a cause of debate in the literature. For instance, since 2015, many authors [38, 41–47] have reported the preference for the sulcus (trans-sulcal), instead of the gyrus (transcortical), as an entry point. They argued that, in theory, the trans-sulcal route minimizes brain injury and reduces the amount of brain traversed to reach the lesion, which could lead to better outcomes. However, there are still no prospective studies on this subject.

Another reason for debate is the method for visualization. For example, in a series of 20 brain neoplasms operated using tubular retractors, our group [42] noted that the cases with incomplete resection were associated with the endoscope use, compared to the cases in which the microscope was used ($p < 0.002$). Our group attributed these findings to the 3D view and fast repositioning granted by the microscope and to the additional space freed up by the absence of the endoscope into the narrow corridor. However, this conclusion must be interpreted with caution since the study is retrospective, has a small sample size, and lacks a control group. Moreover, with the refinement of the existing devices for visualization and the advent of the exoscopes, the results could have been different. Therefore, further studies are still expected to address this issue.

Regarding postoperative imaging changes, there is also some discussion. Raza et al. [48] operated on nine adult patients, and Recinos et al. [33] operated on four pediatric patients, all harboring subcortical brain lesions, and they found no changes in postoperative T2/FLAIR and ADC/diffusion restriction on MRI, except in two cases: one from the adult series, with no clinical significance, and another from the pediatric series, which was a biopsy in a 5-month-old patient with a bulky third ventricle and pineal region tumor. Comparatively, Bander et al. [43] found no increase in FLAIR signal and a nonsignificant increase in DWI signal on postoperative MRI from 20 patients harboring deep-seated brain lesions, showing minimal damage to the surrounding brain parenchyma caused by the retractors. Also, these studies are retrospective and have a small sample size, which requires caution in their interpretation.

## Conclusion

When dealing with subcortical brain lesions, the neurosurgeon faces a challenge: resect the lesion while minimizing collateral injury. In such deep regions, brain retraction is required to maintain an adequate working channel, but it can produce damage, even ischemia, when inappropriately applied. In order to reduce this negative effect, tubular retractors have emerged and evolved from the metal tubes coupled with stereotactic arcs to the transparent plastic conduits to be used with modern frameless navigation system, along with newer neuroimaging systems, revealing the white matter tract anatomy and their relationship with lesions, providing real-time and precise localization, and granting better outcomes. Above all, the use of tubular retractors may be considered minimally invasive surgery as smaller incisions and craniotomies are possible, but even more important, these devices may contribute to the preservation of neurological function.

**Disclosures** Funding Source: No funding was obtained for this manuscript.

**Financial Disclosure** Daniel M. Prevedello is a consultant for Medtronic and Stryker. Daniel M. Prevedello has a royalty agreement with KLS-Martin, Mizuho, and ACE Medical.

# References


1. Zhong J, Dujovny M, Perlin A, Perez-Arjona E, Park H. Brain retraction injury. Neurol Res. 2003;25(8):831–8. https://doi.org/10.1179/016164103771953925.
2. Duffau H. New concepts in surgery of WHO grade II gliomas: functional brain mapping, connectionism and plasticity – a review. J Neuro-Oncol. 2006;79(1):77–115. https://doi.org/10.1007/s11060-005-9109-6.
3. Sarubbo S, De Benedictis A, Merler S, et al. Towards a functional atlas of human white matter. Hum Brain Mapp. 2015;36(8):3117–36. https://doi.org/10.1002/hbm.22832.
4. Koutsarnakis C, Liakos F, Kalyvas AV, et al. The superior frontal Transsulcal approach to the anterior ventricular system: exploring the Sulcal and subcortical anatomy using anatomic dissections and diffusion tensor imaging Tractography. World Neurosurg. 2017;106:339–54. https://doi.org/10.1016/j.wneu.2017.06.161.
5. Jennings JE, Kassam AB, Fukui MB, et al. The surgical white matter chassis: a practical 3-dimensional atlas for planning subcortical surgical trajectories. Oper Neurosurg. 2017;14(5):469–82. https://doi.org/10.1093/ons/opx177.
6. Monroy-Sosa A, Jennings J, Chakravarthi S, et al. Microsurgical anatomy of the vertical rami of the superior longitudinal fasciculus: an intraparietal sulcus dissection study. Oper Neurosurg. 2018:1–13. https://doi.org/10.1093/ons/opy077.
7. Bhattacharyya KB. Godfrey Newbold Hounsfield (1919-2004): the man who revolutionized neuroimaging. Ann Indian Acad Neurol. 2016;19(4):448–50. https://doi.org/10.4103/0972-2327.194414.
8. Kelly PJ, Alker GJ Jr. A method for stereotactic laser microsurgery in the treatment of deep-seated CNS neoplasms. Stereotact Funct Neurosurg. 1980;43(3–5):210–5. https://doi.org/10.1159/000102259.
9. Kelly PJ, Kall BA, Goerss SJ. Computer-interactive stereotactic resection of deep-seated and centrally located Intraaxial brain lesions. Stereotact Funct Neurosurg. 1987;50(1–6):107–13. https://doi.org/10.1159/000100693.
10. Kelly PJ, Goerss SJ, Kall BA. The stereotaxic retractor in computer-assisted stereotaxic microsurgery technical note. J Neurosurg. 1988;69:301–6. https://doi.org/10.3171/jns.1988.69.2.0301.
11. Kelly PJ, Alker GJ. A stereotactic approach to deep-seated central nervous system neoplasms using the carbon dioxide laser. Surg Neurol. 1981;15(5):331–4. https://doi.org/10.1016/0090-3019(81)90158-0.
12. Moshel YA, Link MJ, Kelly PJ. Stereotactic volumetric resection of thalamic Pilocytic Astrocytomas. Neurosurgery. 2007;61(1):66–75. https://doi.org/10.1227/01.NEU.0000255508.43472.5B.
13. Shelden CH, McCann G, Jacques S, et al. Development of a computerized microstereotaxic method for localization and removal of minute CNS lesions under direct 3-D vision. Technical report. J Neurosurg. 1980;52(1):21–7. https://doi.org/10.3171/jns.1980.52.1.0021.
14. Jacques S, Shelden CH, McCann GD, Freshwater DB, Rand R. Computerized three-dimensional stereotaxic removal of small central nervous system lesions in patients. J Neurosurg. 1980;53(6):816–20. https://doi.org/10.3171/jns.1980.53.6.0816.
15. Otsuki T, Jokura H, Yoshimoto T. Stereotactic guiding tube for open-system endoscopy: a new approach for the stereotactic endoscopic resection of intra-axial brain tumors. Neurosurgery. 1990; https://doi.org/10.1227/00006123-199008000-00029.

16. Barlas O. A simple stereotactic retractor for use with the Leksell system. Neurosurgery. 1994;34(2):380–1.
17. Ross DA. A simple stereotactic retractor for use with the Leksell stereotactic system. Neurosurgery. 1993;32(3):475–6. https://doi.org/10.1227/00006123-199303000-00025.
18. Nishihara T, Teraoka A, Morita A, Ueki K, Takai K, Kirino T. A transparent sheath for endoscopic surgery and its application in surgical evacuation of spontaneous intracerebral hematomas. Technical note. J Neurosurg. 2000;92(6):1053–5. https://doi.org/10.3171/jns.2000.92.6.1053.
19. Morgenstern LB, Demchuk AM, Kim DH, Frankowski RF, Grotta JC. Rebleeding leads to poor outcome in ultra-early craniotomy for intracerebral hemorrhage. Neurology. 2001;56(10):1294–9.
20. Jho H-D, Alfieri A. Endoscopic removal of third ventricular tumors: a technical note. Minim Invasive Neurosurg. 2002;45(2):114–9. https://doi.org/10.1055/s-2002-32487.
21. Barlas O, Karadereler S, Mathieson T, Chumas PD. Stereotactically guided microsurgical removal of colloid cysts. Acta Neurochir. 2004;146(11):1199–204. https://doi.org/10.1007/s00701-004-0367-4.
22. Harris AE, Hadjipanayis CG, Lunsford LD, Lunsford AK, Kassam AB. Microsurgical removal of intraventricular lesions using endoscopic visualization and stereotactic guidance. Neurosurgery. 2005;56(1 Suppl):125–32. https://doi.org/10.1227/01.NEU.0000146227.75135.08.
23. Kassam AB, Engh JA, Mintz AH, Prevedello DM. Completely endoscopic resection of intraparenchymal brain tumors. J Neurosurg. 2009;110(1):116–23. https://doi.org/10.3171/2008.7.JNS08226.
24. Ogura K, Tachibana E, Aoshima C, Sumitomo M. New microsurgical technique for intraparenchymal lesions of the brain: Transcylinder approach. Acta Neurochir. 2006;148(7):779–85. https://doi.org/10.1007/s00701-006-0768-7.
25. Jo KW, Shin HJ, Nam DH, et al. Efficacy of endoport-guided endoscopic resection for deep-seated brain lesions. Neurosurg Rev. 2011;34(4):457–62. https://doi.org/10.1007/s10143-011-0319-4.
26. Jo KI, Chung SB, Jo KW, Kong DS, Seol HJ, Shin HJ. Microsurgical resection of deep-seated lesions using transparent tubular retractor: Pediatric case series. Childs Nerv Syst. 2011;27(11):1989–94. https://doi.org/10.1007/s00381-011-1529-3.
27. Yadav YR, Yadav S, Sherekar S, Parihar V. A new minimally invasive tubular brain retractor system for surgery of deep intracerebral hematoma. Neurol India. 2011;59(1):74–7. https://doi.org/10.4103/0028-3886.76870.
28. Ratre S, Yadav YR, Parihar VS, Kher Y. Microendoscopic removal of deep-seated brain Tumors using tubular retraction system. J Neurol Surg Part A Cent Eur Neurosurg. 2016;77(4):312–20. https://doi.org/10.1055/s-0036-1580595.
29. Ichinose T, Goto T, Morisako H, Takami T, Ohata K. Microroll retractor for surgical resection of brainstem cavernomas. World Neurosurg. 2010;73(5):520–2. https://doi.org/10.1016/j.wneu.2010.06.049.
30. Greenfield JP, Cobb WS, Tsouris AJ, Schwartz TH. Stereotactic minimally invasive tubular retractor system for deep brain lesions. Neurosurgery. 2008;63(4 Suppl):334–40. https://doi.org/10.1227/01.NEU.0000334741.61745.72.
31. Dorman JK. Tumor resection utilizing a minimally invasive spinal retractor with a novel cranial adaptor. Minim Invasive Neurosurg. 2008;51(6):358–60. https://doi.org/10.1055/s-0028-1085447.
32. Fahim DK, Relyea K, Nayar VV, et al. Transtubular microendoscopic approach for resection of a choroidal arteriovenous malformation. J Neurosurg Pediatr. 2009;3(2):101–4. https://doi.org/10.3171/2008.11.PEDS08280.
33. Recinos PF, Raza SM, Jallo GI, Recinos VR. Use of a minimally invasive tubular retraction system for deep-seated tumors in pediatric patients. J Neurosurg Pediatr. 2011;7(5):516–21. https://doi.org/10.3171/2011.2.PEDS10515.

34. Waran V, Vairavan N, Sia SF, Abdullah B. A new expandable cannula system for endoscopic evacuation of intraparenchymal hemorrhages. J Neurosurg. 2009;111(United States PT-Journal Article LG-English DC-20091202):1127–30. https://doi.org/10.3171/2009.4.JNS081506.
35. McLaughlin N, Prevedello DM, Engh J, Kelly DF, Kassam AB. Endoneurosurgical resection of intraventricular and intraparenchymal lesions using the port technique. World Neurosurg 2013;79(2 Suppl.):S18.e1–8. https://doi.org/10.1016/j.wneu.2012.02.022.
36. Day JD. Transsulcal parafascicular surgery using brain path® for subcortical lesions. Neurosurgery. 2017;64(1):151–6.
37. Bauer AM, Rasmussen PA, Bain MD. Initial single-center technical experience with the BrainPath system for acute intracerebral Hemorrhage evacuation. Oper Neurosurg. 2017;13(1):69–76. https://doi.org/10.1227/NEU.0000000000001258.
38. Labib MA, Shah M, Kassam AB, et al. The safety and feasibility of image-guided brainpath-mediated transsulcul hematoma evacuation: a multicenter study. Clin Neurosurg. 2017;80(4):515–24. https://doi.org/10.1227/NEU.0000000000001316.
39. Medical V. ViewSite Brain Access System (VBAS). http://www.vycorvbas.com. Accessed April 12, 2018.
40. NICO Corporation/. BrainPath. http://www.niconeuro.com/nico-product-line/. Accessed April 12, 2018.
41. Ding D, Starke RM, Webster Crowley R, Liu KC. Endoport-assisted microsurgical resection of cerebral cavernous malformations. J Clin Neurosci. 2015;22(6):1025–9. https://doi.org/10.1016/j.jocn.2015.01.004.
42. Hong CS, Prevedello DM, Elder JB. Comparison of endoscope- versus microscope-assisted resection of deep-seated intracranial lesions using a minimally invasive port retractor system. J Neurosurg. 2016;124(3):799–810. https://doi.org/10.3171/2015.1.JNS141113.
43. Bander ED, Jones SH, Kovanlikaya I, Schwartz TH. Utility of tubular retractors to minimize surgical brain injury in the removal of deep intraparenchymal lesions: a quantitative analysis of FLAIR hyperintensity and apparent diffusion coefficient maps. J Neurosurg. 2016;124(4):1053–60. https://doi.org/10.3171/2015.4.JNS142576.
44. Habboub G, Sharma M, Barnett GH, Mohammadi AM. A novel combination of two minimally invasive surgical techniques in the management of refractory radiation necrosis: technical note. J Clin Neurosci. 2017;35:117–21. https://doi.org/10.1016/j.jocn.2016.09.020.
45. Scranton RA, Fung SH, Britz GW. Transulcal parafascicular minimally invasive approach to deep and subcortical cavernomas: technical note. J Neurosurg. 2016;125(6):1360–6. https://doi.org/10.3171/2015.12.JNS152185.
46. Sujijantarat N, El Tecle N, Pierson M, et al. Trans-Sulcal Endoport-assisted evacuation of Supratentorial intracerebral Hemorrhage: initial single-institution experience compared to matched medically managed patients and effect on 30-day mortality. Oper Neurosurg. 2017;14(5):524–31. https://doi.org/10.1093/ons/opx161.
47. Weiner HL, Placantonakis DG. Resection of a Pediatric thalamic juvenile Pilocytic astrocytoma with whole brain Tractography. Cureus. 2017;9(10) https://doi.org/10.7759/cureus.1768.
48. Raza SM, Recinos PF, Avendano J, Adams H, Jallo GI, Quinones-Hinojosa A. Minimally invasive trans-portal resection of deep intracranial lesions. Minim Invasive Neurosurg. 2011;54(1):5–11. https://doi.org/10.1055/s-0031-1273734.

# Chapter 6
# Open Approaches to Intraventricular Tumors, Colloid Cysts, and the Subcortical Space


Aditya Kondajji, Prasanth Romiyo, Courtney Duong, Won Kim, and Isaac Yang


## Introduction to Intraventricular Tumors

Intraventricular tumors pose a unique surgical challenge due to their deep location and close association with perforating arteries and complex white matter tracts. One of the earliest descriptions of the treatment of intraventricular tumors comes from Walter E. Dandy's monograph, *Benign Tumors in the Third Ventricle of the Brain: Diagnosis and Treatment* [19]. In this study, Dandy details a series of 21 cases with a mortality of 33%. Since then, there has been substantial research into the intricate neuroanatomy of the ventricles and their surrounding structures. In particular, tractography through diffusion tensor imaging has provided invaluable insight into the multidirectional architecture of white matter tracts [7].

Intraventricular tumors account for only 0.8–1.6% of all intracranial tumors but make up 16% of childhood and adolescent intracranial tumors [1]. These tumors can be broadly classified into primary intraventricular tumors or parenchymal tumors with exophytic growth. Primary intraventricular tumors originate from the lining of the ventricles [11]. This includes the ependymal or subependymal lining, septum pellucidum, choroid plexus, and arachnoid tissue. Parenchymal tumors with exophytic growth arise from regions surrounding the ventricles and grow more than two-thirds into a ventricle [1]. The following eight types of tumors account for more than 90%


A. Kondajji · W. Kim · I. Yang (✉)
Ronald Reagan UCLA Medical Center, Department of Neurosurgery, Los Angeles, CA, USA
e-mail: akondajji@mednet.ucla.edu; wonkim@mednet.ucla.edu; iyang@mednet.ucla.edu

P. Romiyo
Tina & Fred Segal Brain Tumor and Skull Base Research Fellow, Ronald Reagan UCLA Medical Center, Department of Neurosurgery, Los Angeles, CA, USA
e-mail: promiyo@mednet.ucla.edu

C. Duong
David Geffen School of Medicine, Department of Neurosurgery, Los Angeles, CA, USA
e-mail: cqduong@mednet.ucla.edu



© Springer Nature Switzerland AG 2022
G. Zada et al. (eds.), *Subcortical Neurosurgery*,
https://doi.org/10.1007/978-3-030-95153-5_6

of intraventricular neoplasms: choroid plexus papillomas, chordoid plexus carcinomas, meningiomas, ependymomas, subependymomas, subependymal giant cell astrocytomas (SEGA), central neurocytomas, and metastases [1]. As summarized by Agarwal and Kanekar, each of these types of tumors are more likely to appear in certain ventricles [1]. Specifically, 50% of choroid plexus tumors occur in the lateral ventricles, and 40% occur in the fourth ventricle. Meningiomas commonly occur in the atria of the lateral ventricles. Ependymomas occur in the fourth ventricle in >60% of cases, while subependymomas occur in the fourth ventricle in 50–60% of cases and the lateral ventricular margins or septum in 30–40% of cases. SEGAs nearly always occur at the foramen of Monro, and central neurocytomas typically are found at the inferior septum pellucidum and anterior lateral ventricle. Intraventricular metastases account for only 0.9–4.6% of all cerebral metastases and are typically seen in the lateral ventricles [40]. Clinical signs and symptoms are usually secondary to cerebrospinal fluid (CSF) obstruction and elevated intracranial pressure. Infants may present with hydrocephalus, loss of appetite, and irritability [80]. Children and adults present with headache and vomiting with papilledema [22]. The specific location of the tumor may result in additional findings. For example, tumors of the posterior fossa may produce cerebellar dysfunction [1]. It should be noted that seizures and visual changes are not typically associated with intraventricular tumors [1].

## Introduction to Colloid Cysts

In 1858, Heinrich Wallmann identified the first colloid cyst on autopsy in his manuscript titled *Eine colloid cysts im dritten Hirnnventrikl und ein lipom im plexus chorioides* [76]. The first successful operative removal would not occur until 1921 on a young female patient confirmed to have a third ventricular tumor on cerebral pneumography at the Johns Hopkins Hospital by Dandy [18]. Despite accounting for less than 2% of primary brain tumors overall, colloid cysts are now commonly recognized as the most prevalent tumor of the third ventricle causing CSF obstruction of the foramen of Monro [30, 72]. While the majority of colloid cysts are stable and found incidentally on imaging, patients can present with symptoms of obstructive hydrocephalus or even with dementia, and gait disturbances without elevated pressure, similar to normal pressure hydrocephalus [49]. Drop attacks and paradoxical headaches caused by changes in head position have also been described in the literature although this finding has not been proven to be pathognomonic [83]. Of all the possible outcomes associated with colloid cysts, the most feared is sudden death without signs of herniation or hydrocephalus speculated to arise from acute cardiac arrest associated with compression of hypothalamic cardiovascular regulatory centers [45, 75]. For this reason, neurosurgeons favor surgical treatment over conservative modalities such as observation for even asymptomatic colloid cysts when signs of cyst or ventricle enlargement are present [36].

While these benign and congenital tumors have no illustrated genetic loci, familial inheritance has been posited through twin studies and generational reports in the literature [2, 9, 58, 62]. Embryologically, colloid cysts are believed to arise from either endodermal respiratory epithelium or components of the primitive neuroectoderm that give rise to the tela choroidea [41]. These theories are supported by the finding that they are immunohistochemically distinct in profile from choroid plexus epithelium and ependyma [43]. Colloid cysts are composed of an inner mucin-producing epithelial layer that stains PAS positive surrounded by an outer fibrinous layer that forms adhesions to surrounding ventricular structures anchored by a pedicle or broad sessile base [41, 44, 53]. In the overwhelming majority of cases, colloid cysts develop in the anterior portion of the third ventricle although rare cases in the septum pellucidum, retroforniceal region, and velum interpositum have rarely been reported [6]. The classic rostral presentation in the roof of the third ventricle occluding or even protruding through the foramen of Monro to occupy space in the lateral ventricles can easily be identified on CT imaging, in part due to the cyst's proteinaceous contents composed of radiodense calcium ([50]; Fig. 6.1). MR imaging of colloid cysts may provide additional prognostic value as cyst T2

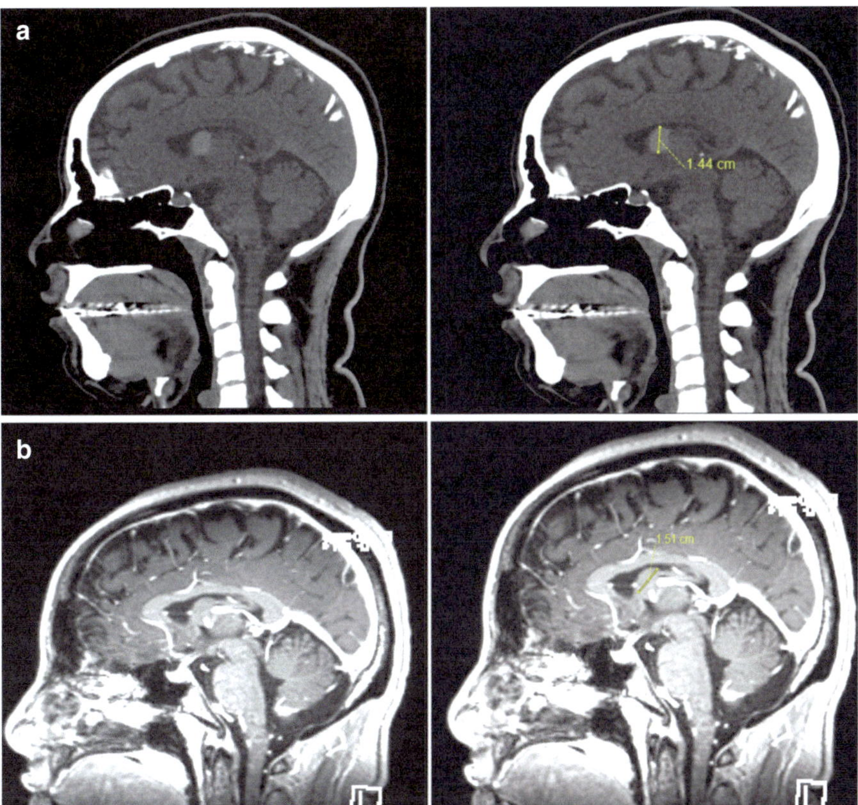



**Fig. 6.1** Colloid cyst shown on sagittal view from CT (**a**) and MR (**b**) imaging. The lesion is more readily appreciated on CT imaging due to its isointense appearance on MR

hyperintensity has been reported to correlate positively with risk of future growth and mass effect symptoms [8, 61]. However, CT scans are preferred as colloid cysts can variably appear isointense on MR imaging [51]. Colloid cysts range from 3 to 40 mm in diameter, with even larger cases reported in the literature [3, 5].

## Anatomy of the Lateral Ventricles

It is necessary to understand the anatomy of the ventricles in order to anticipate the risks and challenges of resecting intraventricular tumors. The lateral ventricles are a pair of curved structures composed of a body, atria, and three horns. These three horns are known as the anterior horn, posterior horn, and inferior horn. Both of the lateral ventricles communicate with the third ventricle through the foramen of Monro. The two lateral ventricles are separated by the thin septum pellucidum. The body of the lateral ventricles lies within the parietal lobe and extends anteriorly from the foramen of Monro to the splenium of the corpus callosum posteriorly [66]. Thus, the roof of the body is formed by the inferior portion of the body of the corpus callosum. The floor of the body is composed, from lateral to medial, of the body of the caudate nucleus, the stria terminalis and thalamostriate vein, the lateral part of the superior surface of the thalamus, and the choroid fissure [68]. The atria have a triangular shape and connect to the body, inferior horn, and posterior horn. The tapetum of the splenium of the corpus callosum forms the roof of the atrium, the floor is formed by the collateral trigone, and the medial wall is formed by the calcar avis of the calcarine fissure [66]. Similarly, the medial wall of the posterior horn is formed by the bulb of the corpus callosum and calcar avis. The floor of the posterior horn is formed by the collateral trigone. The roof and lateral walls are formed by the tapetum and separate the horn from the optic radiations [68]. The inferior horn extends from the atrium and terminates at the amygdala. Its floor is formed by the collateral eminence and hippocampus, with the hippocampus covered by the alveus. The roof of the inferior is formed laterally by the tapetum and medially by the tail of the caudate nucleus and stria terminalis [68]. The anterior horn's anterior wall and roof are bounded by the genu of the corpus callosum, the floor of the horn is formed by the rostrum, and the lateral walls are formed by the head of the caudate nucleus. The medial wall of the frontal horn is formed by the columns of the fornix inferiorly [66].

## Third Ventricular Anatomy

The approach for resection of third ventricular tumors, including colloid cysts, depends on the location, lesion size, and the clinical status of the patient. For instance, the transcortical approach favors tumors that require subchoroidal exposure and provides optimal access to tumors off the anterior third ventricle but would be inappropriate for those in the posterior compartment [27]. This approach is also favored in patients with larger ventricles or preexisting ventricular dilation and is more effective for voluminous tumors [55, 60]. Thorough knowledge of third ventricular anatomy is critical to appreciate the operative risks and tenets that must be at the fore of any open procedures targeting the colloid cysts. The third ventricle is a unilocular, narrow, midline cavity bearing semblance to a funnel in functionality and appearance [77]. The floor of the third ventricle is composed of the mamillary bodies, the infundibulum of the hypothalamus, the posterior perforated substance, and the midbrain tegmentum. The lateral walls are bound by the hypothalamus inferiorly and the thalamus superiorly. *The choroid fissure is located between the thalamus and the body of the fornix and is the site of origin for the choroid plexus.* The posterior wall is made of the pineal body, habenular commissure, pulvinar, posterior commissure, the splenium of the corpus callosum, and the aqueduct of Sylvius at its lowest point. Anteriorly, the third ventricular space is bound by the optic chiasm, lamina terminalis, and the rostrum of the corpus callosum [23, 78].

The roof of the third ventricle, which houses essential vessels, is especially important to spatially envision as colloid cysts frequently form fibrinous adhesions to this region. The roof consists of four layers (Fig. 6.2). The most superior layer is made of the body of the fornix anteriorly, with the posterior aspect encompassing the crura and hippocampal commissure. The next three layers include two thin

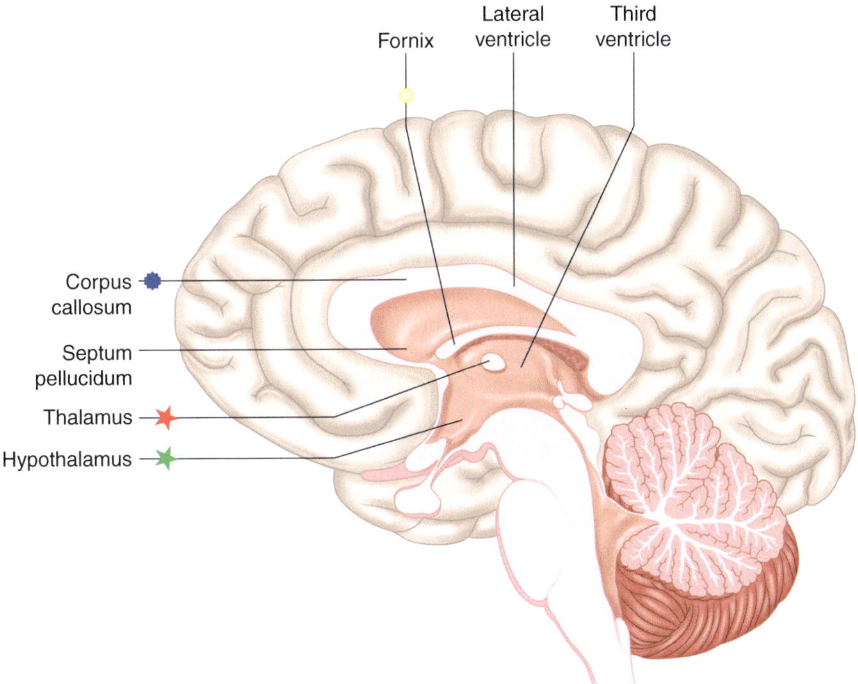


**Fig. 6.2** Third ventricular roof

layers of connective tissue derived from pia mater named tela choroidea, with a layer between them housing blood vessels. The choroid plexus in the roof of the third ventricle is attached to the deep layer of the tela. *The velum interpositum, located between the two layers of the tela, contains the medial posterior choroidal arteries and the internal cerebral veins more anteriorly.* The medial posterior and superior posterior choroidal arteries supply the tela choroidea [64, 82]. The anterior section of the roof of the third ventricle is cannulated by the foramen of Monro. Here, structures like the choroid plexus, medial posterior choroidal artery, internal cerebral vein, anterior septal vein, and thalamostriate vein all converge [26]. The foramen of Monro is accessed in order to debulk and remove colloid cysts in both the transcortical and transcallosal approaches.

## Fourth Ventricle Anatomy

The fourth ventricle is a single, midline structure located anteriorly from the cerebellum and posteriorly from the medulla and pons. The ventricle is pyramid shaped, with the base of the pyramid composed of the dorsal side of the brainstem and the apex of the cone located in the anterior part of the cerebellar vermis [54]. The floor of the fourth ventricle is covered by a single-cell layer of ependyma, and the impressions of cranial nerve nuclei can be appreciated. The longitudinal median sulcus forms the vertical midline of the ventricle. The hypoglossal trigone can be observed at the medullary level, while the colliculus of the facial nerve can be seen at the pontic level [54]. The base of the pyramid is also characterized by four corners, or angles. The two lateral angles are the foramina of Luschka, the upper angle communicates with the aqueduct of Sylvius, and the lower angle continues as the central canal of the medulla and spinal cord. Notably, the obex forms the posterior wall of the lower angle. The apex of the fourth ventricle, the fastigium, is situated in the ventral surface of the cerebellar vermis and is bounded laterally by the cerebellar peduncles, superiorly by the lingula, and inferiorly by the nodule [54]. The superior walls of the fourth ventricle are formed by the superior cerebellar peduncle, while the lower walls are formed by the inferior cerebellar peduncles. Importantly, the lower portion of the roof supports the choroid plexuses of the fourth ventricle which are a set of paired structures that run from the obex to the lateral angles. The foramen of Magendie, a medial opening of the fourth ventricle that communicates with the subarachnoid space through the cisterna magna, is located at the bottom of the inferior medullary velum [54]. Generally speaking, the fourth ventricle is supplied by the basilar artery and cerebellar arteries. Specifically, the superior portion of the fastigium is vascularized by the superior cerebellar artery, which runs through the cerebellar-mesencephalic fissure [63]. The lower portion of the roof and choroid plexus is supplied by the posterior inferior cerebellar artery. The anterior inferior cerebellar artery, located along the cerebellar-pontine fissure, supplies the lateral angles of the base of the ventricle. The base is also supplied by perforating branches of the anterior spinal artery, basilar artery, and P1 of the posterior cerebral artery

[63]. Venous drainage of the fourth ventricle is carried through the veins running with their corresponding arteries [54].

## Open Transcortical, Transventricular, and Intraventricular Approach

Open surgical approaches for colloid cysts have not changed drastically since 1921, with Dandy favoring a posterior transcallosal approach followed by the development of a frontal transcortical approach by Greenwood in 1949 [19, 31]. Mckissock further refined this technique in 1951, paving a path for neurosurgeons to reach deeply located tumors in coordinates surrounded by critical neurovasculature [15]. With the advent of endoscopic technologies, enhanced microsurgical techniques, improved imaging, and reimagined navigation through frameless stereotaxy, the relatively high morbidity associated with early surgeries for these benign lesions has been greatly reduced [69]. Open surgery is now considered the gold standard for the categorical treatment of colloid cysts [56]. Stereotactically guided aspiration has been performed as an alternative to open surgery, but these procedures often fail to completely eradicate the cyst and are noted to have a high rate of recurrence [52]. For tumors of the third ventricle, the transcallosal and transcortical approaches are most often employed. The optimal procedure for removal of colloid cysts should minimize insults to brain parenchyma associated with prolonged retraction. In addition, patient-specific clinical status and ventricular anatomy should be taken into account. For instance, acute management of obtunded patients experiencing obstruction at the foramen of Monro routinely involves bilateral drainage of the lateral ventricles to avoid subfalcine herniation. However, in patients with GCS scores of 14 or 15, ventricular drainage should be deferred to allow for dilation and ease of operation [46]. Permissive dilation is particularly useful in the transcortical approach to the third ventricle.

The initiation of the transcortical approach for removal of colloid cysts begins with neuronavigation, ensuring that the entry pathway directly points toward the foramen of Monro. Once registration is completed, a small frontal burr hole craniotomy is performed with a cruciate dural incision made to reveal the middle frontal gyrus of the nondominant hemisphere, usually on the right side. The left side may be favored if the same-sided ventricle is dilated to a greater extent. Kocher's point, 2.5 cm from the midline and 1 cm anterior to the coronal suture, is then identified [4]. A small resection is made 0.5–1.5 cm lateral to this landmark to allow for passage of a guiding catheter into the frontal horn of the lateral ventricle. Successful insertion of the catheter should bypass the motor strip and nearby eloquent structures including Broca's area and subsequently guide dissection in later steps. In its initial stages, the transcortical approach should feel commonplace as it is a continuation of basic neurosurgical skills. Next, microdissection is performed through the white matter surrounding the catheter to create a 1–2 cm linear cerebrotomy. Minimal cortical opening is performed in order to decrease the likelihood of postoperative epilepsy [41]. Frameless stereotaxy is used throughout this process to ensure that the planned trajectory is maintained (Fig. 6.3).

It is the author's preference to use tubular retractor systems that navigate critical subcortical tracts parafascicularly. Smaller variants of these tools are preferred in order to eliminate unnecessary disruption of adjacent structures. Before setting the retractors, the foramen of Monro must be visualized. A helpful method of triangulating this aperture is to search for the more obvious placement of the choroid plexus and to follow it anteriorly until the point of convergence with the septal and thalamostriate veins. The foramen of Monro lies just anterior to this point. Once identified, the retractors are set [46].

Prior to removing the cyst, which often causes bilateral ventricular dilation due to its position in the anterior third ventricle, a pellucidotomy is performed so that only unilateral shunting is needed postsurgically should the patient develop hydrocephalus [81]. Once completed, the colloid cyst is then targeted. If there is difficulty visualizing the wall of the cyst, the surgeon may opt for a more posterolateral angle to directly view the foramen of Monro. With this line of sight afforded from the lateral ventricle, larger colloid cysts can be immediately identified. Smaller cysts

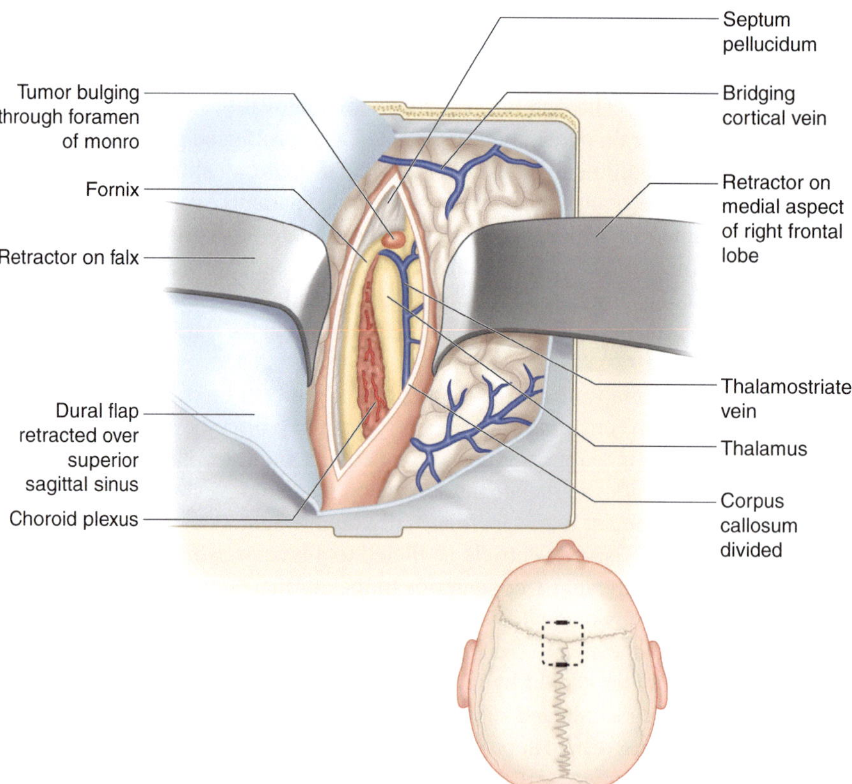


**Fig. 6.3** Transcortical, intraventricular approach

may be obstructed by the choroid plexus which requires readjusting in order to reveal the lesion; however, forniceal integrity must be preserved in order to safeguard the patient from suffering impairments in memory [42]. Any vessels originating from the choroid plexus that feed the colloid cysts are coagulated and then cut. The cyst is then punctured using a ringed curette with its contents carefully aspirated. Any attachments to the roof of the third ventricle or surrounding structures are also coagulated and cut with the cyst and then removed through the foramen of Monro as a whole instead of piecemeal. Using this approach, there is a surgical blind spot as the posterior compartment of the third ventricle may have a small piece of cyst capsule that remains attached. For this reason, an endoscope may be useful for observing the posterior aspect of the third ventricle and the contralateral foramen of Monro [10].

Alternative routes to the intraforaminal approach to the third ventricle have been utilized to reach challenging colloid cysts. The transchoroidal approach was developed to gain access to the velum interpositum and then the bottom layers of the roof of the third ventricle by dissecting through the choroidal fissure, the area between the fornix and the thalamus [37]. Wen et al. have advocated for use of a transchoroidal approach as it takes advantage of microsurgical anatomy by travelling through a naturally occurring cleft. The top layer of the taenia choroidea is dissected through the choroidal fissure to reveal the two internal cerebral veins where further dissection between these vessels can be performed due to lack of bridging veins. This ultimately allows for exposure of the third ventricle after continuing through the bottom layer of taenia choroidea and the choroid plexus [77, 79]. However, this approach risks abruption of blood flow through retraction of the internal veins and the fornix [34]. Subchoroidal and suprachoroidal methods have also been recommended for the resection of colloid cysts. In the subchoroidal approach, the taenia choroidea is opened inferolaterally to the choroid plexus alongside the thalamus. The risk of damaging the thalamostriate vein is greatly increased in this approach as the route to the third ventricle passes within 5–10 mm of the vessel [56]. In the suprachoroidal approach, an incision in the tenia fornices is performed to reveal the internal cerebral veins and the remaining layers of the third ventricular roof. Both routes are performed nonroutinely due to their proximity to the thalamus, fornix, and aforementioned vasculature. However, in select cases, these approaches may be the preferred choice.

## Open Transcallosal, Interhemispheric Approach

The transcallosal approach serves as the counterpart to the transcortical entry in modern neurosurgery. Guided by literature reporting less seizure activity, this interhemispheric craniotomy has grown in favor among colleagues as the preferred route for colloid cyst resection as well as for tumors located within the frontal horn, the body of the lateral ventricle, and the anterior third ventricle [80]. The transcallosal approach begins with adjusting the patient so that the superior sagittal sinus lines up parallel to the floor to leverage gravity retraction for when it becomes necessary to dissociate the sinus and falx away from the ipsilateral hemisphere [16]. A craniotomy anterior to the coronal suture is performed followed by a U-shaped dural incision to uncover the superior sagittal sinus [15, 73]. The sinus is then retracted to allow for access to the midline. Special care is taken to avoid parasagittal bridging veins; however, smaller veins may be sacrificed despite the best efforts. The corpus callosum is then targeted for microdissection after separation of the right superior frontal gyrus from the falx and circumnavigation around larger bridging cortical veins (Fig. 6.4). A 1–2 cm incision is made in the corpus callosum with microdissection performed painstakingly so as to spare the cingulate gyrus and any encountered pericallosal arteries [32]. After entry into the lateral ventricle is achieved, the same routes to the third ventricle used in the transcortical approach can be initiated for colloid cyst removal. For tumors located in the frontal horns and anterior portion of the body, the goal of resection is central enucleation and subsequent peripheral dissection. It can be beneficial to place cotton sponges into the trigone to prevent tumor cells from moving into the occipital and temporal horns [80]. The transcallosal approach is beneficial for patients without hydrocephalus, and recent advances in microsurgery have minimized the risk of vascular damage. Furthermore, the transcallosal approach avoids injury to white matter tracts located within the cortical and subcortical space.

**Fig. 6.4** Transcallosal, interhemispheric approach

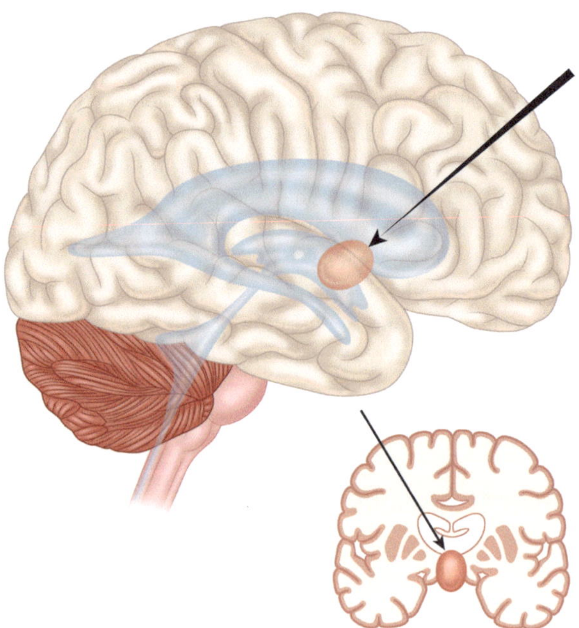

## Pterional Transsylvian Approach

The pterional transsylvian approach is commonly performed for tumors of the temporal horn of the lateral ventricle [80]. The patient is placed in dorsal decubitus position, and a pterional craniotomy is performed at the level of the Sylvian fissure. Likewise, the dura is opened with a central incision along the Sylvian fissure, and the fissure is then opened from the pars opercularis to the inferior frontal gyrus [59]. As the frontal lobe is separated from the temporal lobe, care is taken to mobilize the middle cerebral artery. The Sylvian artery must be displaced to better visualize the limiting sulcus of the insula [59]. A small corticotomy is then performed at the limiting sulcus of the insula behind the limen insulae, affording access to the temporal horn [13].

## Parieto-Occipital Interhemispheric Approach

The parieto-occipital interhemispheric approach may be employed for tumors of the posterior third ventricle, atrium, and occipital horn [80]. The patient is placed in sitting position, and burr holes are made a few millimeters lateral of the midline on the contralateral side of the superior sagittal sinus. Incision of the dura should be performed to preserve the veins draining into the superior sagittal sinus. Dissection is then performed toward the splenium of the corpus callosum. An incision through the precuneal gyrus anterior to the parieto-occipital sulcus is then made, which provides access to the atria and occipital horns.

## Telovelar Approach for the Fourth Ventricle

The median inferior suboccipital cerebellomedullary fissure approach, also known as the telovelar approach, allows access to the fourth ventricle for tumor removal [80]. With the patient in prone position, an incision is made from the C2–C3 spinous processes to the external occipital protuberance, and a burr hole is placed below the protuberance. This ensures that the craniotomy is performed below the transverse sinus. C1 laminectomy may be performed if this improves the working angle, especially when needing to reach the rostral aspects of the fourth ventricle [29]. Subsequently, an opening is made through the vallecula followed by separation of the cerebellar tonsils to access the tonsillouveal sulcus. At this point, the foramen of Magendie, tela choroidea, and inferior medullary velum may be observed. The telovelum is then opened to the level necessary to remove the tumor. This incision allows excellent access to the lateral angles, caudal half of the ventricle, and superolateral recess [29]. The most rostral aspects of the fourth ventricle may be more challenging to access, but as previously stated, C1 laminectomy allows for an improved angle of approach.

## Complications and Controversies

The transcortical and transcallosal approaches to deep regions of the brain are complex and technically challenging procedures with their own inherent risk profiles. Complications shared between them include risk for damage to the thalamostriate vein, septal vein, fornices, and internal cerebral veins. Disruption of the thalamostriate vein can lead to hemorrhagic infarction of the thalamus and basal ganglia, which carries the risk of developing parkinsonism [47]. Damage to this vessel can also cause mutism, hemiplegia, and drowsiness [15]. While early reports advocated for sacrifice of this vein due to its strong collateral support in order to enlarge the foramen of Monro, the degree of collateral support has not been shown to prognosticate which patients would go on to develop postoperative complications [35, 74]. Therefore, active preservation of this structure is paramount. In cases where the colloid cyst projects superiorly to cause lateral separation of the fornices, the interforniceal route had been proposed as an alternative to the third ventricle. This too has fallen by the wayside in contemporary neurosurgical practice after poorer outcomes than initially anticipated result.

The transcallosal route carries unique sequelae as a result of its pathway to the lateral ventricle. Retraction of the cortex for extended periods can lead to postoperative bouts of contralateral leg weakness. However, improvements in microsurgery have minimized the need for prolonged insult. The greatest concern is that of venous infarction due to sacrifice of large cortical bridging veins or drawn-out retraction of the superior sagittal sinus, especially in patients with hypercoagulable states [28, 36, 48]. The likelihood that pericallosal arteries may be damaged is also heightened given that anatomical variants such as one or three pericallosal arteries may exist that are not apparent on preoperative MR imaging [24, 33, 39]. Disconnection syndrome has also been reported although limiting the incision to 2.5 cm or less within the corpus callosum has largely prevented this complication [70]. Furthermore, damage to the supplementary motor cortex or thalamus along the interhemispheric route may also contribute to mutism [57]. In terms of technical difficulty, the transcallosal approach can be disorienting for surgeons with respect to ventricular anatomy as different head placements may be set. Additionally, the working space available through the interhemispheric corridor may be narrower than in the transcortical approach.

In the transcortical approach, technical challenges include less space to maneuver when operating in patients with smaller or less dilated ventricles and the availability of only one foramen of Monro to access the third ventricle. Intraventricular complications related to this approach are the same as in the transcallosal approach except that there is less risk of damaging the fornix and thalamostriate vein (Laidlaw). Edema due to retraction of the cortex in this approach has been associated with contralateral, self-resolving hemiparesis [49]. Conflicting reports have been cited in the literature pertaining to cognitive ramifications arising from cerebrotomy. In 2002, Desai et al. discovered in their single institutional experience that of 30 patients who underwent a transcortical approach for removal of a colloid cyst, 26% had seizures [21]. Another group reported no seizures postoperatively after performing the same approach in 27 patients and corroborated these findings with a literature review revealing a seizure rate of 8.3% across 238 transcortical cases [25]. In direct contrast to commonly held sentiment, Milligan et al. found that out of the 127 patients who had removal of intraventricular lesions, postoperative seizures arose in 25% of those who underwent a transcallosal, interhemispheric approach versus 8% in the transcortical cohort ($P = 0.1$; [55]). These publications showcase the ongoing debate still surrounding the optimal approach to deep lesions of the third ventricle.

Between the transcortical and transcallosal approaches, the larger question looms as to whether endoscopic or microsurgical techniques offer better outcomes for resection of colloid cysts. Connolly et al. found that out of 483 patients, split almost evenly between endoscopic and microsurgical approaches, the seizure rate was 14.7% for the microsurgical group and 5.4% in the endoscopic group ($P = 0.001$). The 30-day readmission rate was also higher for the microsurgical group ($P = 0.015$) [17]. Contrastingly, Brostigen et al. found that there was no statistically significant difference between microsurgery and endoscopic surgery for colloid cysts related to the grade of resection or postoperative complications in 32 consecutive patients [12]. In corroboration with this finding, a more comprehensive meta-analysis of 1278 patients showed that a higher gross total resection rate and lower rate of occurrence was achieved using microsurgical techniques over the endoscopic method in transcranial operations. No significant differences existed in mortality rate between these two groups, but morbidity was higher in the microsurgical cohort [67]. As microsurgical and endoscopic techniques continue to evolve, the march of superiority alternates in stride. Endoscopic techniques that were once considered ineffective at completely removing the cyst wall have now emerged as a compelling option. Microsurgical approaches that previously produced higher seizure rates and mutism are now improved with neurosurgeons reducing retraction on the cortex and minimizing transgressions against eloquent fiber tracts aided by tools such as diffusion tensor imaging [71]. Both approaches can play a cooperative role in the removal of colloid cysts.

For instance, in cases where it is uncertain whether the entire cyst wall was removed *en bloc*, an endoscope can be used to illuminate the operative blind spot. Reciprocally, microsurgical techniques might be employed if the cyst wall is not completely removed by endoscopic procedures alone.

## Approaches to the Subcortical Space

It is possible for intraaxial tumors to lie below the cortical surface but outside the ventricles, within the subcortical space. Broadly speaking, approaches to the subcortical space can be divided into transgyral or transsulcal approaches. Due to the deep-seated nature of these subcortical lesions, it is necessary to traverse through the cortex and surrounding white matter. The use of preoperative imaging, functional magnetic resonance imaging (fMRI), diffusion tensor imaging (DTI), and cortical mapping is therefore employed to minimize damage to eloquent regions [14].

A transgyral approach necessitates performing a corticectomy that will dissect through the overlying pia, gray matter, and white matter until the tumor is reached. It is therefore critical to choose a gyrus that will have minimal impact to the patient. Examples of such gyri include the anterior frontal lobe, superior parietal lobule, and inferior temporal gyrus [14]. This approach avoids damaging sulcal vessels and results in less damage to the subcortical "U" fibers [65].

For a transsulcal approach, the sulcus that is chosen is typically the one that reaches furthest to the lesion while avoiding critical regions. A craniotomy is performed with the dural opening centered over the sulcus. The arachnoid membrane overlying the sulcus is then carefully dissected [20]. Separation of the surround gyri is maintained with dynamic or fixed retraction as a corticectomy is performed to reach the lesion [14]. The transsulcal approach is considered a parafascicular approach since it is performed parallel to the major white matter tracts [38]. Furthermore, traversing the sulcus itself allows for minimal damage to the brain parenchyma although special care must be taken to avoid damaging sulcal vessels.

## Conclusion

Since the first successful removals of colloid cysts and intraventricular tumors in the early 1920s, burgeoning technologic advancements and increasingly innovative techniques have been developed to ensure favorable outcomes for patients. Today, most neurosurgeons opt to perform either the transcortical or transcallosal approach to reach the foramen of Monro and the third ventricle for debulking and removal of colloid cysts, with important advantages and drawbacks to either approach. Conflicting reports of postoperative seizure complication rates recently shifted the operative paradigm to favor the transcallosal approach; however, it is the authors' opinion that the transcortical, transventricular approach is just as safe and effective as the transcallosal, interhemispheric approach for resection of benign colloid cysts. Once inside the lateral ventricle, the intraforaminal route provides the safest corridor for removal of the cyst as it utilizes a naturally occurring cannulation and spares injury to the thalamus, fornix, and thalamostriate vein. Transchoroidal, subchoroidal, and suprachoroidal approaches are not advocated except in experienced hands or cases where the intraforaminal approach would render the planned resection untenable. In addressing the controversy between microsurgical and endoscopic techniques, the effectiveness will ultimately depend on the comfort and skill level of the operator as both technologies have proven successful at achieving the same end result. As a result of these neurosurgical advances, the majority of patients with colloid cysts are completely cured after resection. For intraventricular tumors, the precise location within the ventricular system dictates which approach should be utilized. Generally speaking, the anterior transcallosal, interhemispheric approach is used for frontal horn tumors, the pterional transsylvian approach for temporal horn tumors, the telovar approach for fourth ventricle tumors, and the parieto-occipital interhemispheric approach for tumors of the posterior third ventricle, occipital horn, and atria. Finally, for tumors lying within the subcortical space, transgyral or transsulcal approaches may be used. The choice of approach is largely dependent on whether an eloquent region will be at risk and if the surgeon feels comfortable maneuvering sulcal vessels. Lesions of the subcortical space and ventricular system are deep seated and require a thorough understanding of neuroanatomy in order to appreciate the approach that must be utilized and the risks of such an approach.

# References


1. Agarwal A, Kanekar S. Intraventricular tumors. Semin Ultrasound CT MR. 2016;37(2):150–8.
2. Aggarwal A, Corbett A, Graham J. Familial colloid cyst of the third ventricle. J Clin Neurosci. 1999;6(6):520–2.
3. Agrawal A, Santhi V, Umamaheswara RV. Giant colloid cyst of the third ventricle: challenges in management. Chin Neurosurg J. 2016;2(1):11.
4. Aref M, Martyniuk A, Nath S, Koziarz A, Badhiwala J, Algird A, et al. Endoscopic third ventriculostomy: outcome analysis of an anterior entry point. World Neurosurg. 2017;104:554–9.
5. Armao D, Castillo M, Chen H, Kwock L. Colloid cyst of the third ventricle: imaging-pathologic correlation. Am J Neuroradiol. 2000;21(8):1470–7.
6. Azab WA, Salaheddin W, Alsheikh TM, Nasim K, Nasr MM. Colloid cysts posterior and anterior to the foramen of Monro: anatomical features and implications for endoscopic excision. Surg Neurol Int. 2014;7:5.
7. Basser PJ, Pajevic S, Pierpaoli C, Duda J, Aldroubi A. In vivo fiber tractography using DT-MRI data. Magn Reson Med. 2000;44(4):625–32.
8. Beaumont TL, Limbrick DD, Rich KM, Wippold FJ, Dacey RG. Natural history of colloid cysts of the third ventricle. J Neurosurg. 2016;125(6):1420–30.
9. Benoiton LA, Correia J, Kamat AS, Wickremesekera A. Familial colloid cyst. J Clin Neurosci. 2014;21(3):533–5.
10. Birski M, Birska J, Paczkowski D, Furtak J, Rusinek M, Rudas M, et al. Combination of neuroendoscopic and stereotactic procedures for total resection of colloid cysts with favorable neurological and cognitive outcomes. World Neurosurg. 2016;85:205–14.
11. Boudreau RP. Primary intraventricular tumors. Radiology. 1960;75(6):867.
12. Brostigen CS, Meling TR, Marthinsen PB, Scheie D, Aarhus M, Helseth E. Surgical management of colloid cyst of the third ventricle. Acta Neurol Scand. 2017;135(4):484–7.
13. Campero A, Ajler P, Garategui L, Goldschmidt E, Martins C, Rhoton A. Pterional transsylvian-transinsular approach in three cavernomas of the left anterior mesiotemporal region. Clin

Neurol Neurosurg. 2015;130:14–9. https://doi.org/10.1016/j.clineuro.2014.12.013. PMID: 25576880.
14. Chaichana L. Kaisorn, chapter 22 – transsulcal versus transgyral approaches for subcortical tumors. In: Chaichana K, Quiñones-Hinojosa A, editors. Comprehensive overview of modern surgical approaches to intrinsic brain tumors. Academic Press; 2019. p. 379–91.
15. Cikla U, Swanson KI, Tumturk A, Keser N, Uluc K, Cohen-Gadol A, et al. Microsurgical resection of tumors of the lateral and third ventricles: operative corridors for difficult-to-reach lesions. J Neuro-Oncol. 2016;130(2):331–40.
16. Cohen-Gadol A. Interhemispheric craniotomy. In: Neurosurgical atlas. Neurosurgical Atlas, Inc.; 2016. [cited 2019 Jan 12]. Available from: http://www.neurosurgicalatlas.com/volumes/cranial-approaches/interhemispheric-craniotomy.
17. Connolly ID, Johnson E, Lamsam L, Veeravagu A, Ratliff J, Li G. Microsurgical vs. endoscopic excision of colloid cysts: an analysis of complications and costs using a longitudinal administrative database. Front Neurol. 2017;8:259. Available from: https://www.ncbi.nlm.nih.gov/pmc/articles/PMC5465269/
18. Dandy W. The Johns Hopkins hospital. Bull Johns Hopkins Hosp. 1922;32:562.
19. Dandy W. Benign tumors in the third ventricle of the brain: diagnosis and treatment. Arch Neur Psychiatry. 1935;33(1):242.
20. Day JD. Transsulcal parafascicular surgery using brain path® for subcortical lesions. Neurosurgery. 2017;64(CN_suppl_1):151–6.
21. Desai KI, Nadkarni TD, Muzumdar DP, Goel AH. Surgical management of colloid cyst of the third ventricle—a study of 105 cases. Surg Neurol. 2002;57(5):295–302.
22. Duong H, Sarazin L, Bourgouin P, Vézina JL. Magnetic resonance imaging of lateral ventricular tumours. Can Assoc Radiol J. 1995;46(6):434–42.
23. Duvernoy HM. The human brain: surface, three-dimensional sectional anatomy with MRI, and blood supply. Springer Science & Business Media; 2012. p. 492.
24. Ehni G. Interhemispheric and percallosal (transcallosal) approach to the cingulate gyri, intraventricular shunt tubes, and certain deeply placed brain lesions. Neurosurgery. 1984;14(1):99–110.
25. Eichberg DG, Sedighim S, Buttrick S, Komotar RJ. Postoperative seizure rate after transcortical resection of subcortical brain tumors and colloid cysts: a single surgeon's experience. Cureus. 2018;10(1):e2115. Available from: https://www.ncbi.nlm.nih.gov/pmc/articles/PMC5871436/
26. Fonseca RB, Black PM, Filho HA. Approaches to the third ventricle. Arq Bras Neurocir. 2012;31(1):3–9.
27. Fujii K, Lenkey C, Rhoton AL. Microsurgical anatomy of the choroidal arteries: lateral and third ventricles. J Neurosurg. 1980;52(2):165–88.
28. Garrido E, Fahs GR. Cerebral venous and sagittal sinus thrombosis after transcallosal removal of a colloid cyst of the third ventricle case report. Neurosurgery. 1990;26(3):540–2.
29. Ghali MGZ. Telovelar surgical approach. Neurosurg Rev. 2019;44(1):61–76.
30. Glastonbury CM, Osborn AG, Salzman KL. Masses and malformations of the third ventricle: normal anatomic relationships and differential diagnoses. Radiographics. 2011;31(7):1889–905.
31. Greenwood J. Paraphysial cysts of the third ventricle: with report of eight cases. J Neurosurg. 1949;6(2):153–9.
32. Hendricks B, Cohen-Gadol A. Colloid cyst (transcallosal approach). In: Neurosurgical atlas. Neurosurgical Atlas, Inc.; 2016. Available from: http://www.neurosurgicalatlas.com/volumes/brain-tumors/intraventricular-tumors/third-ventricular-tumors/colloid-cyst/colloid-cyst-transcallosal-approach.
33. Hernesniemi J, Romani R, Dashti R, Albayrak BS, Savolainen S, Ramsey C, et al. Microsurgical treatment of third ventricular colloid cysts by interhemispheric far lateral transcallosal approach—experience of 134 patients. Surg Neurol. 2008;69(5):447–53.
34. Herrmann H-D. Transchoroidal approach to the third ventricle: an anatomic study of the choroidal fissure and its clinical application. Neurosurgery. 1998;42(6):1217–8.

35. Hirsch JF, Zouaoui A, Renier D, Pierre-Kahn A. A new surgical approach to the third ventricle with interruption of the striothalamic vein. Acta Neurochir. 1979;47(3):135–47.
36. Horn EM, Feiz-Erfan I, Bristol RE, Lekovic GP, Goslar PW, Smith KA, et al. Treatment options for third ventricular colloid cystscomparison of open microsurgical versus endoscopic resection. Neurosurgery. 2007;60(4):613–20.
37. Ibáñez-Botella G, Domínguez M, Ros B, De Miguel L, Márquez B, Arráez MA. Endoscopic transchoroidal and transforaminal approaches for resection of third ventricular colloid cysts. Neurosurg Rev. 2014;37(2):227–34. discussion 234
38. Jackson C, Gallia GL, Chaichana KL. Minimally invasive biopsies of deep-seated brain lesions using tubular retractors under exoscopic visualization. J Neurol Surg A Cent Eur Neurosurg. 2017;78(6):588–94. https://doi.org/10.1055/s-0037-1602698. PMID: 28482372.
39. Kapu R, Symss NP, Pande A, Vasudevan MC, Ramamurthi R. Management of pediatric colloid cysts of anterior third ventricle: a review of five cases. J Pediatr Neurosci. 2012;7(2):90–5.
40. Koeller KK, Sandberg GD. Armed forces institute of pathology. From the archives of the AFIP. Cerebral intraventricular neoplasms: radiologic-pathologic correlation. Radiographics. 2002;22(6):1473–505.
41. Kondziolka D, Lunsford LD. Microsurgical resection of colloid cysts using a stereotactic transventricular approach. Surg Neurol. 1996;46(5):485–92.
42. Konovalov AN, Pitskhelauri DI, Shkarubo M, Buklina SB, Poddubskaya AA, Kolycheva M. Microsurgical treatment of colloid cysts of the third ventricle. World Neurosurg. 2017;1(105):678–88.
43. Kuchelmeister K, Bergmann M. Colloid cysts of the third ventricle: an immunohistochemical study. Histopathology. 1992;21(1):35–42.
44. Lach B, Scheithauer BW, Gregor A, Wick MR. Colloid cyst of the third ventricle. A comparative immunohistochemical study of neuraxis cysts and choroid plexus epithelium. J Neurosurg. 1993;78(1):101–11.
45. Lagman C, Rai K, Chung LK, Nagasawa DT, Beckett JS, Tucker AM, et al. Fatal colloid cysts: a systematic review. World Neurosurg. 2017;1(107):409–15.
46. Laidlaw J, Kaye AH. 44 – colloid cysts. In: Kaye AH, Laws ER, editors. Brain tumors. 3rd ed. Edinburgh: W.B. Saunders; 2012. p. 849–63. Available from: http://www.sciencedirect.com/science/article/pii/B9780443069673000442.
47. Lanciego JL, Luquin N, Obeso JA. Functional neuroanatomy of the basal ganglia. Cold Spring Harb Perspect Med. 2012;2(12):a009621. Available from: https://www.ncbi.nlm.nih.gov/pmc/articles/PMC3543080/
48. Lega BC, Yoshor D. Postoperative dural sinus thrombosis in a patient in a hypercoagulable state: case report. J Neurosurg. 2006;105(5):772–4.
49. Little JR, MacCarty CS. Colloid cysts of the third ventricle. J Neurosurg. 1974;40(2):230–5.
50. Maeder PP, Holtås SL, Basibüyük LN, Salford LG, Tapper UA, Brun A. Colloid cysts of the third ventricle: correlation of MR and CT findings with histology and chemical analysis. AJR Am J Roentgenol. 1990;155(1):135–41.
51. Mamourian AC, Cromwell LD, Harbaugh RE. Colloid cyst of the third ventricle: sometimes more conspicuous on CT than MR. Am J Neuroradiol. 1998;19(5):875–8.
52. Mathiesen T, Grane P, Lindquist C, von Holst H. High recurrence rate following aspiration of colloid cysts in the third ventricle. J Neurosurg. 1993;78(5):748–52.
53. Mckissock W. The surgical treatment of colloid cyst of the third ventricle; a report based upon twenty-one personal cases. Brain. 1951;74(1):1–9.
54. Mercier P, Bernard F, Delion M. Microsurgical anatomy of the fourth ventricle. Neurochirurgie. 2018;S0028-3770(18):30067–5.
55. Milligan BD, Meyer FB. Morbidity of transcallosal and transcortical approaches to lesions in and around the lateral and third ventricles: a single-institution experience. Neurosurgery. 2010;67(6):1483–96.
56. Nair S, Gopalakrishnan CV, Menon G, Easwer HV, Abraham M. Interhemispheric transcallosal transforaminal approach and its variants to colloid cyst of third ventricle: technical issues based on a single institutional experience of 297 cases. Asian J Neurosurg. 2016;11(3):292–7.

57. Nakasu Y, Isozumi T, Nioka H, Handa J. Mechanism of mutism following the transcallosal approach to the ventricles. Acta Neurochir. 1991;110(3):146–53.
58. Niknejad HR, Samii A, Shen S-H, Samii M. Huge familial colloid cyst of the third ventricle: an extraordinary presentation. Surg Neurol Int. 2015;6(Suppl 11):S349–53.
59. Park JH, Cho HR, Seung WB, Lee SH, Park YS. The pterional-transsylvian approach for tumor in the temporal horn: a case report. Brain Tumor Res Treat. 2015;3(2):118–21. https://doi.org/10.14791/btrt.2015.3.2.118.
60. Pendl G, Öztürk E, Haselsberger K. Surgery of tumours of the lateral ventricle. Acta Neurochir. 1992;116(2):128–36.
61. Pollock BE, Schreiner SA, Huston J. A theory on the natural history of colloid cysts of the third ventricle. Neurosurgery. 2000;46(5):1077–81. discussion 1081-1083
62. Ravnik J, Bunc G, Grcar A, Zunic M, Velnar T. Colloid cysts of the third ventricle exhibit various clinical presentation: a review of three cases. Bosn J Basic Med Sci. 2014;14(3):132–5.
63. Rhoton AL Jr. Cerebellum and fourth ventricle. Neurosurgery. 2000;47(3 Suppl):S7–27.
64. Rhoton AL. The lateral and third ventricles. Neurosurgery. 2002;51(suppl_4):S1-207–71.
65. Sampath R, Katira K, Vannemreddy P, Nanda A. Quantifying sulcal and gyral topography in relation to deep seated and ventricular lesions: cadaveric study for basing surgical approaches and review of literature. Br J Neurosurg. 2014;28(6):713–6. https://doi.org/10.3109/0268869 7.2014.913771. PMID: 24836819.
66. Scelsi CL, Rahim TA, Morris JA, Kramer GJ, Gilbert BC, Forseen SE. The lateral ventricles: a detailed review of anatomy, development, and anatomic variations. AJNR Am J Neuroradiol. 2020;41(4):566–72.
67. Sheikh AB, Mendelson ZS, Liu JK. Endoscopic versus microsurgical resection of colloid cysts: a systematic review and meta-analysis of 1,278 patients. World Neurosurg. 2014;82(6):1187–97.
68. Shenoy SS, Lui F. Neuroanatomy, ventricular system. In: StatPearls [Internet]. Treasure Island: StatPearls Publishing; 2020.
69. Stachura K, Grzywna E. Neuronavigation-guided endoscopy for intraventricular tumors in adult patients without hydrocephalus. Wideochir Inne Tech Maloinwazyjne. 2016;11(3):200–7.
70. Symss NP, Ramamurthi R, Kapu R, Rao SM, Vasudevan MC, Pande A, et al. Complication avoidance in transcallosal transforaminal approach to colloid cysts of the anterior third ventricle: an analysis of 80 cases. Asian J Neurosurg. 2014;9(2):51.
71. Szmuda T, Słoniewski P, Szmuda M, Waszak PM, Starzyńska A. Quantification of white matter fibre pathways disruption in frontal transcortical approach to the lateral ventricle or the interventricular foramen in diffusion tensor tractography. Folia Morphol (Warsz). 2014;73(2):129–38.
72. Tenny S, Thorell W. Cyst, brain, colloid. In: StatPearls [Internet]. Treasure Island: StatPearls Publishing; 2018. Available from: http://www.ncbi.nlm.nih.gov/books/NBK470314/.
73. Tomasello F, Cardali S, Angileri FF, Conti A. Transcallosal approach to third ventricle tumors: how I do it. Acta Neurochir. 2013;155(6):1031–4.
74. Türe U, Yaşargil MG, Al-Mefty O. The transcallosal—transforaminal approach to the third ventricle with regard to the venous variations in this region. J Neurosurg. 1997;87(5):706–15.
75. Turillazzi E, Bello S, Neri M, Riezzo I, Fineschi V. Colloid cyst of the third ventricle, hypothalamus, and heart: a dangerous link for sudden death. Diagn Pathol. 2012;18(7):144.
76. Wallmann H. Eine Colloidcyste im dritten Hirnventrikel und ein Lipom im Plexus chorioides. Archiv f pathol Anat. 1858;14(3):385–8.
77. Wen HT, Rhoton AL, de Oliveira E. Transchoroidal approach to the third ventricle: an anatomic study of the choroidal fissure and its clinical application. Neurosurgery. 1998;42(6):1205–17.
78. Yamamoto I, Rhoton AL, Peace DA. Microsurgical anatomy of the third ventricle: part 2. In: Brock M, editor. Modern neurosurgery 1. Berlin, Heidelberg: Springer Berlin Heidelberg; 1982. p. 205–14. https://doi.org/10.1007/978-3-662-08801-2_24.
79. Yasargil MG. Transchoroidal approach to the third ventricle: an anatomic study of the choroidal fissure and its clinical application. Neurosurgery. 1998;42(6):1218–9.

80. Yaşargil MG, Abdulrauf SI. Surgery of intraventricular tumors. Neurosurgery. 2008;62(6 Suppl 3):1029–40. https://doi.org/10.1227/01.neu.0000333768.12951.9a. discussion 1040-1. PMID: 18695523
81. Zhou JJ, Mooney MA, Farber SH, Bohl MA, Little AS, Nakaji P. Bedside iohexol ventriculography for patients with obstructive colloid cysts: a protocol to identify auto-fenestration of the septum pellucidum. World Neurosurg. 2018;122:e279–84.
82. Zohdi A, Elkheshin S. Endoscopic anatomy of the velum interpositum: a sequential descriptive anatomical study. Asian J Neurosurg. 2012;7(1):12–6.
83. Zohrevandi B, Monsef Kasmaie V, Asadı P, Tajik H. Third ventricle colloid cyst as a cause of sudden drop attacks of a 13-year-old boy. Emerg (Tehran). 2015;3(4):162–4.

# Chapter 7
# Traditional Open and Neuro-Endoscopic Approaches to Intraventricular Pathology

Joshua Prickett, Cristian Gragnaniello, Juan Altafulla, and Zachary N. Litvack

## Introduction

Lesions located within the ventricular system of the brain have long represented some of the most technically challenging targets for the surgeon. With the introduction of the operating microscope, the dedicated ventricular endoscope, and now subcortical access ports, there have been significant refinements in instrumentation and technique to minimize the morbidity of surgical approach. Regardless of which instruments and technique is chosen, a basic understanding of the established options for approaching the ventricular system is key to planning and executing a safe and effective operation. We review the well-documented approaches (both microsurgical and endoscopic) to the supratentorial ventricular system, providing the reader with a framework for choosing an approach based on surgical target and intervening eloquent tissue. This same framework, with some modification to account for primarily trans-sulcal approaches, can be used to plan a port-based surgery.

Intraventricular tumors make up less than 10% of intracranial neoplasms. Based on modern series of lateral ventricular lesions, the most common lesions are high-grade glial neoplasms, followed by meningioma, ependymoma, as well as pilocytic

J. Prickett
Aiken Regional Medical Centers, Department of Surgery, Aiken, SC, USA

C. Gragnaniello
Department of Neurosurgery, UT Health San Antonio, San Antonio, TX, USA
e-mail: gragnaniello@uthscsa.edu

J. Altafulla
Jose Domingo de Obaldia Hospital, Department of Surgery, Panama, Panama

Z. N. Litvack (✉)
Neuroscience Institute, Swedish Medical Center, Seattle, WA, USA
e-mail: zachary.litvack@swedish.org

© Springer Nature Switzerland AG 2022
G. Zada et al. (eds.), *Subcortical Neurosurgery*,
https://doi.org/10.1007/978-3-030-95153-5_7

and grade two astrocytomas. Less common were subependymal giant cell astrocytoma (SEGA), subependymoma, central neurocytoma, choroid plexus papilloma and carcinoma, ganglioglioma, and primitive neuroectodermal tumor (PNET). Common lesions in the third ventricle include colloid cysts and craniopharyngioma. In total, 65% were benign and 35% malignant [6].

In the infancy of neurosurgery, ventricular lesions were both difficult to diagnose and nearly impossible to approach. One of the first known successful intraventricular operations occurred in 1910 (although it wasn't reported until long after by medical historians), when Victor Lespinasse, a Chicago urologist, used a cystoscope to perform endoscopic fulguration of choroid plexus to treat hydrocephalus in two infants. One of the infants died and the other survived for 5 years [14]. Until the advent of air ventriculography (1918) and pneumoencephalography (1919), both by Walter Dandy, there were a few objective studies that could reliably confirm intraventricular pathology [16]. Dandy is widely considered the father of ventricular neurosurgery, having reported the first successful removal of a colloid cyst in 1921. He furthermore is credited with adaptation of Lespinasse' technique to routinely perform ventriculoscopy for management of hydrocephalus and removal of tumors as early as 1922 [23].

Throughout the years, technology has advanced to allow increasingly less invasive routes to intraventricular pathology. These evolved from more traditional approaches including transcortical and trans-sulcal as well as approaches through the anatomic barriers of the ventricular system such as the lamina terminalis and the corpus callosum. Over the past century, we have benefitted from a welcome refinement of ventricular exposures – from the extensive openings required by Dandy in the 1920s due to reliance on overhead lighting and the naked eye to ever smaller openings enabled through the introduction of the operative microscope in the 1950s, followed by the evolution of the Hopkins rod-lens endoscope and now the introduction of port-based intracranial surgery (Fig. 7.1).

## Open Approaches to the Lateral Ventricles

### General Principles

Pathology within the ventricular system is, by definition, within the deepest areas of the brain. Any surgical approach must be designed around being minimally disruptive to the normal tissue separating the surgeon from the pathology, choosing a location that traverses tissue which can potentially be (in part) sacrificed while also choosing a location that minimizes the depth to target. In this section, we discuss the "standard" approaches which have withstood the test of time. Collective experience has shown us that prolonged or forceful retraction of normal brain can result in

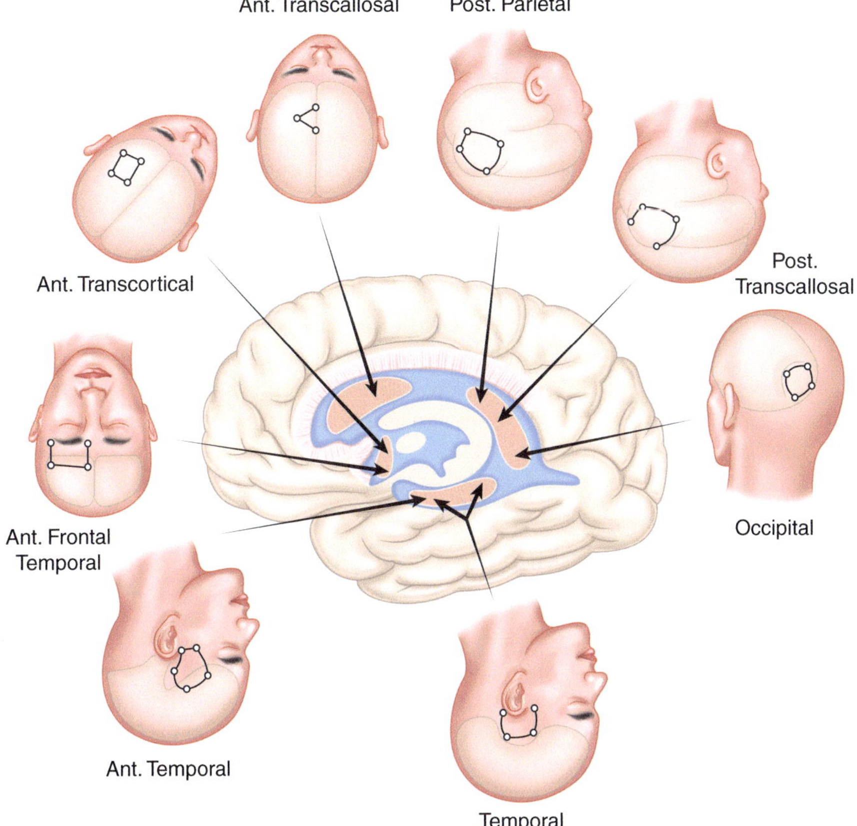


**Fig. 7.1** Approaches to the ventricular system via traditional open routes based on target location. (With permission from Antunes [1])

direct trauma, and both ischemic and shear injury may result in unfavorable neurologic outcomes. One technique which has been popularized is that of "retractorless surgery" or "dynamic retraction" which trades fixed blade retractors for intermittent retraction with either the shaft of the suction of bipolar or a handheld retractor blade in order to limit injury due to prolonged retraction [25]. Another component of retractorless surgery is positioning the patient and head to take advantage of gravity (which exerts an infinitely distributed force as opposed to the point force of a retractor). For example, a lesion might be better approached via a contralateral transfalcine approach, using the lateral position, which utilizes gravity to deliver tumor into the field of view (Table 7.1).

**Table 7.1** Approaches to the ventricular system based on location of lesion

| Target location | Approach |
|---|---|
| Target location | Approach |
| Frontal horn | Frontal transcortical or trans-sulcal |
| Body | Anterior interhemispheric transcallosal |
| Temporal horn | Temporal transcortical or trans-sulcal |
| Atrium | Parietal transcortical or trans-interparietal sulcus |
| | Precuneus approach |
| | Posterior interhemispheric transcallosal |
| Occipital horn | Posterior transcortical or POIP |
| Anterior third ventricle | Translamina terminalis |
| | Frontal transcortical transforaminal |
| | Anterior interhemispheric transcallosal transforaminal |
| | Anterior interhemispheric interforniceal |
| Posterior third ventricle | Expanded transforaminal |
| | Posterior interhemispheric transcallosal |
| | Supracerebellar |

## *Transcortical Approaches to the Lateral Ventricles*

The lateral ventricles can be reached via a perpendicular approach from nearly any area of cortex [8]. An understanding of functional neuroanatomy, along with functional MRI and diffusion tractography, can assist with determining an operative corridor that avoids major neurological morbidity. Although other adjuncts are available, including awake craniotomy and neurophysiological cortical and subcortical mapping, these are largely unnecessary as it is rare for there to be both a singular approach to an intraventricular target and for that approach to be through a highly eloquent area.

For pathology within the frontal horns of the lateral ventricle, the typical approach is ipsilateral, either via direct corticectomy (middle frontal gyrus) or via a transsulcal approach (superior frontal sulcus). This is typically performed with the patient in a relatively neutral supine position, in order to both preserve normal anatomic alignment as well as limit injury to the superior or middle gyri "falling into" the operative corridor. A coronal plane linear incision or "U" flap may be utilized, with the incision and planned craniotomy centered 1–2 cm anterior to the coronal suture. Either the middle frontal gyrus is coagulated and incised or the superior frontal sulcus arachnoid is opened, and the operative corridor is progressively deepened in a perpendicular fashion until encountering the ependyma of the ipsilateral frontal horn. Intraoperative neuronavigation can assist with determining trajectory. Alternatively, a ventricular catheter or brain needle can be passed into the ventricle, and upon return of CSF, bipolar cautery and suction used to follow this to enter the frontal horn. Once the lateral ventricle is entered, the pathology may be addressed or one may continue the trajectory through the foramen of Monro in order to address pathology within the anterior third ventricle. This approach is somewhat limited in normal or small-sized ventricles, and performing corticectomy carries a reported 4–8% risk of inducing seizures [17]. As discussed further below, the transchoroidal route may be used to expand access to the anterior and middle of the third ventricle.


## *Anterior Interhemispheric Transcallosal Approach*

Alternatively, an anterior interhemispheric transcallosal approach may be chosen for targets within the frontal horn and anterior third ventricle. The patient may be positioned supine as above or in a lateral position to take advantage of gravity retraction (Fig. 7.2). CSF diversion through lumbar drainage may help to facilitate this. The dura is opened with a flap based on the superior sagittal sinus that may be gently retracted contralaterally by placing proximal sutures to allow a more favorable approach angle. The mesial frontal lobe is followed along the falx into the interhemispheric fissure. The interhemispheric fissure arachnoid is split, and the pericallosal and callosomarginal arteries are identified. The approach into the fissure is progressively deepened until the avascular white fibers of the corpus callosum come into view. One common mistake is to dissect on one side of both callosal arteries, thus placing the surgeon on a trajectory to mistake the cingulate for the corpus callosum. A 2–3 cm callosotomy is made with electrocautery and suction. Typically, the ventricle is entered within a centimeter of depth. At this point, landmarks including the foramen of Monro, choroid plexus, and thalamostriate and septal veins are used to determine which ventricle has been entered. These landmarks may not be immediately visible, and exploration should be angled anteriorly. If no landmarks are visible, it is possible to have entered a cavum septum pellucidum. Once the ventricle is entered, the pathology may be addressed in similar fashion as via a transcortical or trans-sulcal approach. This approach does not carry the same risk of seizures as a transcortical approach.

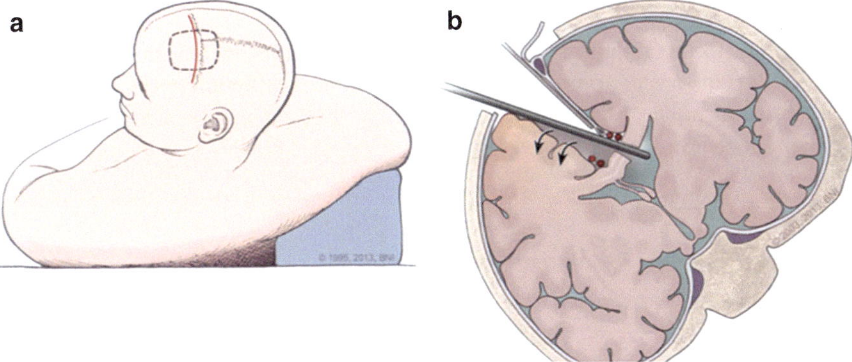

**Fig. 7.2** Cranial-lateral positioning (**a**) and approach (**b**) for an interhemispheric fissure approach to the contralateral ventricle with gravity retraction. (With permission from Zaidi et al. [29])

## Posterior Interhemispheric and Transcortical Approaches to the Atrium and Trigone

Similar to the anterior hemispheric approach to the frontal horn, pathology in the posterior body and atrium may be approached via a posterior interhemispheric transcallosal approach. However, this approach can be severely limited by bridging veins around the central sulcus which cannot be sacrificed without risking venous infarct of primary motor and/or sensory cortex.

To bypass the bridging vein limitation of a posterior interhemispheric transcallosal approach, a more occipito-polar interhemispheric approach was first proposed by Yasargil [27]. The parasplenial-precuneus or parietal-occipital interhemispheric precuneal approach (POIPA) provides access to the trigone and mesial atrium and occipital horns as well as the posterior and medial thalamus and pulvinar. The angle of attack is quite limited, and the approach is technically demanding. A variant contralateral transfalcine POIPA approach been described to improve the angle of attack and visualization [12]. This approach carries with it an increased risk of postoperative (transient) visual deficit due to retraction and potential disconnection of calcarine structures.

Most commonly, lesions of the posterior body of the lateral ventricle are accessed transcortically or via the intraparietal sulcus at the "key point" as described by Ribas [20] (Fig. 7.3). This trans-sulcal approach is similar to that used for port-based cases as described elsewhere in this text. The main risk with this approach is injury to the dominant angular gyrus if an entry point too inferior/ventral is chosen. Injury to, or disconnection of, the dominant angular gyrus can result in Gerstmann syndrome (agraphia, acalculia, finger agnosia, and right/left confusion).

## Transcortical and Trans-Sulcal Approaches to the Temporal Horn

Approaches to the temporal horn include anterior and lateral transtemporal transcortical or trans-sulcal approaches through the middle temporal gyrus or the superior temporal sulcus. The temporal horn may also be approached via anterior temporal lobectomy.

## Complications in Choosing an Approach to the Lateral Ventricles

A lesion within lateral ventricle may be best approached from the contralateral side to achieve early vascular control or to better preserve eloquent tissues. When both sides would be of equivalent risk, a right-sided approach is generally preferred. In

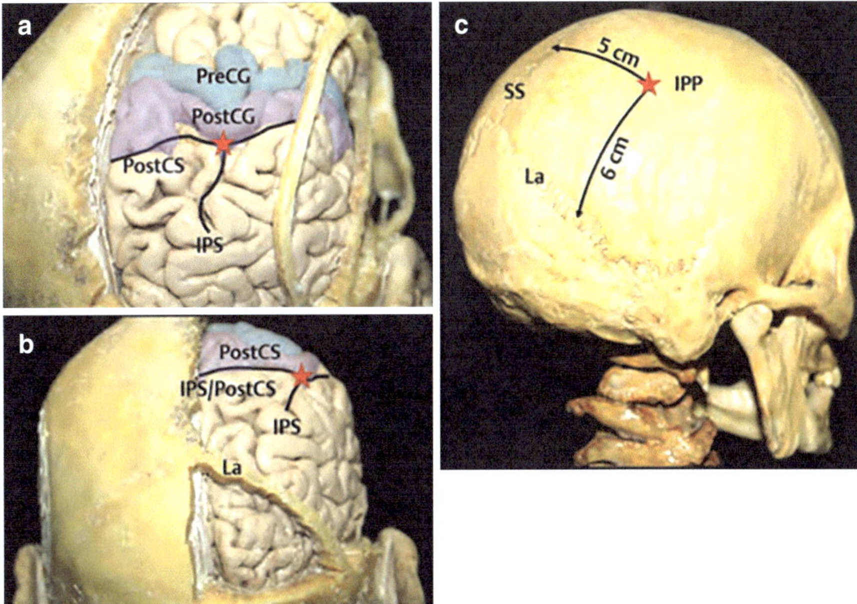


**Fig. 7.3** Location of key sulcal/gyral points as described by Fernandez Cornejo. Intraparietal sulcus and postcentral sulcus intersection point (IPS/PCS). (**a**) Intersection of the intraparietal sulcus (IPS) and the postcentral sulcus (PCS). (**b**) IPS/PCS (posterior view). (**c**) The intraparietal point (IPP) is located underneath a point 6 cm anterior to the lambda (La) and 5 cm lateral to the sagittal suture (SS). Abbreviations: IPP intraparietal point, IPS intraparietal sulcus, IPS/PostCS intraparietal sulcus and postcentral sulcus intersection point, La lambda, PostCS postcentral sulcus, PostCG postcentral gyrus, PreCG precentral gyrus, SS sagittal sulcus. (With permission from Fernandez Cornejo [9])

the series by D'Angelo et al., the incidence of postoperative seizures was zero with transcallosal approaches to the lateral ventricle compared to 5.9% in the transcortical approaches [6]. Conversely in another series, the transcallosal approach carried a 4.4-fold increase in the incidence of postoperative seizures [17]. Making an incision within the body of the corpus callosum, as well as limiting size and posterior extent of incision, helps to limit the complication of disconnection syndrome. Disconnection syndrome is most common with transection of the splenium and consists of apraxia, akinetic mutism with apathy, fixed gaze, incontinence, and right-left confusion [13]. This is distinct from cerebellar mutism that results from the disruption of connectivity between deep cerebellar nuclei and medial frontal and cingulate regions [15].

## Approaches to the Third Ventricle

### *Transcallosal-Expanded Transforaminal Transvenous/ Transchoroidal Route*

This route uses the approach described above to access the lateral ventricle but then further expands the foramen of Monro by incising the tela choroidea to provide a larger working corridor to access the anterior and middle third ventricle. Upon entering the lateral ventricle, the septal vein is identified and is coagulated and divided proximal to the thalamostriate vein (which must be preserved). The taenia thalami is then expanded and the choroidal fissure incision extended in continuity with the foramen and expand the operative corridor. This technique carries a risk of injury to the thalamostriate vein, potential stroke, as well as risk of anterograde amnesia secondary to forniceal injury.

### *Transcallosal Interforniceal*

This approach utilizes the avascular plane in the midline of the roof of the third ventricle. This approach is ideal in patients with a cavum septum pellucidum, which provides a natural plane of dissection between the two fornices. The septum is split in the midline following callosotomy until the forniceal fibers are identified. The fornices are separated in the midline, and the corridor between the internal cerebral veins and posterior choroidal arteries is utilized to enter the roof of the third ventricle via the velum interpositum (Fig. 7.4). There is significant risk of anterograde amnesia with bilateral forniceal injury from dissection and/or retraction. There is also risk to both the thalamostriate and internal cerebral veins.

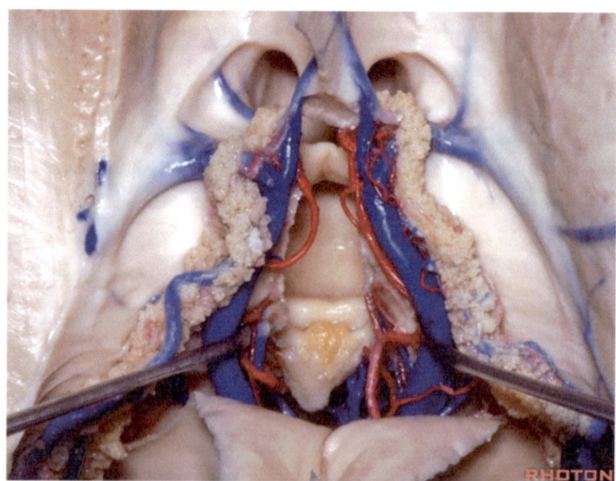

**Fig. 7.4** View of the floor of the third ventricle achieved via an interhemispheric interforniceal approach to the third ventricle. (Courtesy of the Rhoton Collection, American Association of Neurological Surgeons (AANS)/Neurosurgical Research and Education Foundation (NREF))

## *Translamina Terminalis*

This approach is typically reserved for pathology involving the anterior third ventricle. The approach can be done via a subfrontal route, an anterolateral route with a supraorbital or pterional craniotomy, or a transsphenoidal route. One historically under-recognized complication of this approach is cerebral salt-wasting and/or diabetes insipidus. The lamina contains the organum vasculosum, a circumventricular organ devoid of blood-brain barrier which is sodium sensitive and has efferent connections to both arginin-vasopressin (AVP)-rich neurons of the hypothalamus and sympathetic outflow [7]. Surgical transection of the lamina results in both diminished secretion of AVP and loss of complex hypothalamic-renal signaling to reabsorb sodium during urine production.

## *Infratentorial Supracerebellar Approach to the Posterior Third Ventricle*

Pathology of the posterior third ventricle, which comes to the ependymal surface in the posterior wall of the third ventricle at the tectal plate and pineal recess, may be best approached via the infratentorial supracerebellar approach. Preoperative sagittal imaging should be consulted to ensure there is a favorable slope to the tentorium (a more shallow slope to the tentorium is favorable). At the surgeon's preference, positioning may be either in the sitting or the prone (Concorde) position. Regardless of positioning, this is a technically demanding approach requiring a suboccipital craniotomy or craniectomy that exposes and skeletonizes the transverse sinus near the torcula. More traditional open approaches expose the sinuses bilaterally to permit a dural incision crossing the occipital sinus and flap based on the transverse sinuses to expose both cerebellar hemispheres. More recently, unilateral paramedian keyhole approaches (with or without endoscopic assistance) have been successfully described [30]. The cerebellum is gently retracted inferiorly or with gravity assistance, and the singular precentral cerebellar vein is divided. This reveals the thickened arachnoid of the quadrigeminal plate cistern, which is opened to reveal the plate itself and a corridor under the confluence of the internal cerebral and basal veins (of Rosenthal) to the posterior third ventricle (Fig. 7.5).

## Microscopic Versus Endoscopic-Assisted Keyhole Approaches

Any of the aforementioned approaches may be augmented by endoscopic assistance. Doing so permits a smaller craniotomy as well as improved visualization by providing better light at the depths of the surgical field and off-axis viewing with the use of angled endoscopes. However, use of endoscopes in a surgical keyhole can

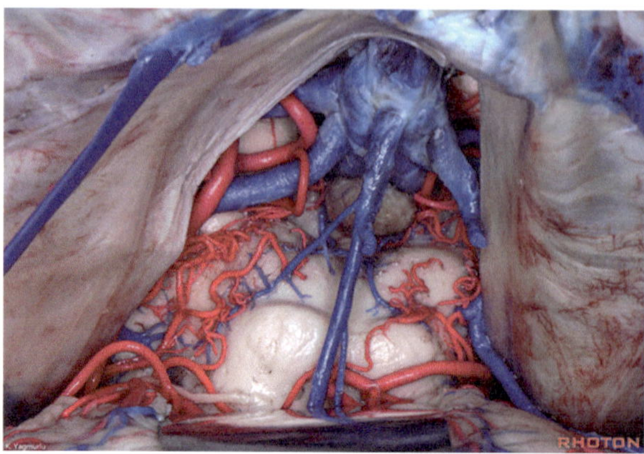

**Fig. 7.5** View of the quadrigeminal plate at the tentorial incisura afforded by an infratentorial supracerebellar approach. The singular midline precentral cerebellar vein is seen in the middle of the field and may be sacrificed with low risk for postoperative complication. (Courtesy of the Rhoton Collection, American Association of Neurological Surgeons (AANS)/Neurosurgical Research and Education Foundation (NREF))

take an already technically demanding approach (such as a supracerebellar infratentorial approach) and make it even more so. An understanding of the regional anatomy and preparation to convert to a larger open approach if necessary are vital.

## Purely Endoscopic Approaches to the Ventricular System

Endoscopic approaches to the ventricles have been gaining popularity as technology improved since the late 1970s when Fukushima reported the biopsy of an intraventricular tumor and Powell few years later described the removal of a colloid cyst with purely endoscopic technique [10, 19, 26]. Endoscopes have been used for a variety of different indications in ventricular surgery including CSF diversion (third ventriculostomy, septum pellucidotomy, shunt placement, aqueductoplasty) and tumor biopsy or excision [2–5, 23]. Due to their utility in managing disorders of CSF circulation, pediatric neurosurgeons developed and adopted endoscopic ventricular techniques more rapidly and widely than their other colleagues.

The choice of the type of endoscope depends on the experience of the operator and surgical goals. The characteristics of the two main types of ventricular endoscopes, the rigid and the flexible, are shown in Fig. 7.6 and summarized in Table 7.2 [17, 19, 21]. Rigid scopes (for the most part) offer superior image resolution and contrast, along with larger working channels and a wider variety of surgical instruments.

Purely endoscopic removal of solid intraventricular masses requires careful patient selection based on size, location, expected firmness, and blood supply of the lesion. When considering a lesion is larger than 2–2.5 cm, there is little advantage

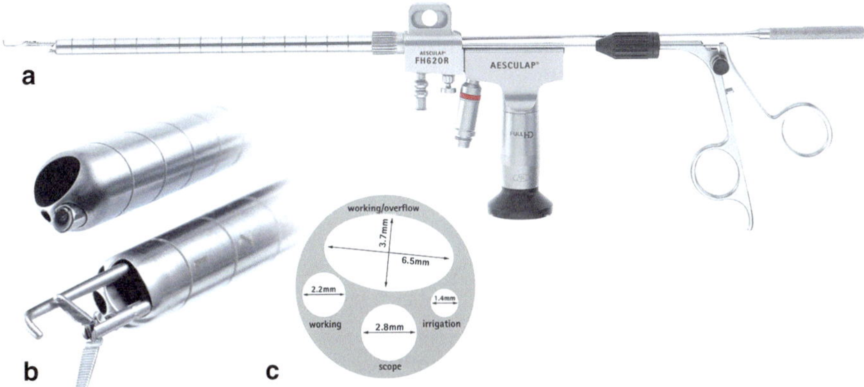



**Fig. 7.6** *Top* – Example of a rigid endoscope with multiple working channels. *Bottom* – Example of a flexible videoendoscope with (**a**) camera sensor, (**b**) LED light, and (**c**) 1 mm working channel. Adapted from Nakaji et al. (with permission from Gaab [11])

**Table 7.2** Endoscopic versus microscopic approach to ventricles

| Approach | Advantages | Disadvantages | Complications |
|---|---|---|---|
| Microscopic | Familiar bimanual neurosurgical techniques employed with stereoscopic vision Ability to use fluorescent adjuncts/ ICG with filter | Lighting decreased at depths Viewing angles are limited by the opening into the ventricle, and expansion of foramen and retraction can lead to neurologic sequelae | Higher rate of postop seizures (4.3%, higher in transcortical approaches) |
| Endoscope w/ single working channel | Physiologic medium Improved visualization or critical structures Ability to visualize the roof of the third with angled lens | 2D view in a fluid medium Specialized instrumentation Requires assistant surgeon or rigid holder Single-axis surgery Steep learning curve | Higher rate of IVH and need for shunting postop |
| Endoscope w/ dual port | Physiologic medium Bimanual surgery | 2D view in a fluid medium Specialized instrumentation Requires assistant surgeon or rigid holder (three hands) More traumatic | |
| Flexible endoscope | Able to reach areas such as temporal horns and posterior third ventricle not possible with rigid | Single-axis surgery Specialized instrumentation and limited by need for flexibility and width of port Steep learning curve | |

in performing a purely endoscopic approach compared to microscopic and/or tubular approaches. If the approach is for tissue biopsy, with or without CSF diversion, a single burr hole approach is typically sufficient for both biopsy and ventriculocisternostomy, although a flexible scope will minimize subcortical shear injury compared to a rigid scope. Flexible endoscopes are more versatile for management of hydrocephalus, permitting access to the entire supratentorial choroid from frontal to temporal horns via single transcortical approach for fulguration of the choroid plexus. This requires a steeper learning curve as the vertical orientation of the image is rotated continuously through the procedure. Only recently with the advent of "camera on a chip" CMOS sensors that flexible scopes have historically suffered from poor image quality.

Selection of an entry point and surgical trajectory for rigid scopes mirrors that of transcortical open approaches. Many consider it safer to cannulate the ventricle first with a ventricular catheter or Peel-Away sheath. Neuronavigation is frequently recommended, especially in cases of slit ventricles or severely distorted ventricular anatomy. One advantage of the Peel-Away sheath is that it minimizes the trauma from repeated "stabbing" movements of the rigid scope and provides additional egress of CSF to prevent hyperinflation of the ventricles. No matter what type of endoscope is chosen for the approach, with one or two portals for instruments, there should always be a portal for irrigation and for fluid outflow to avoid increases in pressure in the ventricular system.

Bleeding during endoscopic ventricular procedures is usually well managed with warm lactated Ringer's irrigation and time, but in cases of sustained bleeding, bipolar coagulation or pressure from an inflatable balloon can be of assistance. Additionally, the endoscope itself can be used to tamponade bleeding or "trap" the bleeder in the rigid sheath. If bleeding is brisk and not manageable with these techniques, a "dry field" could be obtained by exchanging air for CSF. It is critical to inject air through the working channel and drive out CSF (as opposed to aspirating CSF and creating negative pressure within the cranium).

## Conclusions

Management of intraventricular pathology is technically challenging due to the limitations of visualization and constraints of surgical degrees of freedom associated with long working depths. Our understanding of the functional anatomy of fiber tracts and the cerebral connectome has expanded exponentially with improved imaging modalities. In parallel, our ability to measure the impact of iatrogenic injury to these connections has improved with modern neurocognitive assessment. As a result, surgeons are faced with an increasingly limited number of "safe" corridors due to the need to account for functional subcortical anatomy. Maximizing surgical results from these limited corridors has led to a "best of both worlds" approach explored in the remainder of this book, combining open techniques with single shaft (endoscopic) instrumentation and exoscopic visualization.

# References


1. Antounes JL. Management of tumors of the anterior third and lateral ventricles. In: Sindou M, editor. Practical handbook of neurosurgery. Wien: Springer-Verlag; 2009.
2. Balossier A, et al. Endoscopic versus stereotactic procedure for pineal tumour biopsies: comparative review of the literature and learning from a 25-year experience. Neurochirurgie. 2015;61:146–54.
3. Balossicr A, Blond S, Rcyns N. Endoscopic versus stereotactic procedure for pineal tumor biopsies: focus on overall efficacy rate. World Neurosurg. 2016;92:223–8. https://doi.org/10.1016/j.wneu.2016.03.088.
4. Birski M, Birska J, Paczkowski D, Furtak J, Rusinek M, Rudas M, Harat M. Combination of neuroendoscopic and stereotactic procedures for total resection of colloid cysts with favorable neurological and cognitive outcomes. World Neurosurg. 2016;85:205–14.
5. Cohen-Gadol A. Transcallosal interforniceal approach. Retrieved electronically from https://doi.org/10.18791/nsatlas.v4.ch05.5.3.3.
6. D'Angelo VA, Galarza M, Catapano D, Monte V, Bisceglia M, Carosi I. Lateral ventricle tumors: surgical strategies according to tumor origin and development—a series of 72 cases. Neurosurgery. 2008;62(suppl_3):ONS–36–45. https://doi.org/10.1227/01.NEU.0000333772.35822.37.
7. Delpire E, Gagnon KB. Water homeostasis and cell volume maintenance and regulation. Curr Top Membr. 2018;81:3–52. https://doi.org/10.1016/bs.ctm.2018.08.001. Review. PubMed PMID: 30243436; PubMed Central PMCID: PMC6457474
8. Ellenbogen RG. Transcortical surgery for lateral ventricular tumors. Neurosurg Focus. 2001;10(6):1–13.
9. Fernandez Cornejo V, et al. Anatomical landmarks and cranial anthropometry. In: Gagliardi F, Gragnaniello C, Mortini P, Caputy A, editors. Operative cranial neurosurgical anatomy. New York: Thieme; 2019.
10. Fukushima T. Endoscopic biopsy of intraventricular tumors with the use of a ventriculofiberscope. Neurosurgery. 1978;2(2):110–3.
11. Gaab MR. Neuroendoscopic technology. In: Torrez-Corzo JG, Rangel-Castilla L, Nakaji P, editors. Neuroendoscopic surgery. New York: Thieme; 2016.
12. Geyik M, Erkutlu I, Alptekin M, Gezgin I, Mizrak A, Pusat S, Gok A. Parieto-occipital interhemispheric precuneal approach to the lesions of the atrium: experience with 66 patients. Turk Neurosurg. 2017;27(3):325–32. https://doi.org/10.5137/1019-5149.JTN.16296-15.1.
13. Geschwind N. Disconnexion syndromes in animals and man, Brain. 1965;88(2):237.
14. Grant JA. Victor darwin lespinasse: a biographical sketch. Neurosurgery. 1996;39(6):1232–3. https://doi.org/10.1097/00006123-199612000-00030.
15. Lee S, Na YH, Moon HI, Tae WS, Pyun SB. Neuroanatomical mechanism of cerebellar mutism after stroke. Ann Rehabil Med. 2017;41(6):1076–81.
16. Lutters B, Koehler PJ. Cerebral pneumography and the 20th century localization of brain tumours. Brain. 2018;141(3):927–33. https://doi.org/10.1093/brain/awy031.
17. Milligan BD, Meyer FB. Morbidity of transcallosal and transcortical approaches to lesions in and around the lateral and third ventricles: a single-institution experience. Neurosurgery. 2010;67(6):1483–96. https://doi.org/10.1227/NEU.0b013e3181f7eb68.
18. Perneczky A. Tumors of the lateral and third ventricle: removal under endoscope-assisted keyhole conditions. Neurosurgery. 2005;57(4 Suppl):302–11.
19. Powell MP, Torrens MJ, Thomson JL, Horgan JG. Isodense colloid cysts of the third ventricle: a diagnostic and therapeutic problem resolved by ventriculoscopy. Neurosurgery. 1983;13(3):234–7.
20. Ribas GC, Yasuda A, Ribas EC, Nishikuni K, Rodrigues AJ. Surgical anatomy of microneurosurgical sulcal key points. Neurosurgery. 2006;59(suppl_4):ONS–177–211. https://doi.org/10.1227/01.NEU.0000240682.28616.b2.

21. Sampath R, Vannemreddy P, Nanda A. Microsurgical excision of colloid cyst with favorable cognitive outcomes and short operative time and hospital stay: operative techniques and analyses of outcomes with review of previous studies. Neurosurgery. 2010;66(2):368–75. https://doi.org/10.1227/01.NEU.0000363858.17782.82.
22. Sawaya R. Immediate morbidity and mortality associated with transcallosal resection of tumors of the third ventricle. J Clin Neurosci. 2010;17(7):830–6.
23. Scarff JE. Endoscopic treatment of hydrocephalus: description of a Ventriculoscope and preliminary report of cases. Arch Neurol Psychiatry. 1936;35(4):853–61. https://doi.org/10.1001/archneurpsyc.1936.02260040163011.
24. Sheikh AB, Mendelson ZS, Liu JK. Endoscopic versus microsurgical resection of colloid cysts: a systematic review and meta-analysis of 1278 patients. World Neurosurg. 2014;82(6):1187–97. https://doi.org/10.1016/j.wneu.2014.06.024.
25. Spetzler RF, Sanai N. The quiet revolution: retractorless surgery for complex vascular and skull base lesions. J Neurosurg. 2012;116(2):291–300. https://doi.org/10.3171/2011.8.JNS101896. PubMed PMID: 21981642
26. Wilson DA, Fusco DJ, Wait SD, Nakaji P. Endoscopic resection of colloid cysts: use of a dual-instrument technique and an anterolateral approach. World Neurosurg. 2013;80(5):576–83.
27. Yasargil MG: Microneurosurgery: Microneurosurgery of CNS Tumors. Stuttgart, Georg Thieme Verlag, 1996:IVB:pp 38–42, 56–57, 63–65, 313–318, 320–323.
28. Yaşargil MG, Abdulrauf SI. Surgery of intraventricular tumors. Neurosurgery. 2008;62(suppl_3):SHC1029–41. https://doi.org/10.1227/01.NEU.0000316427.57165.01.
29. Zaidi HA, Chowdhry SA, Nakaji P, Abla AA, Spetzler R. Contralateral interhemispheric approach to deep-seated cavernous malformations: surgical considerations and clinical outcomes in 31 consecutive cases. Neurosurgery. 2014;75(1):80–6. https://doi.org/10.1227/NEU.0000000000000339.
30. Zaidi HA, Elhadi AM, Lei T, Preul MC, Little AS, Nakaji P. Minimally invasive endoscopic supracerebellar-infratentorial surgery of the pineal region: anatomical comparison of four variant approaches. World Neurosurg. 2015;84(2):257–66. https://doi.org/10.1016/j.wneu.2015.03.009.

# Chapter 8
# Trans-sulcal, Channel-Based Parafascicular Surgery: Basic Concepts and a General Overview

Sean P. Polster, David Satzer, and Julian Bailes

## Introduction

Subcortical mass lesions present a unique challenge for neurosurgical resection. The lesions are deep and distort delicate anatomy [1]. Operations that access deep locations are associated with morbidity. Access routes are limited and are often entered via corticotomy where a corridor is created with blunt fixed retractor blades. Utilizing bipolar forceps, the white matter is splayed to provide straight-line access to the deep anatomy and ultimately a lesion. It is likely that this maneuver for access damages the cortical surface of the brain as well as the subcortical white matter tracts.

It is hypothesized that the maneuvers of access contribute to cortical and fiber track disruption [2]. From the large trials in intracerebral hemorrhage, we can infer that sometimes access to deep lesions can result in morbidity that offsets the potential benefit [3, 4]. With the advent of minimally invasive surgery, reducing the "cost" of access has been a growing area of research and innovation with great potential.

Deep subcortical lesions present unique challenges as they are near critical vascular structures, can be difficult to reach (working distance), have reduced visibility, and are associated with higher complication rates and morbidity. This problem was historically addressed by the ideological advent of retractorless surgery. This improved upon the potential of cortical disruption by removing fixed square retractor blades but has not addressed all facets of tumor surgery in order to have a

S. P. Polster · D. Satzer
University of Chicago, Department of Neurosurgery, Chicago, IL, USA
e-mail: spolster@uchicago.edu; David.Satzer@uchospitals.edu

J. Bailes (✉)
NorthShore University Health Systems, Department of Neurosurgery, Evanston, IL, USA
e-mail: JBailes@northshore.org


G. Zada et al. (eds.), *Subcortical Neurosurgery*,
https://doi.org/10.1007/978-3-030-95153-5_8

maximal impact. The neurosurgeon's armamentarium has been aggressively pursuing innovations that attempt to allow better access for improved outcomes. Pragmatic clinical trials will be necessary to validate innovations if they are to have a meaningful impact.


## The Problem

If we borrow some insight from trials on intracranial hemorrhage (ICH), we can suggest cortical disruption, or access is a factor in the value of addressing subcortical lesions. Currently, no robust trial exists or is ongoing outside of those for ICH. The many historical trials on ICH have attempted to address the role of surgery. The Surgical Treatment of ICH (STICH) trial was performed to compare early surgery versus conservative treatment for patients with supratentorial ICH. This was a large international multicenter prospectively randomized clinical trial. More than 400 patients were randomized to either surgical or medical management. However, the STICH trial failed to show a superiority of surgical management over medical treatment alone [3]. Post hoc analysis described a subset of superficial hematomas (within 1 cm of the cortical surface) that could benefit from surgery; this was tested in the subsequent trial, STICH II, where superficial ICH patients were randomly assigned to early surgery versus best medical management. The results revealed that surgery does not grant an outcome advantage (functional or mortality) [4]. Currently, we are awaiting the results and analysis of ENRICH and the forthcoming next iteration of CLEAR/ MISTIE trials to better understand the value of improved surgical techniques which aim to defray the theorized cost of open surgery. The MISTIE trials have set a precedent that procedural competence is important, and achieving volume reduction to a threshold is needed for functional improvement. With catheter-based hematoma evacuation, a mortality benefit was finally realized in MISITE III [5]. However, only those who reached ICH reduction to $\leq 15$ mL (or >70% of clot removed) realized a functional benefit to mRS 0-3. The lesson to glean from this is that less invasive surgeries have trended toward improved outcomes likely because they distort less normal anatomy (or maximally restore the remaining anatomy or penumbra of surrounding tissue) [6]. It is unclear if technical adjuncts, such as the NICO product line, will aid in these important factors, but enthusiasm is high. Other potential technical adjuncts are in the pipeline, each leveraging a reduction in the cortical disruption of open surgery. How this knowledge within the setting of ICH will translate to other fields of neuro-oncology has yet to be determined.

The evolution of subcortical surgery has occurred over the past few decades with advances in microsurgery technique, understanding of anatomy, image guidance/ planning systems, and technical adjuncts. The most recent and widely adapted systems utilize all of these advancements in a system-based approach.

## Corridors Within the Brain

G. Yaşargil pioneered the modern era of microsurgery by applying technical mastery and a recognition that *"the subarachnoid space and in particular, the cisterns, provide a natural pathway for dissection that preserves all important brain structures…."* [7] This methodology requires exceptional skill to apply to all pathologies deep in the brain and still produce some limitation for subcortical lesions. However, this idea and mastery of knowledge is the foundation of modern surgery and lies the foundation for the next generation of innovation. Understanding the white matter tracts and cortical map allows us to address subcortical lesions in a similar fashion, by utilizing parafascicular pathways and sulcal corridors.

Over the last decade, retractors, either fixed or dynamic, have been used, each requiring a selective skill set with its respective inherent drawbacks. It was not until Kelly et al. published the first report of utilizing a tubular retractor system [8], which aimed to allow minimally invasive access utilizing image guidance to preserve normal surrounding anatomy to subcortical lesions. This method was hypothesized to result in less cortical and white mater track disruption compared to fixed square retractor blades. In this endeavor, they require special instruments with increased working distance and the utilization of multiple modalities such as a stereotactic frame, image guidance, and laser ablation instruments. This idea has been leveraged in the modern day with continued use of tubular retractors, ports, endoscopes, catheters, and laser fibers. Again, all requires a multimodal approach to understand fiber tracts and cortical anatomy.

## Transcortical Approach

Transcortical minimally invasive surgery, either open or by endoport-assisted technology, requires subcortical access via one of two approaches: (1) trans-sulcal or (2) trans-gyral. In some cases, surface or functional anatomy will dictate one over another. However, theoretical consideration should be made when selecting these approaches [9]. In a trans-sulcal approach, the gyral banks can provide stability for an endoport while preserving both the superficial vasculature and the vessels located at the depth of the sulcus [10]. The fiber tract disruption is typically from encountering what has been termed the "plis de passage" forming anatomical bridges from one gyrus to another constituting the gyral continuum [11] but, in practice, has not been a problem. However, minimal disruption of these connections can help to avoid approach-related morbidity. The major risks of a trans-sulcal approach related to vascular injury or parenchymal trauma related to excessive retraction, again with consequences highly depending on location. The advantage comes from an overall less disruption of tissue [12–14] (Fig. 8.1a–d). Trans-gyral approaches sacrifice the gyrus up front and risk deficits that correspond to the anatomical location, the advantage in the preservation of cortical veins, if subpial movement is unavailable.

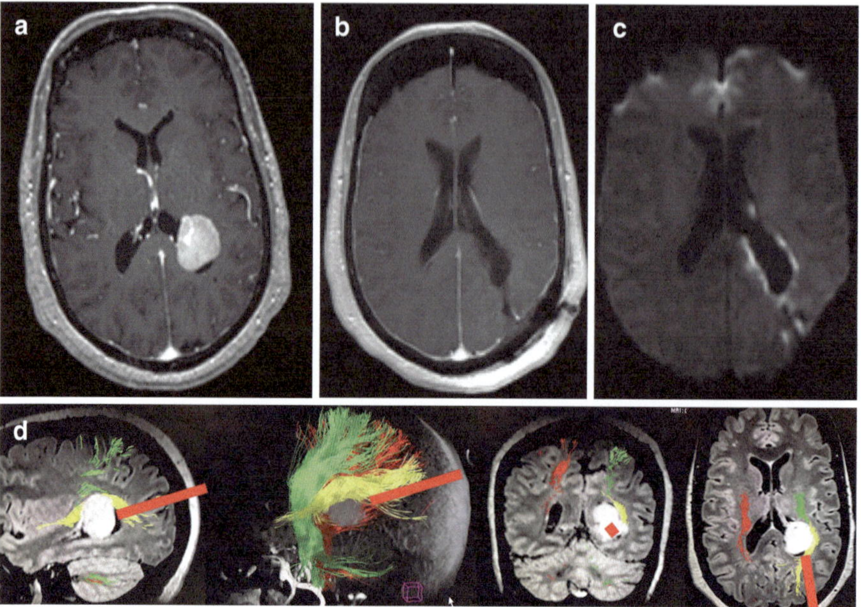

**Fig. 8.1** Illustrative case of a trans-sulcal parafascicular approach to the ventricular atrium for meningioma resection in a 63-year-old female. Magnetic resonance imaging of (**a**) T1 post contrast showing enhancement of a left ventricular meningioma and (**b**) subsequent post-resection T1 post contrast imaging with gross total resection and approach cavity with (**c**) diffusion-weighted imaging showing minimal restriction along operative corridor. (**d**) Diffuse tensor imaging superimposed with red bar showing preoperative planning negotiating the optic radiations

Preoperative consideration of anatomy, imaging, pathology, and baseline functional deficits can all aid in method selection [15]. Once an entry method is chosen, subcortical parafascicular tracts which run both perpendicular and parallel to entry need to be considered.

## Parafascicular Approach

To use the parafascicular approach in a practical setting, the surgeon needs to understand the target and the entry point of the proposed intervention. These two points while considering the intervening fascicular tracts are the foundation of minimizing disruption [16]. The target point is dictated by the pathology with entry points selected as those that (1) allow for the shortest distance to access and (2) transgress the least eloquent anatomy. The first point is addressed by understating the patient and the pathology at hand. Operating on a high-grade glioma versus intraventricular meningioma has inherent difference, considering preoperative deficits and expected outcomes are all part of preoperative planning and patient selection that is individualized to the patient and the pathology. Selecting an entry point that is near the lesion goes hand in hand with transgressing the least amount of eloquent anatomy. This is done with the aid of preoperative planning software, cortical mapping techniques (electrophysiological and ultrasound, possibly MEG), and more recently with tractography (diffuse tensor imaging). Cranial navigation systems have begun incorporating these into operating packages that greatly enhance the surgeon's understanding of white matter tracts.

Minimally disruptive parafascicular surgery requires the surgeon to know the location of major white matter tracts in order to minimize the risks associated with accessing and resecting deep-seated lesions. Some centers, including clinical trials such as MISTIE and ENRICH, restrict the surgeon to a discrete set of surgical trajectories known to avoid major subcortical tracts based on aggregate anatomic knowledge [6, 17, 18]. In order to expand the number of surgical corridors in a patient-specific manner, some surgeons have utilized tractography with diffusion tensor imaging (DTI) to identify major white matter pathways. DTI measures anisotropy to detect the type of large, organized white matter tracts that should be avoided in parafascicular surgery. DTI has some well-known limitations that affect intraoperative use. Generation of DTI maps is operator-dependent and significantly affected by factors such as seed placement and voxel geometry. When white matter tracts are interrupted, for example, in the case of infiltrative primary brain tumors, it can be difficult to distinguish tract infiltration from edema.

## Technical Adjuncts for Parafascicular Surgery

Tubular retraction (endoport) systems have been designed to provide a working channel to deep-seated brain lesions while avoiding trauma associated with extensive dissection and retraction with blunt retractor blades (Fig. 8.2). Damage from direct mechanical injury and ischemia to the surrounding white matter, along with

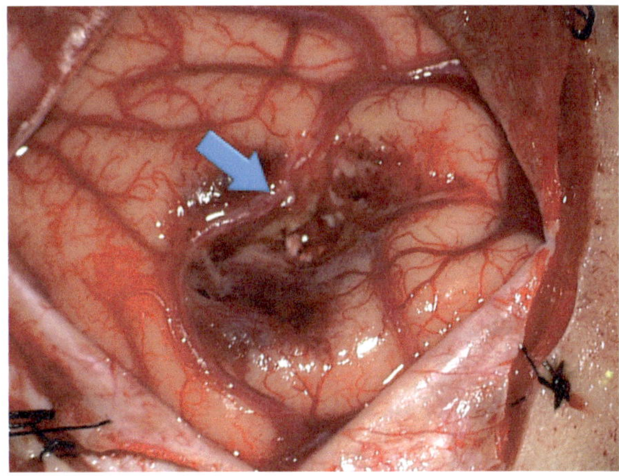

**Fig. 8.2** Operative photograph showing tubular retractor removal with preservation of both the gyral banks and the immediate superficial vessel (arrow) (same case as in Fig. 8.1)

"tissue creep" around a fixed, steel retractor which can obscure the exposure, are the primary drawbacks. In contrast with blunt unidirectional retraction, tubular retractor devices radially distribute pressure on adjacent tissue, thereby reducing trauma to the brain parenchyma [19]. The most commonly used tubular retractor is the BrainPath(R) device (Nico Corp, Indianapolis, Indiana). The system consists of a range of retractor sheaths measuring 11.0–13.5 mm in diameter and 50–75 mm in length, as well as a sharp-tipped obturator used for retractor insertion which accommodates the StealthSystem (Medtronic, Dublin, Ireland) neuronavigation (or similar platform) probe. Following craniotomy and small dural opening (sized to accommodate retractor diameter), the arachnoid is opened and the BrainPath retractor is inserted under image guidance. Once inserted to target, the obturator is removed and the tubular retractor sheath is secured with a shepherd's hook attached to a retractor system (e.g., Greenberg(R) or Budde(R) retractor).

A number of methods have been used to enhance visualization down narrow working channels to deep subcortical lesions. The surgical microscope is familiar to all neurosurgeons and is used by many surgeons in conjunction with the endoport, but the microscope is limited by depth of field and illumination. Endoscopes can improve visualization by bringing the light source closer to the surgical field and can provide high-resolution images of the working area but occupy a significant part of the working space within the endoport and require either an assistant or the use of one of the operator's hands. Alternatively, the lens and illumination source can be brought far from the surgical field in the form of an exoscope. The VITOM(R) exoscope (Karl Storz Endoscopy America Inc., El Segundo, California) is commonly used with the BrainPath(R) system and can be mounted on a mechanical arm. High-definition exoscope cameras offer a greater depth of field than is permitted by a traditional surgical microscope. Furthermore, exoscopes allow more uniform illumination throughout the endoport working area as the illumination cones out on the surgical field rather than coning in as does a surgical microscope (Fig. 8.3a, b).

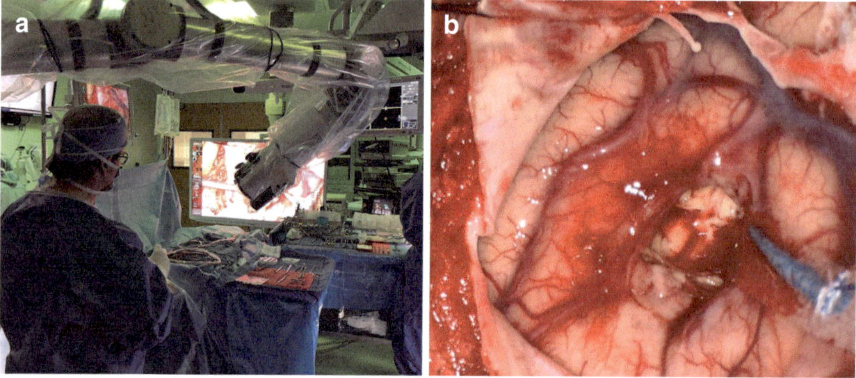

Fig. 8.3 (a) Master surgeon utilizing dynamic retraction for subcortical mass resection via a transsulcal parafascicular approach with exoscope technology. (b) Operative photograph showing preservation of gyral banks and superficial vessels

However, both endoscopic and exoscopic technologies introduce a new learning curve and are only recently migrating to 3D technologies, leading some surgeons to continue to favor the traditional microscope.

Standard microsurgical instruments can be used in the endoport working channel. For many, bipolar cautery and variable suction are the workhorse of tubular retractor-based subcortical surgery. Specialized, low-profile, multifunctional instruments have been designed for use in this setting. For example, the Nico Myriad(R) instrument is a side-cutting, aspirating device engineered for use down the narrow working channel of the BrainPath(R) retractor sheath. General useful features of instrumentation used in endoport-assisted subcortical surgery include multiple functionality (e.g., suction and resection features) and malleable instrument shafts.

## Future Directions

Parafascicular surgery represents a key component as the state-of-the-art neurosurgical procedures for subcortical lesions. Advancements in technology are coming about in the neuro-oncology space with better instruments and improved imaging and platform technologies. In intracerebral hemorrhage, clinical trials are allowing us to better understand deep brain disruption and methods for subcortical and ventricular access. Taken together, the lessons learned from clinical trials with technological innovations will further improve neurosurgery and the reaming frontier of subcortical lesions.

## References


1. Nishiyama K. From exoscope into the next generation. J Korean Neurosurg Soc. 2017;60(3):289–93.
2. Axer M, Amunts K, Grassel D, et al. A novel approach to the human connectome: ultra-high resolution mapping of fiber tracts in the brain. NeuroImage. 2011;54(2):1091–101.
3. Mendelow AD, Gregson BA, Fernandes HM, et al. Early surgery versus initial conservative treatment in patients with spontaneous supratentorial intracerebral haematomas in the International Surgical Trial in Intracerebral Haemorrhage (STICH): a randomised trial. Lancet. 2005;365(9457):387–97.
4. Mendelow AD, Gregson BA, Rowan EN, Murray GD, Gholkar A, Mitchell PM. Early surgery versus initial conservative treatment in patients with spontaneous supratentorial lobar intracerebral haematomas (STICH II): a randomised trial. Lancet. 2013;382(9890):397–408.
5. Hanley DF, Thompson RE, Rosenblum M, et al. Efficacy and safety of minimally invasive surgery with thrombolysis in intracerebral haemorrhage evacuation (MISTIE III): a randomised, controlled, open-label, blinded endpoint phase 3 trial. Lancet. 2019;393(10175):1021–32.
6. Awad IA, Polster SP, Carrión-Penagos J, et al. Surgical performance determines functional outcome benefit in the minimally invasive surgery plus recombinant tissue plasminogen activator for intracerebral hemorrhage evacuation (MISTIE) procedure. Neurosurgery. 2019;84(6):1157–68.

7. Yasargil MG. Microsurgery – volume I: microsurgical anatomy of the basal cisterns and vessels of the brain, diagnostic studies, general operative techniques and pathological considerations of the intracranial aneurysms. New York: Thieme; 1987.
8. Kelly PJ, Goerss SJ, Kall BA. The stereotaxic retractor in computer-assisted stereotaxic microsurgery. Technical note. J Neurosurg. 1988;69(2):301–6.
9. Spena G, Garbossa D, Panciani PP, Griva F, Fontanella MM. Purely subcortical tumors in eloquent areas: awake surgery and cortical and subcortical electrical stimulation (CSES) ensure safe and effective surgery. Clin Neurol Neurosurg. 2013;115(9):1595–601.
10. Latini F, Ryttlefors M. Rethinking the standard trans-cortical approaches in the light of superficial white matter anatomy. Neural Regen Res. 2015;10(12):1906–9.
11. Byrne RW. Functional mapping of the cerebral cortex. Springer; 2016.
12. Wright J, Chugh J, Wright CH, et al. Laser interstitial thermal therapy followed by minimal-access transsulcal resection for the treatment of large and difficult to access brain tumors. Neurosurg Focus. 2016;41(4):E14.
13. Zhou H, Miller D, Schulte DM, et al. Transsulcal approach supported by navigation-guided neurophysiological monitoring for resection of paracentral cavernomas. Clin Neurol Neurosurg. 2009;111(1):69–78.
14. Valkanov S, Valkanov P. Using of transsulcal microsurgical approach in surgical treatment of intracerebral lesions- literature review. Trakia J Sci. 2014;3:304–8.
15. D'Angelo VA, Galarza M, Catapano D, Monte V, Bisceglia M, Carosi I. Lateral ventricle tumors: surgical strategies according to tumor origin and development–a series of 72 cases. Neurosurgery. 2005;56(1 Suppl):36–45. discussion 36-45
16. Ture U, Yasargil MG, Friedman AH, Al-Mefty O. Fiber dissection technique: lateral aspect of the brain. Neurosurgery. 2000;47(2):417–26. discussion 426-417
17. Fam MD, Hanley D, Stadnik A, et al. Surgical performance in minimally invasive surgery plus recombinant tissue plasminogen activator for intracerebral hemorrhage evacuation phase III clinical trial. Neurosurgery. 2017;81(5):860–6.
18. ENRICH: early MiNimally-invasive removal of intracerebral hemorrhage (ICH) (ENRICH). 2019; https://clinicaltrials.gov/ct2/show/NCT02880878.
19. Ogura K, Tachibana E, Aoshima C, Sumitomo M. New microsurgical technique for intraparenchymal lesions of the brain: transcylinder approach. Acta Neurochir. 2006;148(7):779–85. discussion 785

# Chapter 9
# Trans-sulcal, Channel-Based Parafascicular Surgery for Subcortical and Intraventricular Lesions: Instruments and Technical Considerations


Mohamed A. R. Soliman, Claudio Cavallo, Sirin Gandhi, Xiaochun Zhao, and Mohamed A. Labib


## Introduction and Historical Background

Brain lesions located in the subcortical, periventricular, and intraventricular areas are challenging from a surgical standpoint as they are associated with potential high morbidity rates secondary to white matter tract injury [1]. Moreover, deep-seated lesions can be assessed only through narrow surgical corridors which prevent adequate intraoperative visualization. Traditionally, fixed blade retractors were used to facilitate access to deep lesions [2]. The edges of these retractors may exert a significant constant pressure on the surrounding fiber tracts that may lead to retraction-induced ischemia [3]. In addition, this iatrogenic injury can be aggravated by the repeated entry of surgical instruments into the surgical field. Due to the abovementioned limitations, the results of this conventional technique have not been considered satisfactory and have encouraged the development of new advances.


M. A. R. Soliman (✉)
Faculty of Medicine, Department of Neurosurgery, Cairo University, Cairo, Egypt

Department of Neurosurgery, Jacobs School of Medicine and Biomedical Science, University at Buffalo, New York, NY, USA
e-mail: moh.ar.sol@kasralainy.edu.eg

C. Cavallo
Vanderbilt University Medical Center, Department of Neurosurgery, Nashville, TN, USA
e-mail: Claudio.cavallo@vumc.org

S. Gandhi
St. Joseph's Hospital and Medical Center, Department of Surgery, Phoenix, AZ, USA

X. Zhao
OU Health, Department of Neurosurgery, Oklahoma City, OK, USA
e-mail: Xiaochun-Zhao@ouhsc.edu

M. A. Labib
Department of Neurosurgery, University of Maryland Medical Center, Baltimore, MD, USA



© Springer Nature Switzerland AG 2022  121
G. Zada et al. (eds.), *Subcortical Neurosurgery*,
https://doi.org/10.1007/978-3-030-95153-5_9

Kelly et al. were the first to report the use of tubular retractors in 1987 with a stereotactic technique assisted by thin-walled hollow cylinders [4]. Several methods have been described to access intracranial lesions in deep locations while attempting to decrease the associated morbidity. Modern endoport-assisted systems employ a progressive dilatation mechanism which gradually expand the surgical corridor and consequently limit the white matter tracts transection [5, 6]. These devices have been used in either a trans-sulcal or trans-gyral fashion. The advantage of the trans-sulcal approach is mainly related to a shorter working distance which in turn might contribute in further minimizing the damage to the white matter tracts. In addition, the trans-sulcal technique engages the U-fibers which contribute less to the projection and association fibers which run in the gyrus [7]. This technique might contribute to reducing the amount of viable brain tissue that must be traversed to gain access to the deep-located lesions. In this chapter, we discuss the use of channel-based tubular retraction devices through the trans-sulcal parafascicular approach.

## Surgical Indications

### Patient Selection

Accessing selected deep subcortical lesions using channel-based tubular retractors through a trans-sulcal parafascicular approach is a potentially viable alternative to traditional transcortical microneurosurgery [7].

This innovative surgical technique is appropriate for both primary and secondary subcortical neoplastic lesions, as well as lesions which are vascular and infective in nature. Intraparenchymal hemorrhage and selected intraventricular and deep cerebellar lesions can also be considered [8]. Cerebral lesions reaching the cortical surface are not ideal for this surgical approach, whereas subcortical lesions located at any depth into the brain parenchyma can be potentially treated with the trans-sulcus tubular retractor technique.

### Preoperative Preparation and Planning

Radiological workup is critical to better evaluate the role of this technique for the management of subcortical brain lesions. The preoperative imaging workup essential for surgical planning usually consists of several MRI sequences including T1-weighted with and without contrast and T2-weighted MRI, DWI, and DTI with tractography (Fig. 9.1).

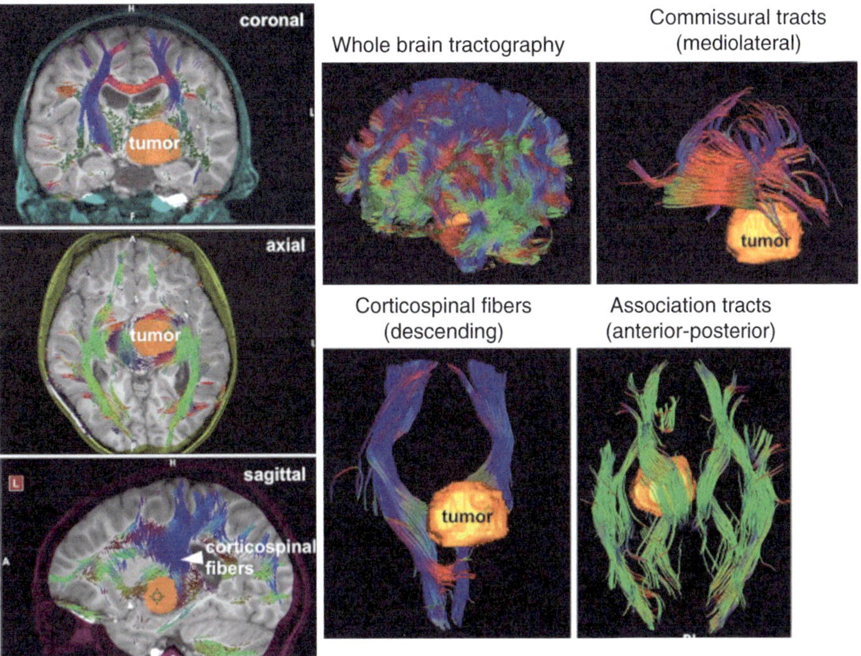


**Fig. 9.1** Spatial relation of the tumor to the white matter tract [1]

A careful review of the imaging findings and cortical anatomy is important in the planning of the trans-sulcal parafascicular approach. Ideally, cannulation with the tubular retractor should be performed as parallel as possible to white matter tracts in order to minimize surgical morbidity (Fig. 9.2). Moreover, the surgical trajectory of cannulation should be dictated by the orientation of the long axis of the lesion and should be preferably planned separately on the T1 contrast and DTI images rather than on a single fused image [9].

DWI imaging helps to determine the lesion's water content which reflects the texture and density of the pathological tissue. This characteristic is relevant as it affects the desired depth of cannulation.

## Instrumentation

There is a variety of channel-based retractors that can be used for the trans-sulcal parafascicular approach. These endoports can be categorized into the following: peel-away catheters, oval-shaped retractors, and circular-shaped retractors.

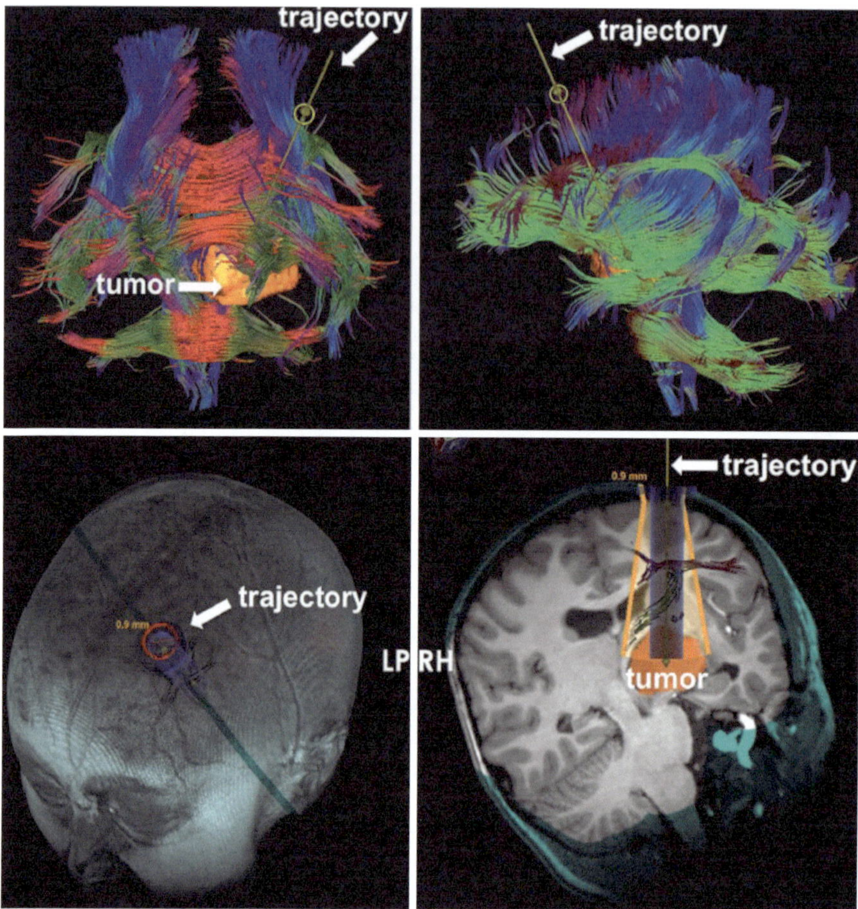


**Fig. 9.2** Planning the surgical corridor [1]

## The Peel-Away Catheters (Medtronic™)

These tubular devices share an analogous design with the peel-away central line catheters, and they represent the least disruptive endoport-assisted option [7]. They have a maximal diameter of 8 mm, and they can be inserted into the brain parenchyma through a burr hole [7]. Their therapeutic application is mainly limited for lesions in the cerebral ventricles as a clear fluid medium is required [7]. Intraoperative visualization is provided by the use of endoscopes which prevent a bimanual technique. The limited working-channel area might compromise the intraoperative maneuverability, and it can consequently make the procedure more challenging from a surgical perspective.

## *Oval-Shaped Retractors*

Oval-shaped retractors represent another type of channel-based access systems. They are advantageous because they have a greater width than the circular retractors, which allows the bimanual techniques and better maneuverability [10]. However, these retractors have a blunt tip, and their *most commonly used diameter* is 1.7 cm, which can make it difficult to work through the trans-sulcal approach and can cause disruption of the white matter tracts because of inequivalent radial retraction [11–13].

## *ViewSite ™ (Vycor Medical, Bohemia, NY)* (Fig. 9.3a)

The ViewSite™ is a tubular retractor specifically designed for intracranial use. Each retractor consists of two parts: the obturator and the retractor. This device is made out of transparent plastic, and its retractor shape is a slightly tapered cylinder with

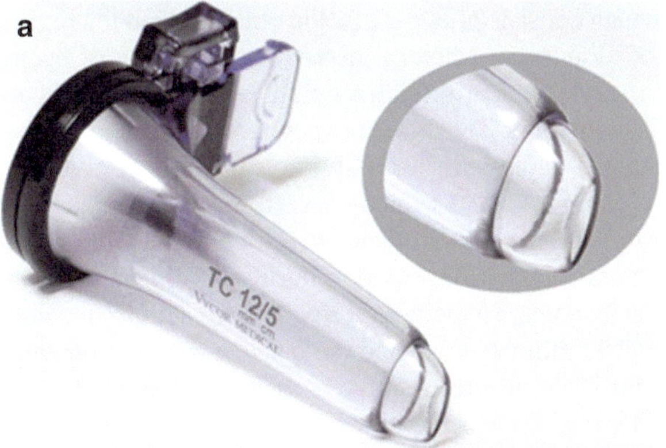


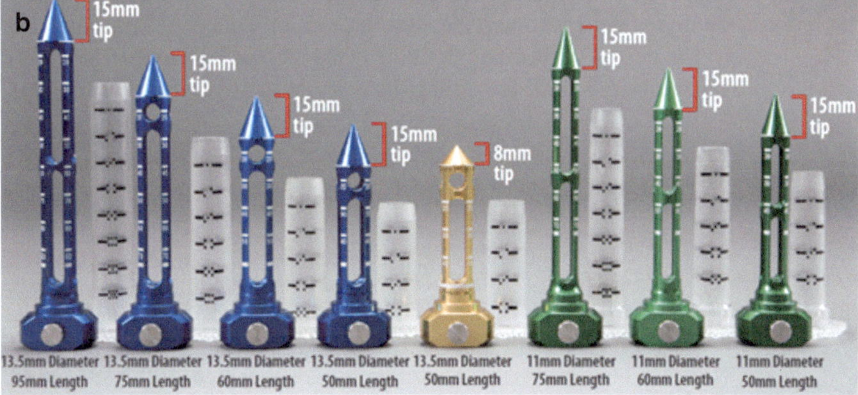


**Fig. 9.3**  Channel-based retractors. (**a**) ViewSite™, (**b**) BrainPath®

an ovoid or circular cross section. It is available in a variety of widths (12–28 mm) and lengths (3–7 cm) [14]. The most commonly used width is 17 mm [2, 14]. The retractor's outer edge is slightly wider, and its outer part is attached to a flat tab that may serve as a handle for insertion and manipulation or can be used for attaching it to a retraction arm. The obturator extends a few millimeters beyond the distal end of the retractor and is tapering down to a very narrow flat surface. There is a very small opening at the distal tip of the obturator that allows blood or cerebrospinal fluid to exit. In addition, this tip can accommodate the tip of the navigation probe during insertion of the retractor system [11–13].

## Circular-Shaped Retractors

Circular retractors are another versatile version of endoports which apply an equivalent radial force to the surrounding brain parenchyma and white fiber tracts. Despite the fact that they allow bimanual instrumentation, their smaller width (13.5 mm) limits the surgical freedom and the maneuverability of instruments [13].

The BrainPath® (Nico Corp, Indianapolis, Indiana) (Fig. 9.3b) is a particular type of circular-shaped retractor which consists of two parts: the obturator and the retractor. The obturator is made of aluminum, whereas the retractor is made of cyclic olefin copolymer, a frosted material which minimizes light reflection and allows visualization of the surrounding anatomy. The retractor is cylindrical in shape with a circular cross section. This channel-based retractor is available in a variety of widths (11.5–13.5 mm) and lengths (5–9.5 cm) which can be selected depending on the size and location of the target lesion. Both the obturator and retractor present depth markings for reference on their shafts to assist the surgeon during the procedure. The distal end of the obturator has a conical shape with a rounded tip and no opening. The obturator tip extends 7.5–15 millimeters beyond the distal end of the retractor, and it acts as a "blunt" dissector when inserted into the brain parenchyma [13].

The obturator has a blunt, tapered tip which can gently dilate the opening on the cerebral sulcus once applied on the arachnoid. The obturator is advanced through the brain parenchyma with its outer sheath to prevent any abrasion or trapping of cortical tissue. The design of the obturator allows the navigation probe to be locked into it to provide real-time guidance during the cannulation phase [11–13].

## Intraoperative Real-Time Imaging

A specially designed ultrasound probe (Hitachi Aloka, Wallingford, CT, USA) (Fig. 9.4) can be used to help localize lesions and their proximity to vascular structures during surgery, especially for deep and small lesions. The probe is 12–14 mm in diameter. The ultrasound probe is used during the advancement of the retractor to localize the lesion. It can guide the trajectory and retractor depth, which allows

**Fig. 9.4** The specially designed ultrasound probe (Hitachi Aloka, Wallingford, CT, USA)

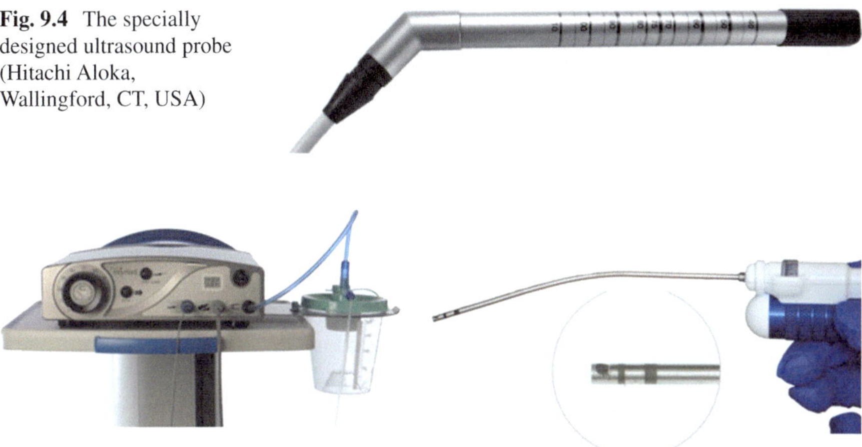

**Fig. 9.5** NICO Myriad® Device

real-time visualization during the advancement of the retractor and active correction of the trajectory until the lesion is centered within the ultrasound image. After resection of the lesion, ultrasound can characterize the extent of resection or the need for further resection [7].

## *Automated Lesion Resection Devices*

In case of a firm, high-density, non-resectable lesion, an automated resection device such as ultrasonic aspirator or a NICO Myriad® device is another useful adjunct to debulk the lesion. However, the relatively high profile of currently available ultrasonic aspirator devices makes them less attractive to employ within small tubular channels [12, 13].

The NICO Myriad® (Nico Corp) (Fig. 9.5) device is a minimally invasive system that is designed for intracranial soft tissue removal with either direct, endoscopic, or microscopic visualization. The system consists of a high-speed reciprocating inner cannula inside an outer cannula and an electronic suction control. The device relies on a side-mouth cutting and aspiration opening found 0.6 mm from the blunt dissector tip. A foot pedal controls the activation of the cutting blade, and it regulates the intensity of the suction aspiration. If needed, the aspiration opening can be rotated via a control button on the handpiece, and the shaft can be slightly bent gently. Tissue samples may be harvested from the collection chamber with minimal crushing by the device, which promotes tissue preservation. The device is available in a variety of widths (11–19 G) and lengths (10–31 cm). The main advantage of this device is the design of the handpiece which allows better visualization of the surgical field through the channel-based retractor. Moreover, the NICO Myriad facilitates access to tumors which are hard to reach with conventional surgical instruments, and it assists in pathological tissue removal without generating further heat [15].

## Technical Considerations

### *Anesthesia*

The channel-based retractor technique can be used in concert with several different anesthetic protocols including the traditional general anesthesia or awake craniotomy with conscious sedation. The latter is mainly selected depending on the location of the lesion and the preoperative patient's clinical conditions.

### *Patient Position*

Once anesthesia has been induced, the patient is positioned supine, prone, lateral, or park bench according to the preoperative plan. Subsequently, the patient's head is immobilized by a Mayfield head holder or Sugita frame. Some surgeons dissuade from using mannitol in order to prevent the collapse of the subarachnoid spaces and decrease the effect of the brain shift [16].

### *Intraoperative Navigation*

With the use of the image guidance three-dimensional space navigation system, registration is performed. The preplanned surgical route is confirmed, and the entry point is marked on the scalp. The small incision is then planned accordingly.

### *Surgical Procedure*

The skin incision and craniotomy are centered along the preplanned surgical trajectory over the targeted lesion. Following the skin incision, the scalp is retracted with blunt retractors or scalp hooks, and a small craniotomy is performed. It is advisable before opening the dura to use ultrasound to confirm the location of sulcus of interest that will be traversed. The dural opening is usually performed in a cruciate fashion. In case of brain tumors, it is recommended to open the dura more extensively to allow maximal flexibility of the sulcus. On the contrary, in case of intracerebral hemorrhage, the dural opening is only slightly larger in size than the retractor diameter in order to form a pressure seal, which propels the extrusion of the hematoma into the retractor. Dural flaps are tacked up by sutures, and appropriate hemostasis is performed before bringing the microscope or exoscope into the field. The use of intraoperative somatosensory-evoked potential (SSEP) and motor-evoked potential (MEP) is recommended especially when there an involvement of the corticospinal tracts for lesions in eloquent areas [7]. Using the navigation probe, the preplanned surgical trajectory and entry point are confirmed and adjusted if necessary. The arachnoid is opened over the sulcus (approximately 3–6 mm). Subsequently, the appropriate retractor length is selected based on the surgical trajectory analysis on the preoperative MRI. Retractors with a length a few millimeters longer than the preplanned trajectory from the cortical surface are recommended as they decrease the risk of unintended cortical laceration and provide more room for manipulation of the retractor. Using navigation guidance, the retractor is advanced through the arachnoid opening into the sulcus until it reaches the preplanned target depth. The tip of the obturator is usually beyond the distal rim of the retractor; therefore, the sheath is advanced 15 millimeters over the obturator as this is the distance between the retractor and the obturator tip. The obturator is then removed while the sheath is secured in place through a special hook that attaches it into a conventional articulated snake retractor system. Intraoperative visualization down the endoport can be achieved either with an extracorporeal exoscope [17, 18] or a surgical microscope [19].

Generally, there are two ways of cannulation depending on the water content of the lesion on the DWI sequence:

1. *Deep cannulation:* The retractor can be placed within the lesion to allow a resection in an inside-out fashion. The resection can be stopped at white matter interface. This technique is usually recommended for soft and/or less dense lesions such as high-grade gliomas and intracerebral hematomas. Deep cannulation is contraindicated for lesions with firm consistency as it may cause the rolling of the lesion outside the field of the retractor and difficulty in localizing it.

2. *Superficial cannulation:* The retractor is placed at the surface of the lesion which is exposed by removing a white matter cuff over it at the interface between the pathological tissue and the viable brain parenchyma or white fiber tracts. This technique is usually recommended for firm and/or dense lesions, such as cerebral metastases. It is ideal to excise this type of lesions *en bloc* to avoid spillage of malignant cells in cases of metastasis [20]. However, a piecemeal resection for metastatic lesions has been described by other authors [11].

## *Resection of the Lesion or Evacuation of the Hematoma*

The standard technique for the excision of the lesion with the channel-based approach consists of the bimanual use of suction, microscissors, and bipolar cautery. A similar technique can be used for evacuating intracerebral hematoma. If the lesion is larger than the retractor diameter or the source of bleeding is beyond the retractor scope, the viewing angle can be adjusted. The tubular retracted can be swiveled, and the procedure can also be assisted by an angled endoscope to inspect circumferentially within the surgical field. In this way, a more distant source of bleeding, for example, can be identified and residual tumor tissue can be resected. Gross total resection is mostly dependent on the size and location of the lesion as well as the surgical technique. According to our personal experience, bayoneted surgical instruments are the most effective in the relatively small working space offered by the endoport. Both ultrasonic aspirators or side-cutting aspirators (Myriad® from NICO Corporation) can be helpful during surgical resection of the lesion.

## *Hemostasis and Closure*

Once the lesion is excised, hemostasis is achieved by controlling any bleeding vessels with the use of low-intensity bipolar electrocautery forceps. Hemostatic agents such as Floseal® (Baxter) can be used for small diffuse bleeding. Subsequently, the surgical cavity is filled with saline or lactated Ringer's solution, and the retractor is slowly withdrawn. If any additional source of bleeding is identified, the surgeon should stop removing the retractor and hemostasis should again be achieved. It is ideal to do several rounds of irrigation with saline. A small piece of hemostatic agent (SURGICEL® (Johnson & Johnson Patient Care; New Brunswick, NJ) or GELFOAM®) is placed over the exposed brain. The dura is closed in a watertight fashion, and the bone flap is put back in place and secured. The galea and skin are closed in the usual fashion.

## Overview of Clinical Studies

A comprehensive literature review of the channel-based trans-sulcal approach for subcortical deep-seated lesions identified 21 articles published in peer-reviewed journals (Table 9.1). These clinical studies used a variety of endoport devices including tubular/oval retractors, BrainPath, and VBAS (ViewSite Brain Access System). The electronic search was conducted on several relevant international databases, including PUBMED (Medline), EMBASE, and the Web of Science database for articles in English which specified the number of patients enrolled. Studies

**Table 9.1** Systematic review of patients operated upon by trans-sulcal, channel-based parafascicular

| Author, date | Number of patients | Retractor system | Pathology | Complication rate (%) | Extent of resection |
|---|---|---|---|---|---|
| Ritsma et al. [21], 2014 | 1 | BrainPath | Intracerebral hematoma (temporal) | 100% Recurrent bleeding and reoperation but return of the patient to the normal function | Complete evacuation |
| Kassam et al. [9], 2015 | 13 | BrainPath | GBM (6) Intracerebral hematoma (4) Abscess (1) Metastasis (1) Pilocytic astrocytoma (1) | 15.% Postoperative hematoma (1) DVT (1) | ICH complete evacuation (50%) Evacuation >85% (50%) Tumors not specified |
| Przybylowski et al. [19], 2015 | 11 | BrainPath | Intracerebral hematoma | 27.3% Death due to rebleeding (patient has chronic coagulopathy due to severe alcoholic cirrhosis) (1) Pneumonia, renal failure, and esophageal perforation (1) Duodenal perforation and UGIB (1) | >85% (63.6%) |
| Amenta et al. [22] 2016 | 1 | BrainPath | Cavernoma (thalamus) | Transient weakness for 12 h | Complete excision |
| Chen et al. [23], 2016 | 6 | BrainPath | Traumatic hematoma | None | >90% evacuation |
| Eliyas et al. [24], 2016 | 20 | BrainPath | Colloid cyst (5) Low grade glioma (5) Metastasis (3) Subependymoma (3) Meningioma (2) Central neurocytoma (1) Lymphoma (1) | 15% Short-term memory loss (transient) (2) Transient weakness (1) | GTR (75%) |

(continued)

**Table 9.1** (continued)

| Author, date | Number of patients | Retractor system | Pathology | Complication rate (%) | Extent of resection |
|---|---|---|---|---|---|
| Labib et al. [17], 2016 | 39 | BrainPath | Intracerebral hematoma | 15.4% Respiratory failure (2) Rebleeding (1) Persistent hemiplegia (1) DVT (1) Pneumonia and Cl. difficile (1) | >90 (72%) |
| Bauer et al. [18], 2017 | 9 | BrainPath (9) | Intracerebral hematoma | 22.2% Respiratory failure and hypernatremia | >85% evacuation (100%) |
| Chen et al. [25], 2017 | 1 | BrainPath | Fungal infection | 0% | GTR |
| Day et al. [16], 2017 | 49 | BrainPath | Gliomas (23) Metastasis (20) Intracerebral hematoma (6) | 18.3% Postoperative hemorrhage (2) Transient neurologic deficit (3) Permanent neurologic deficit (2) New infarct (1) Mortality (1) | GTR of tumors (79.1%) Complete evacuation of hematoma (83%) |
| Eichberg et al. [8], 2017 | 20 | VBAS (7) BrainPath (13) | Metastasis (9) Colloid cyst (6) GBM (2) Melanoma (1) Radiation necrosis (1) Subependymoma (1) | 10% Transient short-term memory deficit (1) Postoperative stroke of unclear etiology in POD 1 (1) | GTR (90%) |
| Jackson et al. [13], 2017 | 11 | BrainPath | GBM (3) Anaplastic astrocytoma (3) Demyelinating disease (2) Lymphoma (2) Metastasis (1) | 0% | Not specified |
| Sujijantara et al. [26], 2017 | 16 | BrainPath | Intracerebral hematoma | Mortality (family withdrawal) (1) Postoperative seizures (2) Unrelated medical problems (pneumonia, UTI, cardiac complications) (13) | >85% evacuation (87.5%) |

**Table 9.1** (continued)

| Author, date | Number of patients | Retractor system | Pathology | Complication rate (%) | Extent of resection |
|---|---|---|---|---|---|
| Weiner et al. [1], 2017 | 1 | BrainPath | Pilocytic astrocytoma | 100% Transient increased weakness and newly developed oculomotor palsy | GTR |
| Witek et al. [27], 2017 | 1 | BrainPath | AVM | 0% | Total excision |
| Akbari et al. [28], 2018 | 10 | BrainPath | Metastasis (4) GBM (3) Anaplastic astrocytoma (1) Low-grade glioma (2) | 40% Postoperative permanent increased weakness (1) Postoperative transient increased weakness (2) Pulmonary embolism and death (1) | GTR (80%) |
| Bakhsheshian et al. [11], 2018 | 25 | BrainPath | Metastasis | 4% Hemiparesis and subsequent DVT | GTR (80%) |
| Iyer et al. [12], 2018 | 14 | BrainPath | GBM (11) Anaplastic astrocytoma (3) | 7.1% Postoperative permanent increased weakness (1) | Excision >85% (100%) |
| Goren et al. [29], 2018 | 6 | BrainPath | Cavernoma | 16.7% Wound dehiscence (1) | Complete excision (100%) |
| Sindelar et al. [30], 2018 | 1 | BrainPath | Intracerebral and intraventricular bleed | Neurologically improved and no complications | >90% removal of the hematoma |
| Bander et al. [31], 2019 | 18 | BrainPath | Glioma (16) Lymphoma (2) | 5.6% Postoperative minor hematoma (1) | Not mentioned |

describing a transcortical approach or lacking details on complication and the extent of resection (EOR) of the tumor or evacuation of hematoma were not included. Overall, 273 patients underwent a channel-based trans-sulcal approach. There were 93 intracerebral hematomas (6 traumatic and 1 associated with intraventricular hemorrhage), 78 gliomas, 63 metastases, 11 colloid cysts, 7 cavernomas, 5 lymphomas, 4 subependymomas, 2 meningiomas, 2 pilocytic astrocytoma, 2 demyelinating lesions, 1 central neurocytoma, 1 abscess, 1 fungal infection, 1 melanoma, 1 radiation necrosis, and 1 AVM. Patient diagnosis, complications, and extent of evacuation or excision are reported in Table 9.1.

The ability to evacuate more than 85–90% of ICH was achieved in 80.6% of cases, whereas the gross total resection (GTR) rate of brain lesions was 82%. The complication rate was higher in the intracerebral hematoma group (15.6%) compared to other pathologies (9.4%).

Complications reported included transient neurologic deficits (2.9%), permanent neurologic deficits (motor weakness or cranial nerve deficit) (2.9%), bleeding requiring additional surgery (1.8%), DVT (1.5%), transient short-term memory loss (1.1%), respiratory failure (1.1%), death (1.1%) (one of the patients was because the family asked for care withdrawal), postoperative seizures (0.7%), minor hematoma (0.7%), pulmonary embolism (0.4%), new infarct (0.4%), and wound dehiscence (0.4%). Other medical complications represented 6.6% of the overall complications and included pneumonia, upper gastrointestinal bleeding, duodenal perforation, esophageal perforation, urinary tract infection, cardiovascular problems, and renal failure.

A randomized, multicenter clinical trial ENRICH (Early MiNimally-invasive Removal of ICH) began in December 2016. This study compares early surgical hematoma evacuation (<24 h) using BrainPath versus standard medical management for ICH. Three hundred patients will be recruited in at least 15 medical centers.

# References

1. Weiner HL, Placantonakis DG. Resection of a pediatric thalamic juvenile pilocytic astrocytoma with whole brain tractography. Cureus. 2019;9(10):e1768. Available from: https://www.ncbi.nlm.nih.gov/pmc/articles/PMC5724810/
2. Recinos PF, Raza SM, Jallo GI, Recinos VR. Use of a minimally invasive tubular retraction system for deep-seated tumors in pediatric patients: technical note. J Neurosurg Pediatr. 2011;7(5):516–21.
3. Andrews RJ, Bringas JR. A review of brain retraction and recommendations for minimizing intraoperative brain injury. Neurosurgery. 1993;33(6):1052–64.
4. Kelly PJ, Goerss SJ, Kall BA. The stereotaxic retractor in computer-assisted stereotaxic microsurgery: technical note. J Neurosurg. 1988;69(2):301–6.
5. Ogura K, Tachibana E, Aoshima C, Sumitomo M. New microsurgical technique for intraparenchymal lesions of the brain: transcylinder approach. Acta Neurochir. 2006;148(7):779–85.
6. Nagatani K, Takeuchi S, Feng D, Mori K, Day JD. High-definition exoscope system for microneurosurgery: use of an exoscope in combination with tubular retraction and frameless neuronavigation for microsurgical resection of deep brain lesions. No Shinkei Geka. 2015;43(7):611–7.
7. Gassie K, Wijesekera O, Chaichana KL. Minimally invasive tubular retractor-assisted biopsy and resection of subcortical intra-axial gliomas and other neoplasms. J Neurosurg Sci. 2018;62(6):682–9.
8. Eichberg DG, Buttrick S, Brusko GD, Ivan M, Starke RM, Komotar RJ. Use of tubular retractor for resection of deep-seated cerebral tumors and colloid cysts: single surgeon experience and review of the literature. World Neurosurg. 2018;112:e50–60.
9. Kassam AB, Labib MA, Bafaquh M, Ghinda D, Fukui MB, Nguyen T, Corsten M. Part II: an evaluation of an integrated systems approach using diffusion-weighted, image-guided, exoscopic-assisted, transsulcal radial corridors. Innovative Neurosurg. 2015;3(1–2):25–33.

Available from: https://www.degruyter.com/view/j/ins.2015.3.issue-1-2/ins-2014-0012/ins-2014-0012.xml

10. Marenco-Hillembrand L, Alvarado-Estrada K, Chaichana KL. Contemporary surgical management of deep-seated metastatic brain tumors using minimally invasive approaches. Front Oncol. 2018;8:198–204. Available from: https://www.frontiersin.org/articles/10.3389/fonc.2018.00558/full

11. Bakhsheshian J, Strickland BA, Jackson C, Chaichana KL, Young R, Pradilla G, et al. Multicenter investigation of channel-based subcortical trans-sulcal exoscopic resection of metastatic brain tumors: a retrospective case series. Oper Neurosurg. 2019;16(2):159–66.

12. Iyer R, Chaichana KL. Minimally invasive resection of deep-seated high-grade gliomas using tubular retractors and Exoscopic visualization. J Neurol Surg A Cent Eur Neurosurg. 2018;79(4):330–6.

13. Jackson C, Gallia GL, Chaichana KL. Minimally invasive biopsies of deep-seated brain lesions using tubular retractors under exoscopic visualization. J Neurol Surg A Cent Eur Neurosurg. 2017;78(6):588–94.

14. Raza SM, Recinos PF, Avendano J, Adams H, Jallo GI, Quinones-Hinojosa A. Minimally invasive trans-portal resection of deep intracranial lesions. Minim Invasive Neurosurg. 2011;54(1):5–11.

15. Dlouhy BJ, Dahdaleh NS, Greenlee JDW. Emerging technology in intracranial neuroendoscopy: application of the NICO myriad: technical note. Neurosurg Focus. 2011;30(4):E6.

16. Day JD. Transsulcal parafascicular surgery using brain path® for subcortical lesions. Neurosurgery. 2017;64(CN_suppl_1):151–6.

17. Labib MA, Shah M, Kassam AB, Young R, Zucker L, Maioriello A, et al. The safety and feasibility of image-guided BrainPath-mediated transsulcal hematoma evacuation: a multicenter study. Neurosurgery. 2017;80(4):515–24.

18. Bauer AM, Rasmussen PA, Bain MD. Initial single-center technical experience with the BrainPath system for acute intracerebral hemorrhage evacuation. Oper Neurosurg. 2017;13(1):69–76.

19. Przybylowski CJ, Ding D, Starke RM, Webster Crowley R, Liu KC. Endoport-assisted surgery for the management of spontaneous intracerebral hemorrhage. J Clin Neurosci. 2015;22(11):1727–32.

20. Patel AJ, Suki D, Hatiboglu MA, Rao VY, Fox BD, Sawaya R. Impact of surgical methodology on the complication rate and functional outcome of patients with a single brain metastasis. J Neurosurg. 2015;122(5):1132–43.

21. Ritsma B, Kassam A, Dowlatshahi D, Nguyen T, Stotts G. Minimally invasive subcortical parafascicular transsulcal access for clot evacuation (Mi SPACE) for intracerebral hemorrhage. Case Rep Neurol Med. 2014;2014:102307. Available from: https://www.hindawi.com/journals/crinm/2014/102307/abs/.

22. Amenta PS, Dumont AS, Medel R. Resection of a left posterolateral thalamic cavernoma with the Nico BrainPath sheath: case report, technical note, and review of the literature. Interdiscip Neurosurg. 2016;5:12–7.

23. Chen JW, Paff MR, Abrams-Alexandru D, Kaloostian SW. Decreasing the cerebral edema associated with traumatic intracerebral hemorrhages: use of a minimally invasive technique. In: Applegate RL, et al., editors. Brain edema XVI: translate basic science into clinical practice, vol. 121. Acta Neurochirurgica Supplement; 2016. p. 279–84.

24. Eliyas JK, Glynn R, Kulwin CG, Rovin R, Young R, Alzate J, et al. Minimally invasive transsulcal resection of intraventricular and periventricular lesions through a tubular retractor system: multicentric experience and results. World Neurosurg. 2016;90:556–64.

25. Chen Y-N, Omay SB, Shetty SR, Liang B, Almeida JP, Ruiz-Treviño AS, et al. Transtubular excisional biopsy as a rescue for a non-diagnostic stereotactic needle biopsy—case report and literature review. Acta Neurochir. 2017;159(9):1589–95.

26. Sujijantarat N, Tecle NE, Pierson M, Urquiaga JF, Quadri NF, Ashour AM, et al. Transsulcal endoport-assisted evacuation of supratentorial intracerebral hemorrhage: initial single-

institution experience compared to matched medically managed patients and effect on 30-Day mortality. Oper Neurosurg. 2018;14(5):524–31.

27. Witek AM, Moore NZ, Sebai MA, Bain MD. BrainPath-mediated resection of a ruptured subcortical arteriovenous malformation. Oper Neurosurg. 2018;15:32–8.

28. Akbari SHA, Sylvester PT, Kulwin C, Shah MV, Somasundaram A, Kamath AA, et al. Initial experience using intraoperative magnetic resonance imaging during a trans-sulcal tubular retractor approach for the resection of deep-seated brain tumors: a case series. Oper Neurosurg. 2019;16(3):292–301.

29. Goren O, Griessenauer CJ, Bohan CO, Berry CM, Schirmer CM. Minimally invasive parafascicular surgery for resection of cerebral cavernous malformations utilizing image-guided BrainPath system. Oper Neurosurg. 2019;17(4):348–53. Available from: https://academic.oup.com/ons/advance-article/doi/10.1093/ons/opy389/5253304.

30. Sindelar BD, Patel V, Chowdhry S, Bailes JE. A case report in hemorrhagic stroke: a complex disease process and requirement for a multimodal treatment approach. Cureus. 2019;10(7):e2976. Available from: https://www.ncbi.nlm.nih.gov/pmc/articles/PMC6138459/.

31. Bander ED, Jones SH, Pisapia D, Magge R, Fine H, Schwartz TH, et al. Tubular brain tumor biopsy improves diagnostic yield for subcortical lesions. J Neuro-Oncol. 2019;141(1):121–9.

# Chapter 10
# Standard Parafascicular Approaches to Subcortical Regions

J. Manuel Revuelta Barbero, David Bray, and Gustavo Pradilla

## Abbreviations

| | |
|---|---|
| AF | Arcuate fasciculus |
| CF | Cingulate fasciculus |
| DTI | Diffusion tensor imaging |
| FAT | Frontal aslant tract |
| IFOF | Inferior fronto-occipital fascicle |
| ILF | Inferior longitudinal fascicle |
| MRI | Magnetic resonance imaging |
| NIHSS | National Institute of Health Stroke Score |
| OR | Optic radiations |
| SFS | Superior frontal sulcus |
| SLF | Superior longitudinal fasciculus |

J. M. R. Barbero
Department of Neurosurgery, Emory University, Atlanta, GA, USA
e-mail: jmrevuelta@emory.edu

D. Bray
Department of Neurosurgery, Emory University School of Medicine, Atlanta, GA, USA
e-mail: dbray3@emory.edu

G. Pradilla (✉)
Neurological Surgery, Emory University School of Medicine, Atlanta, GA, USA
e-mail: gpradil@emory.edu

© Springer Nature Switzerland AG 2022
G. Zada et al. (eds.), *Subcortical Neurosurgery*,
https://doi.org/10.1007/978-3-030-95153-5_10

# Introduction

Surgical access to subcortical brain lesions remains challenging due to limited visualization, narrow corridors for instrument maneuverability, and the delicate nature of the cortical and subcortical structures at risk. It is difficult to maintain optimal field magnification, illumination, and focal length while maneuvering instruments in a deep, subcortical field within narrow corridors. The success of minimally-invasive neurological surgery hinges upon effective utilization of modern neuroimaging for diagnosis and preoperative patient and approach selection, intimate knowledge of subcortical anatomy, delicate microsurgical technique, and adequate utilization of adjuvant techniques to preserve functionality and maximize safe resection.

Transsulcal access points are used to safely navigate the subcortical white matter while providing maximal exposure for safe and thorough resection of the targeted lesion. Minimally-invasive surgical techniques strive to minimize trauma to surrounding tissues and protect white matter fascicles, preserve neurological function, and reduce iatrogenic morbidity. Traditional transsulcal approaches to deep lesions required the use of operative microscopy often coupled to fixed blade retractors, which could injure the cortical and subcortical structures due to hypoperfusion or direct mechanical trauma [1–4]. Previously developed tubular retractors designed to circumvent these challenges have seen greater improvements and adoption in recent years propelled by developments in high-definition endoscopy, exoscopic visualization systems, and port-based surgery assisted by neuronavigation [5–7]. These minimally-invasive techniques have heretofore been employed for intracerebral hemorrhage evacuation [7, 8] and neoplasm biopsy and resection [9–11], especially in lesions with low-to-moderate vascularity and smaller than 5 cm.

Transsulcal-parafascicular corridors to subcortical and intraventricular lesion have been previously described based upon cadaveric, functional MRI, and diffusion tensor imaging (DTI) studies [12–15]. Precise knowledge and understanding of the pathological displacement of normal subcortical structures is necessary to select the ideal operative corridor for a specific lesion [7, 16]. Preoperative DTI is a useful tool for such planning, albeit subject to imaging artifact due to perilesional edema [17, 18]. In these cases, surgeons may employ neurophysiological adjuncts such as cortical and subcortical motor mapping to reduce neurological injury.

In this chapter, we will use illustrative cases to describe anatomical and DTI considerations related to the white matter fibers involved in standard parafascicular approaches to subcortical regions. We will also describe surgical nuance and common neurological complications possible with these approaches.

# Parafascicular Surgical Corridors

Standard convention classifies the various approaches (i.e., anterior, posterior, and lateral) to subcortical regions in relation to the entry point employed to reach the target. Ideal trajectories to deep targets remain parallel to major fiber tracts to minimize vector loading. The paramount principle of minimally-invasive surgery is to avoid or reduce fiber tract transgression.

## *Anterior Corridor*

This transsulcal-parafascicular approach allows for access to the subcortical frontal lobe, the frontal horn of lateral ventricles, and the third ventricle. It is considered the "gate access" to the anterior basal ganglia including the caudate nucleus, putamen, and external capsule, and it is commonly employed for hemorrhage evacuation in these locations.

### Representative Clinical Case

A 74-year-old woman, with a history of hypertension and diabetes mellitus type 2, presented to our institution with an intraparenchymal hemorrhage. On neurological evaluation, the patient had a dense left hemiparesis and National Institute of Health Stroke Score (NIHSS) of 27. CT and MRI were performed demonstrating a right intraparenchymal hemorrhage in the basal ganglia (Fig. 10.1a–d). A complete hemorrhage evacuation by transfrontal access via a supraorbital "eyebrow" craniotomy using a tubular retractor system (BrainPath® system, NICO Corporation, Indianapolis, USA) was achieved (Fig. 10.1e–g). The patient was discharged on the third day to an acute rehabilitation center with GCS 15, NIHSS 8, and mRS 2. At 3 months follow-up, the patient presented an NIHSS of 3 and mRS of 1.

### Anatomical, DTI Relevant Landmarks, and Special Considerations

The anterior corridor spreads from the most anterior point of the superior frontal sulcus (SFS) to its intersection with the precentral sulcus and supplementary motor area. This point is known as the *posterior coronal point* [19]. The forehead crease and eyebrow incisions offer good access for anterior approaches since they frequently coincide with this entry point in most patients.

The most relevant white matter tracts implicated in the transfrontal access are the association fibers known as the superior longitudinal fasciculus (SLF) laterally and the cingulate fasciculus (CF) medially. Normally, the SLF runs just deep to the U-fibers, connecting portions of the frontal lobe with occipital and temporal areas. The CF follows its trajectory from the cingulate gyrus to the entorhinal cortex. It is associated with motivational and emotional aspects of behavior and working memory.

The SFS separates the superior from the middle frontal gyrus and has been divided into three segments in its anterior-to-posterior length [20]. The posterior and middle segments (also known as proximal/middle) cover an extension from the precentral sulcus to a point situated 3 cm anterior to the coronal suture. The trajectories offered by those segments may endanger the frontal aslant tract (FAT), the

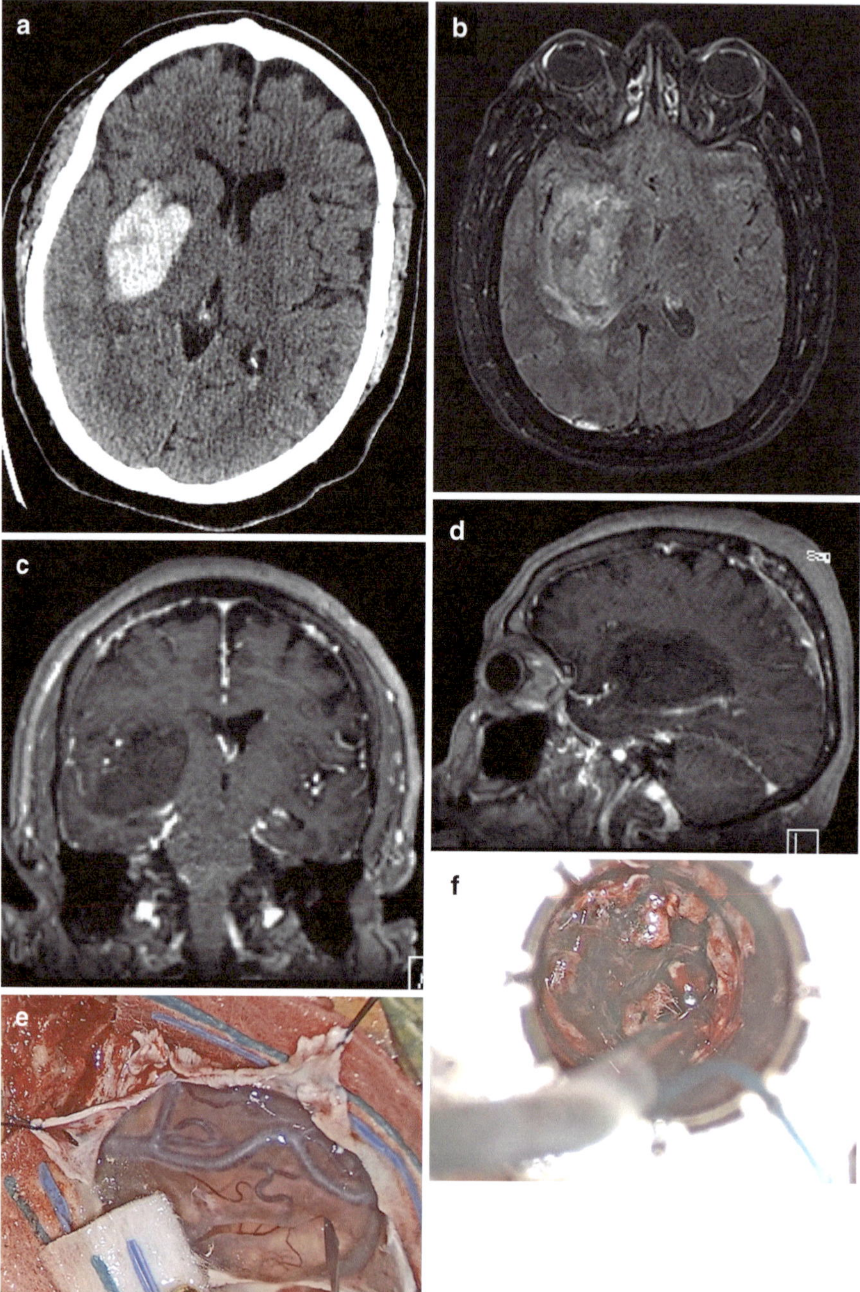

**Fig. 10.1** Preoperative imaging (**a**. CT; **b–d**. MRI) reveals a right intraparenchymal hemorrhage in the basal ganglia. Intraoperative view, after dural and arachnoid opening (**e**), and exoscope-enhanced view through the port (**f**). Postoperative CT demonstrated complete intraparenchymal hemorrhage evacuation (**g**). Illustrative artwork showing the integration of tractography, transulcal access (A), port-based access (B), exoscopic visualization (C), and resection for anterior basal ganglia hemorrhages and posterior thalamic lesions (D)

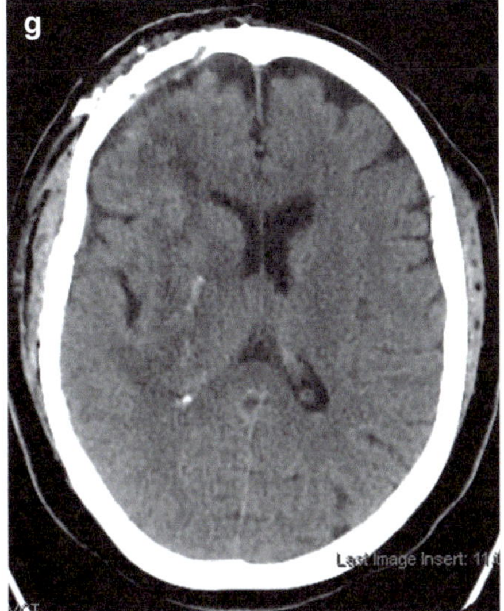


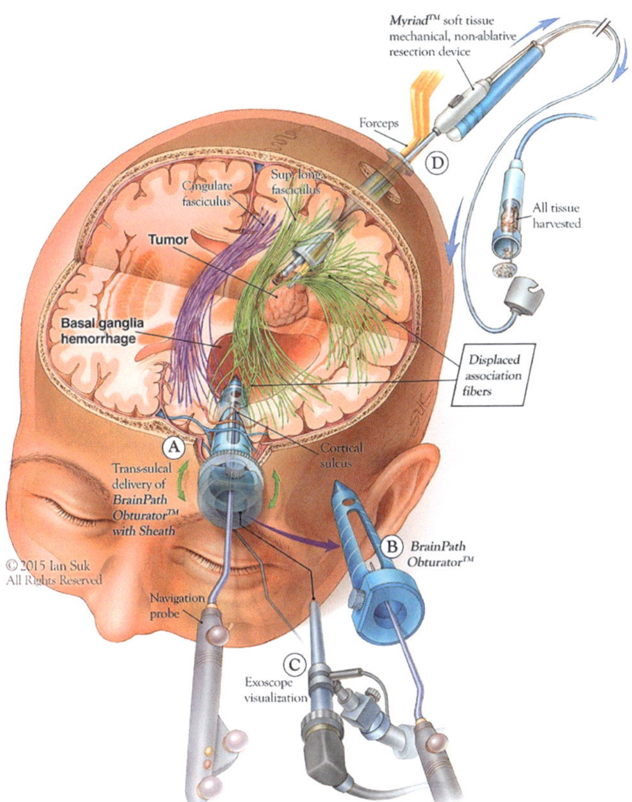


**Fig. 10.1** (continued)

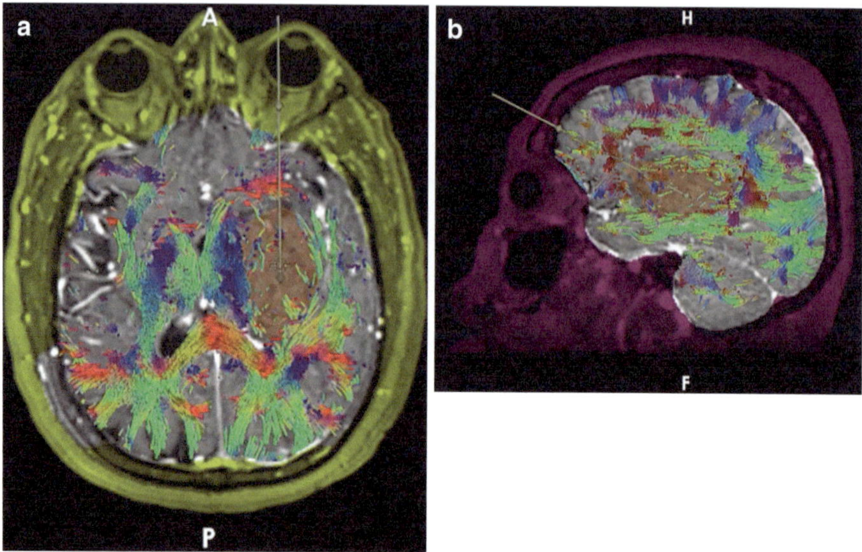

**Fig. 10.2** DTI reveals expansion of the anterior corridor as consequence of the white matter tract displacement secondary to pathology. (**a**) Axial view showing the LSF lateral and the CF medial. (**b**) Sagital view showing the trajectory along the long axis of the hematoma

intermediate segments of SLF, and the CF which may result in potential speech disabilities, apraxia, and supplementary motor area syndrome [21, 22]. We prefer to avoid transgression of the posterior two-thirds of SFS without an awake craniotomy to reliably avoid injury to anatomical speech centers [20, 23]. The most anterior SFS segment extends from the anterior limit of the middle SFS segment to the orbital crest, offering a safe entry point along the long axis of SLF and CF fascicles, and away from the FAT [20]. This corridor can be often expanded secondary to pathology (Fig. 10.2).

It is critical to avoid injury to the anterior white matter tracts; SLF injury is associated with ideomotor apraxia and spatial neglect [24, 25], and CF damage can result in psychiatric disorders and behavioral changes [26, 27].

## *Posterior Corridor*

This corridor provides safe and direct access to the lateral ventricles, especially to the atrium and the peri-atrial region.

### Representative Clinical Case

A 69-year-old female with a past medical history of hypertension presented with confusion and suffered a fall striking her head with brief loss of consciousness. Upon arrival, her neurological examination was unremarkable, but her initial head

CT revealed a left parietal hypodensity. A subsequent brain MRI with contrast confirmed the presence of an enhancing mass with central necrosis and minimal intratumoral hemorrhage centered within the left median parietal lobe with adjacent T2 FLAIR hyperintensity that extended to the occipital lobe and crossed the midline along the splenium, most consistent with a high-grade glioma (Fig. 10.3). Tractographic analysis revealed a safe entry point at the parieto-occipital sulcus, and she underwent a left parieto-occipital craniotomy for resection of the lesion using a 75 mm BrainPath system with robotic-guided exoscopic visualization under electrophysiologic monitoring with somatosensory- and motor-evoked potentials. A

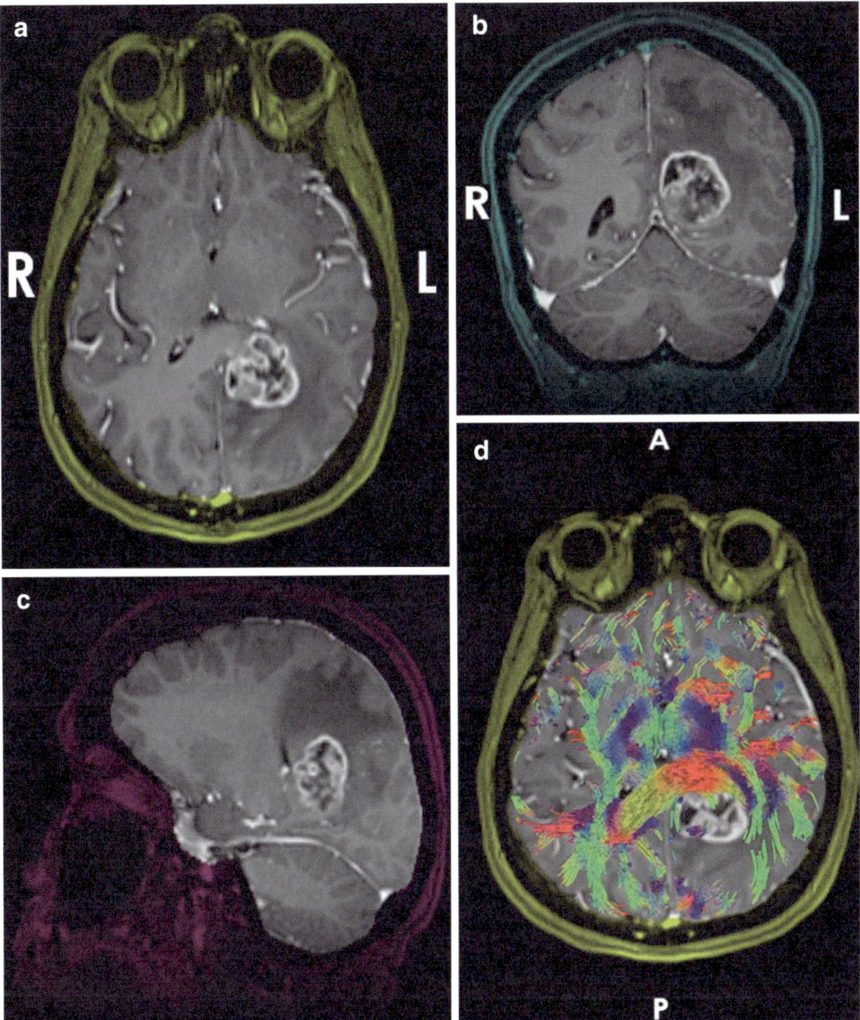

**Fig. 10.3** Preoperative imaging (**a–c**. MRI; **d–f**. DTI) reveals a left parieto-occipital mass with contrast enhancement. Postoperative imaging demonstrated gross total resection with a small trajectory and minimal changes to the surrounding normal tissue (**g–i**)

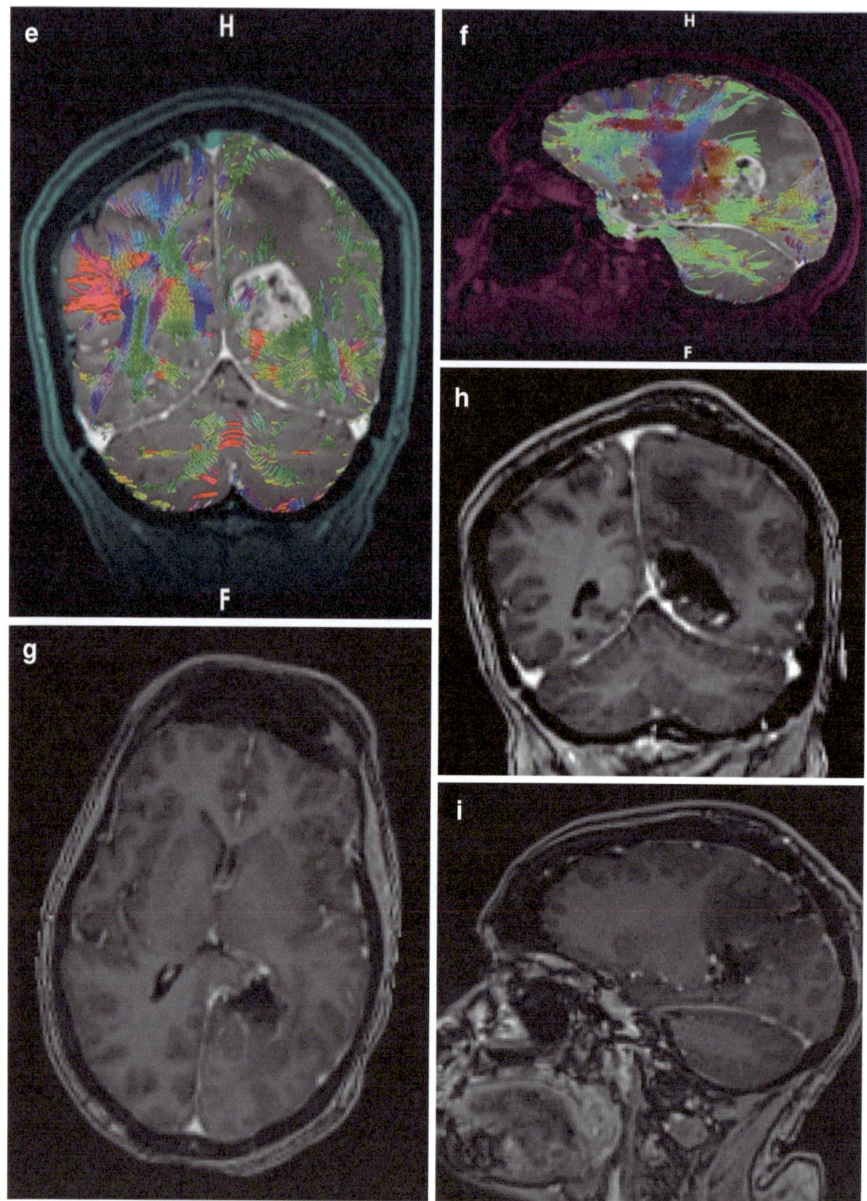

**Fig. 10.3** (continued)

gross total resection was achieved without any neurological deficits, and the patient was discharged home on postoperative day 3 in good condition. Pathology revealed an IDH, wild-type, WHO grade IV glioblastoma, and she underwent postoperative radiation and chemotherapy with no evidence of recurrence at the 18-month follow-up MRI.

**Anatomical, DTI Relevant Landmarks, and Special Considerations**

The posterior corridor is accessed through the parieto-occipital and intraparietal sulcus, spanning from the posterior margin of the primary sensory fibers to the optic radiations. Both sulci have an oblique direction, pointing at their deepest point toward the occipital horn and the atrium, respectively [28, 29]. The subcortical complex surrounding the atrium was described as a temporoparietal fiber association area and involves a hub of multiple fiber tracts [30]. The main fiber tracts involved in this corridor are the *optic radiations* (OR) large association fibers in the occipital lobe running laterally to the atrium and along the roof and in the lateral edge of the temporal horn toward the calcarine sulcus [31], the *arcuate fasciculus* (AF) connecting the inferior frontal regions and posterior temporal regions with a critical role in language [32], and the *vertical rami of the SLF*, ascending association fibers that connect the dorsal portion of SLF to the parietal lobe [33, 34]. With DTI, the vertical rami of the SLF is represented by blue fibers as a result of its rostrocaudal trajectory [34]. These fibers associate the parietal lobes and control different cognitive functions such as working memory and visual-spatial orientation [35, 36]. These relationships could explain the variety of neurological presentations reported as consequences of parietal lobe dysfunction, particularly in visual and language deficits [37–39].

Others have proposed the *anterior segment of intraparietal sulcus* as an ideal transparietal access [19]. An exhaustive DTI study showed that this access point should not be used to the atrium as there is theoretical increased risk of postoperative neurological deficit [40]. Instead, the middle segment of the intraparietal sulcus may be the safest surgical access to the atrium of the lateral ventricle [41]. It is critical to remember that occipital lobe tumors can medially displace the optic radiations, which may necessitate selecting another access point or surgical corridor. Intraparietal and parieto-occipital sulci offer access to the medial and lateral subcortical regions surrounding the optic radiations [34].

## *Lateral Corridor*

Several *association, projection,* and *commisural* fibers intersect with traditional access corridors to subcortical pathology due to the perpendicular orientation of critical white matter tracts rendering the lateral corridor as suboptimal for accessing most subcortical lesions. In selected cases, however, it represents the best way to protect deflected fibers displaced by the pathology in question. In these cases, awake testing and intraoperative mapping techniques are often needed to avoid tract injury and further neurological deficits.

## Representative Clinical Case

A 70-year-old female with a previous history of breast adenocarcinoma status post mastectomy, radiation, and chemotherapy presented with a mild expressive aphasia, headaches, and mild right-sided weakness. A comprehensive evaluation with head, chest, abdominal, and pelvic CT scans showed a left temporal hyperdensity and no additional masses suggestive of other systemic metastases. A subsequent MRI with contrast confirmed the presence of a 2.5 cm mostly solid lesion located in the superior temporal gyrus centered in the posterior third of the temporal lobe with extensive vasogenic edema. Tractography showing displacement of the arcuate fasciculus superiorly and dorsally. Her Karnofsky Performance status was >70, and she underwent an awake left temporal craniotomy with speech and motor subcortical mapping utilizing a 60 mm BrainPath port under robotic-assisted exoscopic visualization. The patient had an uneventful postoperative course, and her speech and motor deficits improved significantly by postoperative day 5. She was discharged to rehabilitation on postoperative day 6 and underwent postoperative stereotactic radiosurgery to the cavity as well as systemic chemotherapy. No evidence of regional recurrence was seen at the 2-year follow-up MRI (Fig. 10.4).

## Anatomical, DTI Relevant Landmarks, and Special Considerations

The lateral aspect of the cerebral hemisphere can be divided into two halves by a line traversing in the axial plane. The upper half is comprised of the SLF and a neurofascicular hub complex of the intersection of seven different temporoparietal fiber tracts [30, 42]. Three different white matter tracts create the inferior half of the subcortical anatomy of the lateral segment of the cerebral hemisphere. These tracts include the inferior fronto-occipital fascicle (IFOF), connecting the orbitofrontal with occipital cortices (language, particularly lexical and semantic processing of the speech) [43, 44]; the *inferior longitudinal fascicle* (ILF), connecting temporal with occipital cortices (visuospatial analysis) [43, 45]; and the OR (previously described). The posterior aspects of these three white matter tracts form the sagittal stratum [16]. More anteriorly, at the temporal stem, the *uncinate fascicle* (UF), OR, IFOF, and the ILF comprise a neural network hub [46]. The UF, AF, and the vertical rami of the SLF are association tracts between the superior and inferior aspects of the subcortical structures of the lateral cerebral hemisphere. Specifically, the UF, a hook-shaped fiber tract traveling from the amygdala, surrounds the limen insulae and spread across the frontal-parietal lobes, connecting memory and limbic structures; injury can cause psychiatric dysfunction [47, 48]. The AF originates in the inferior frontal lobe, surrounds the sylvian fissure, and connects to the superior and middle temporal gyri. The AF transmits language function, and its injury can cause conduction aphasia [31, 49].

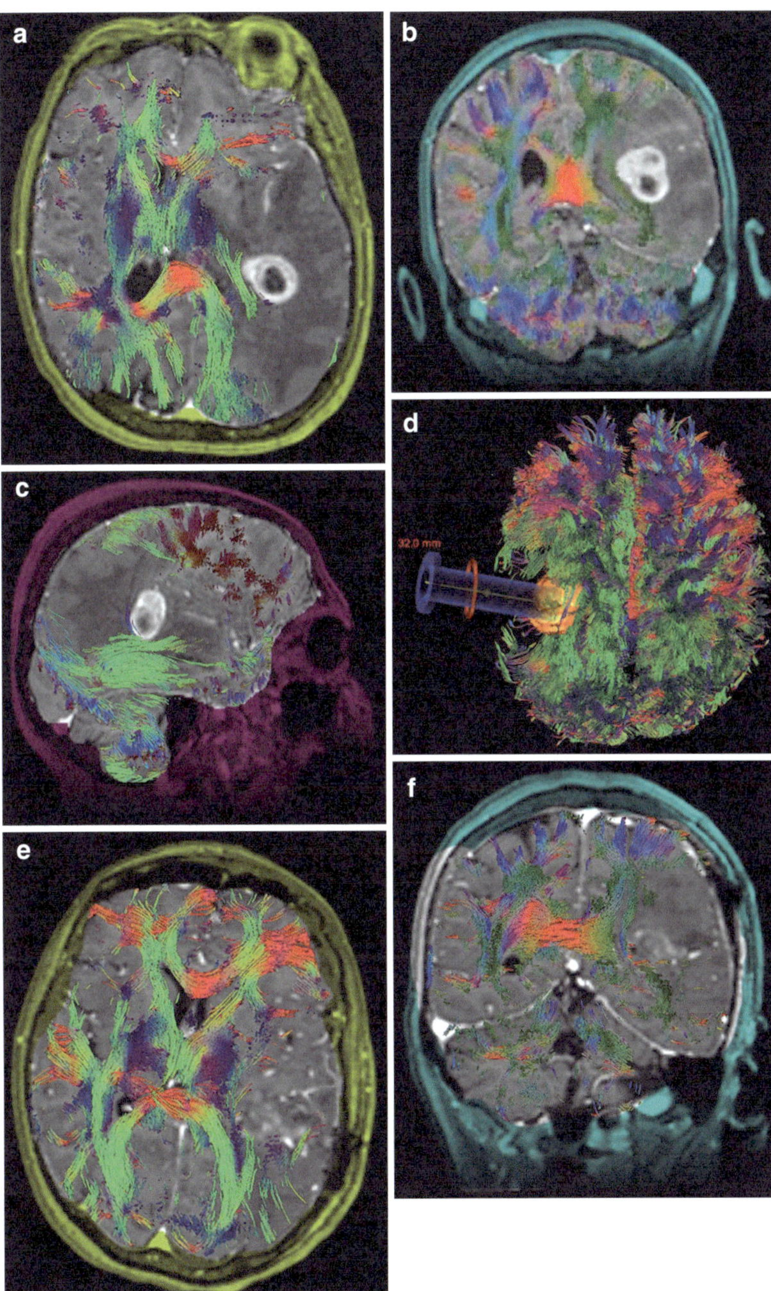

**Fig. 10.4** Preoperative imaging reveals a left parietal mass with contrast enhancement and white matter tracts (**a**–**c**). Planning phase allows construction of a surgical trajectory that clearly avoids critical white matter fibers (**d**). Postoperative imaging demonstrated gross total resection (**e**–**g**)

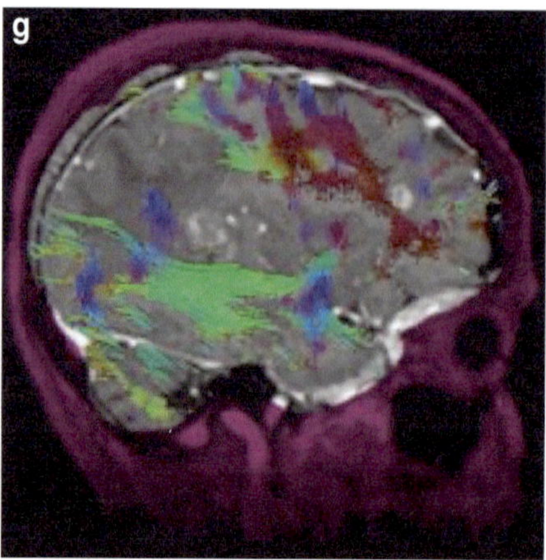


**Fig. 10.4** (continued)

Due to the high density of multiple eloquent fiber tracts, we usually reserve use of the lateral corridor for superficial lesions. Careful preoperative DTI tract analysis and awake cortical/subcortical mapping are two additional modalities that help to preserve neurological function when traversing the lateral cerebral hemisphere.

## Conclusion

Surgical access to subcortical brain lesions represents a challenge where neurosurgeons must preserve each patient's neurological function by respecting normal anatomy and protecting surrounding brain tissue. Minimally-invasive transsulcal-parafascicular standard approaches proved to be safe in subcortical lesions treatment. The employ of delicate microsurgical technique, detailed knowledge of subcortical anatomy, and utilization of modern neuroimaging play a critical role.

## References


1. Geffen G, Walsh A, Simpson D, Jeeves M. Comparison of the effects of transcortical and transcallosal removal of intraventricular tumours. Brain. 1980;103(4):773–88.
2. Kelly PJ, Goerss SJ, Kall BA. The stereotaxic retractor in computer-assisted stereotaxic microsurgery. Technical note. J Neurosurg. 1988;69(2):301–6.
3. Yasargil MG, Cravens GF, Roth P. Surgical approaches to "inaccessible" brain tumors. Clin Neurosurg. 1988;34:42–110.
4. Solaroglu I, Beskonakli E, Kaptanoglu E, Okutan O, Ak F, Taskin Y. Transcortical-transventricular approach in colloid cysts of the third ventricle: surgical experience with 26 cases. Neurosurg Rev. 2004;27(2):89–92.

5. Engh JA, Lunsford LD, Amin DV, Ochalski PG, Fernandez-Miranda J, Prevedello DM, et al. Stereotactically guided endoscopic port surgery for intraventricular tumor and colloid cyst resection. Neurosurgery. 2010;67(3 Suppl Operative):ons198–204; discussion ons-5.

6. Recinos PF, Raza SM, Jallo GI, Recinos VR. Use of a minimally invasive tubular retraction system for deep-seated tumors in pediatric patients. J Neurosurg Pediatr. 2011;7(5):516–21.

7. Labib MA, Shah M, Kassam AB, Young R, Zucker L, Maioriello A, et al. The safety and feasibility of image-guided BrainPath-mediated transsulcul hematoma evacuation: a multicenter study. Neurosurgery. 2017;80(4):515–24.

8. Bauer AM, Rasmussen PA, Bain MD. Initial single-center technical experience with the BrainPath system for acute intracerebral hemorrhage evacuation. Oper Neurosurg (Hagerstown). 2017;13(1):69–76.

9. Kassam AB, Engh JA, Mintz AH, Prevedello DM. Completely endoscopic resection of intraparenchymal brain tumors. J Neurosurg. 2009;110(1):116–23.

10. Nagatani K, Takeuchi S, Feng D, Mori K, Day JD. High-definition exoscope system for microneurosurgery: use of an exoscope in combination with tubular retraction and frameless neuronavigation for microsurgical resection of deep brain lesions. No Shinkei Geka. 2015;43(7):611–7.

11. Eliyas JK, Glynn R, Kulwin CG, Rovin R, Young R, Alzate J, et al. Minimally invasive transsulcal resection of intraventricular and periventricular lesions through a tubular retractor system: multicentric experience and results. World Neurosurg. 2016;90:556–64.

12. Flores BC, Whittemore AR, Samson DS, Barnett SL. The utility of preoperative diffusion tensor imaging in the surgical management of brainstem cavernous malformations. J Neurosurg. 2015;122(3):653–62.

13. Bander ED, Jones SH, Kovanlikaya I, Schwartz TH. Utility of tubular retractors to minimize surgical brain injury in the removal of deep intraparenchymal lesions: a quantitative analysis of FLAIR hyperintensity and apparent diffusion coefficient maps. J Neurosurg. 2016;124(4):1053–60.

14. Soares JM, Magalhaes R, Moreira PS, Sousa A, Ganz E, Sampaio A, et al. A Hitchhiker's guide to functional magnetic resonance imaging. Front Neurosci. 2016;10:515.

15. Day JD. Transsulcal parafascicular surgery using BrainPath® for subcortical lesions. Neurosurgery. 2017;64(CN_suppl_1):151–6.

16. Jennings JE, Kassam AB, Fukui MB, Monroy-Sosa A, Chakravarthi S, Kojis N, et al. The surgical white matter chassis: a practical 3-dimensional atlas for planning subcortical surgical trajectories. Oper Neurosurg (Hagerstown). 2018;14(5):469–82.

17. Nimsky C, Ganslandt O, Hastreiter P, Wang R, Benner T, Sorensen AG, et al. Intraoperative diffusion-tensor MR imaging: shifting of white matter tracts during neurosurgical procedures--initial experience. Radiology. 2005;234(1):218–25.

18. Nimsky C, Ganslandt O, Merhof D, Sorensen AG, Fahlbusch R. Intraoperative visualization of the pyramidal tract by diffusion-tensor-imaging-based fiber tracking. NeuroImage. 2006;30(4):1219–29.

19. Ribas GC, Yasuda A, Ribas EC, Nishikuni K, Rodrigues AJ, Jr Surgical anatomy of microneurosurgical sulcal key points. Neurosurgery. 2006;59(4 Suppl 2):ONS177–210; discussion ONS-1.

20. Monroy-Sosa A, Chakravarthi SS, Fukui MB, Kura B, Jennings JE, Celix JM, et al. White matter-governed superior frontal sulcus surgical paradigm: a radioanatomic microsurgical study-part I. Oper Neurosurg (Hagerstown). 2020;19(4):E343–E56.

21. Gungor A, Baydin S, Middlebrooks EH, Tanriover N, Isler C, Rhoton AL Jr. The white matter tracts of the cerebrum in ventricular surgery and hydrocephalus. J Neurosurg. 2017;126(3):945–71.

22. Baker CM, Burks JD, Briggs RG, Smitherman AD, Glenn CA, Conner AK, et al. The crossed frontal aslant tract: a possible pathway involved in the recovery of supplementary motor area syndrome. Brain Behav. 2018;8(3):e00926.

23. Koutsarnakis C, Liakos F, Kalyvas AV, Skandalakis GP, Komaitis S, Christidi F, et al. The superior frontal transsulcal approach to the anterior ventricular system: exploring the sulcal and subcortical anatomy using anatomic dissections and diffusion tensor imaging tractography. World Neurosurg. 2017;106:339–54.
24. Shinoura N, Suzuki Y, Yamada R, Tabei Y, Saito K, Yagi K. Damage to the right superior longitudinal fasciculus in the inferior parietal lobe plays a role in spatial neglect. Neuropsychologia. 2009;47(12):2600–3.
25. Jang SH, Jang WH. Ideomotor apraxia due to injury of the superior longitudinal fasciculus. Am J Phys Med Rehabil. 2016;95(8):e117–20.
26. Yucel M, Wood SJ, Fornito A, Riffkin J, Velakoulis D, Pantelis C. Anterior cingulate dysfunction: implications for psychiatric disorders? J Psychiatry Neurosci. 2003;28(5):350–4.
27. Fornito A, Yucel M, Wood SJ, Bechdolf A, Carter S, Adamson C, et al. Anterior cingulate cortex abnormalities associated with a first psychotic episode in bipolar disorder. Br J Psychiatry. 2009;194(5):426–33.
28. Ribas GC. The cerebral sulci and gyri. Neurosurg Focus. 2010;28(2):E2.
29. Alves RV, Ribas GC, Parraga RG, de Oliveira E. The occipital lobe convexity sulci and gyri. J Neurosurg. 2012;116(5):1014–23.
30. Martino J, da Silva-Freitas R, Caballero H, Marco de Lucas E, Garcia-Porrero JA, Vazquez-Barquero A. Fiber dissection and diffusion tensor imaging tractography study of the temporoparietal fiber intersection area. Neurosurgery. 2013;72(1 Suppl Operative):87–97; discussion -8.
31. Yagmurlu K, Vlasak AL, Rhoton AL, Jr. Three-dimensional topographic fiber tract anatomy of the cerebrum. Neurosurgery. 2015;11 Suppl 2:274–305; discussion.
32. Ivanova MV, Isaev DY, Dragoy OV, Akinina YS, Petrushevskiy AG, Fedina ON, et al. Diffusion-tensor imaging of major white matter tracts and their role in language processing in aphasia. Cortex. 2016;85:165–81.
33. Kamali A, Sair HI, Radmanesh A, Hasan KM. Decoding the superior parietal lobule connections of the superior longitudinal fasciculus/arcuate fasciculus in the human brain. Neuroscience. 2014;277:577–83.
34. Monroy-Sosa A, Jennings J, Chakravarthi S, Fukui MB, Celix J, Kojis N, et al. Microsurgical anatomy of the vertical rami of the superior longitudinal fasciculus: an intraparietal sulcus dissection study. Oper Neurosurg (Hagerstown). 2019;16(2):226–38.
35. Grefkes C, Fink GR. The functional organization of the intraparietal sulcus in humans and monkeys. J Anat. 2005;207(1):3–17.
36. Luckmann HC, Jacobs HI, Sack AT. The cross-functional role of frontoparietal regions in cognition: internal attention as the overarching mechanism. Prog Neurobiol. 2014;116:66–86.
37. Culham JC, Kanwisher NG. Neuroimaging of cognitive functions in human parietal cortex. Curr Opin Neurobiol. 2001;11(2):157–63.
38. Sanai N, Martino J, Berger MS. Morbidity profile following aggressive resection of parietal lobe gliomas. J Neurosurg. 2012;116(6):1182–6.
39. Andersen RA, Andersen KN, Hwang EJ, Hauschild M. Optic ataxia: from Balint's syndrome to the parietal reach region. Neuron. 2014;81(5):967–83.
40. Jang SH, Kim SH, Kwon HG. The safe area in the parieto-occipital lobe in the human brain: diffusion tensor tractography. World Neurosurg. 2015;83(6):982–6.
41. Koutsarnakis C, Liakos F, Kalyvas AV, Liouta E, Emelifeonwu J, Kalamatianos T, et al. Approaching the atrium through the intraparietal sulcus: mapping the sulcal morphology and correlating the surgical corridor to underlying fiber tracts. Oper Neurosurg (Hagerstown). 2017;13(4):503–16.
42. De Benedictis A, Duffau H, Paradiso B, Grandi E, Balbi S, Granieri E, et al. Anatomo-functional study of the temporo-parieto-occipital region: dissection, tractographic and brain mapping evidence from a neurosurgical perspective. J Anat. 2014;225(2):132–51.
43. Catani M, Jones DK, Donato R, Ffytche DH. Occipito-temporal connections in the human brain. Brain. 2003;126(Pt 9):2093–107.

44. Saur D, Kreher BW, Schnell S, Kummerer D, Kellmeyer P, Vry MS, et al. Ventral and dorsal pathways for language. Proc Natl Acad Sci U S A. 2008;105(46):18035–40.
45. Ffytche DH, Blom JD, Catani M. Disorders of visual perception. J Neurol Neurosurg Psychiatry. 2010;81(11):1280–7.
46. Rubino PA, Rhoton AL Jr, Tong X, Oliveira E. Three-dimensional relationships of the optic radiation. Neurosurgery. 2005;57(4 Suppl):219–27; discussion -27.
47. Kier EL, Staib LH, Davis LM, Bronen RA. MR imaging of the temporal stem: anatomic dissection tractography of the uncinate fasciculus, inferior occipitofrontal fasciculus, and Meyer's loop of the optic radiation. AJNR Am J Neuroradiol. 2004;25(5):677–91.
48. Baydin S, Gungor A, Tanriover N, Baran O, Middlebrooks EH, Rhoton AL Jr. Fiber tracts of the medial and inferior surfaces of the cerebrum. World Neurosurg. 2017;98:34–49.
49. Kamali A, Flanders AE, Brody J, Hunter JV, Hasan KM. Tracing superior longitudinal fasciculus connectivity in the human brain using high resolution diffusion tensor tractography. Brain Struct Funct. 2014;219(1):269–81.

# Chapter 11
# Trans-sulcal, Minimally Invasive Parafascicular Surgery for Brain Metastases


Joshua Bakhsheshian, Ben Allen Strickland, and Gabriel Zada


## Abbreviations

| | |
|---|---|
| DTI | Diffusion tensor imaging |
| FAT | Frontal aslant tract |
| GTR | Gross total resection |
| ILF | Inferior longitudinal fasciculus |
| LITT | Laser-induced thermal therapy |
| MIPS | Minimally invasive parafascicular surgery |
| MRI | Magnetic resonance imaging |
| RPA | Recursive partitioning analysis |
| SLF | Superior longitudinal fasciculus |
| SRS | Stereotactic radiosurgery |
| STR | Subtotal resection |


J. Bakhsheshian (✉)
University of Southern California, Department of Neurosurgery, Los Angeles, CA, USA
e-mail: Joshua.bakhsheshian@med.usc.edu

B. A. Strickland
Los Angeles County General Hospital, Department of Neurosurgery, Los Angeles, CA, USA
e-mail: ben.strickland@med.usc.edu

G. Zada
Keck Hospital, Neurological Surgery, Los Angeles, CA, USA
e-mail: gzada@usc.edu



© Springer Nature Switzerland AG 2022
G. Zada et al. (eds.), *Subcortical Neurosurgery*,
https://doi.org/10.1007/978-3-030-95153-5_11

# Introduction

Brain metastases are the most common central nervous system neoplasms, and their incidence continues to rise with improvements in diagnostic modalities and systemic treatments [1]. Treatment options include various combinations of chemotherapy, stereotactic radiosurgery (SRS) or whole brain radiation therapy, laser-induced thermal therapy (LITT), or craniotomy for surgical resection [2–7].

Prior class I studies have shown greater survival and functional independence with surgical resection of solitary brain metastasis followed by radiation therapy versus those treated with radiation therapy alone [4–6]. Surgery is typically reserved for patients with control of their primary cancer, good neurologic function, and a symptomatic lesion that is often solitary and accessible.

The majority of brain metastases occur at the gray-white junction, which is accessible due to close juxtaposition to the cerebral cortex or cerebellar hemisphere. However, the subset of brain metastases, referred to as deep-seated subcortical lesions, are found within or adjacent to critical white matter tracts, basal ganglia, and thalamus. These lesions are typically treated using stereotactic radiosurgery (SRS) because of the increased associated risk in surgical morbidity. However, there is no preferred treatment option for these subcortical deep-seated metastases when they are larger and are associated with mass effect and significant vasogenic edema. These lesions may not be ideal candidates for radiosurgery alone due to delayed treatment effects, large tumor volumes with significant edema, dependence on corticosteroids, and the lack of tissue availability for molecular analyses.

Recent advancements in minimally invasive parafascicular surgery (MIPS) have aimed to minimize insult to healthy cortical and subcortical tissue through the use of tubular-based retractors and integrated surgical planning based on diffusion tensor imaging of subcortical fascicles. Multiple case series have demonstrated that utilization of a trans-sulcal MIPS approach is a safe and feasible surgical option for the resection of carefully selected metastatic brain lesions [8–11]. The current chapter reviews considerations for using this surgical technique, patient selection, current evidence regarding outcomes, and potential limitations.

# Patient Selection

Multiple treatment options are available and should be carefully considered for patients with brain metastases [6, 12–14]. Intervention in cancer patients depends on overall performance status, predicted survival time, recursive partitioning analysis (RPA) class, medical comorbidities, and patient preferences, among numerous other factors. For patients with larger brain metastases whom are not ideal candidates for radiosurgery (larger tumor volumes, surrounding vasogenic edema, and/or long-term corticosteroid dependence), options may include surgical resection or laser-induced thermal therapy (LITT) [6, 15]. Patients with large (>2 cm), isolated, deep-seated metastatic lesions with associated mass effect may be considered suitable candidates for a trans-sulcal MIPS approach followed by adjuvant SRS. This approach is advantageous when the lesion is found in subcortical critical white matter tracts or nearby basal ganglia and thalamus. These surgical candidates are typically in RPA class I (age <65 years, KPS ≥70, controlled primary cancer, and no extracranial metastases) or RPA class II (age >65 years, KPS ≥70, uncontrolled primary cancer, and/or extracranial metastases) [4, 5]. In some cases, patients can present with suspected brain metastases without a known primary cancer or tumors observed with CT or PET imaging. Melanoma is a classic example of an occult cancer that may present with brain metastasis. In these cases, an additional indication for surgery would be for tissue diagnosis to guide subsequent treatment.

## Surgical Planning and Approach

In patients with subcortical brain metastases, the surgical goal should be maximal safe tumor resection with avoidance of new neurologic deficits. Generally, all cases can be performed under general endotracheal anesthesia with intraoperative neurophysiologic monitoring. In select cases, MIPS can be used during awake craniotomy with mapping for tumors arising in or near eloquent speech or motor regions. Depending on the modalities that will be utilized, SSEP and MEP monitoring and cortical/subcortical speech and motor mapping should be planned for. The patient's head is placed in a Mayfield skull clamp while trying to keep the head in a neutral plain to facilitate orientation. The craniotomy should be centered on the desired sulcus, thus allowing for a trans-sulcal, MIPS approach to minimize potential injury to adjacent eloquent cortical and subcortical areas. Functional and DTI sequences should be used to plan a trajectory parallel to key subcortical tracts including the corticospinal tract, optic radiations, cingulate gyrus, superior longitudinal fasciculus (SLF), inferior longitudinal fasciculus (ILF), arcuate fasciculus, frontal aslant tract (FAT; association fibers of the supplementary motor area complex), and other key white matter tracts. Surgical planning based on a prespecified entry and target point, as well as trajectory, may not be the shortest route to the subcortical mass, but may utilize a longer route to avoid or be in parallel with critical tracts in order to avoid shear injury to these fascicles. When planning an approach and target point for docking and navigation, a deep or surface docking approach may be selected. For most tumors without associated hematomas, we recommend docking on the surface of the tumor. Navigational guidance can assist with planning an ideal skin incision (~4 cm), craniotomy (~3 cm), dural opening (14 mm), and sulcal identification (Fig. 11.1). Minimal diuresis is required for these operations.

Following the craniotomy, the dura is opened in a cruciate fashion. At this point, the exoscope (Karl Storz Endoscopy, Tuttlingen, Germany, or Synaptive Medical, Toronto, Canada) can be brought into the field for operative visualization [16, 17], which can be secured to a pneumatic holder (Karl Storz Endoscopy, Tuttlingen, Germany) or other type of holder for visualization and mobilization. The selected

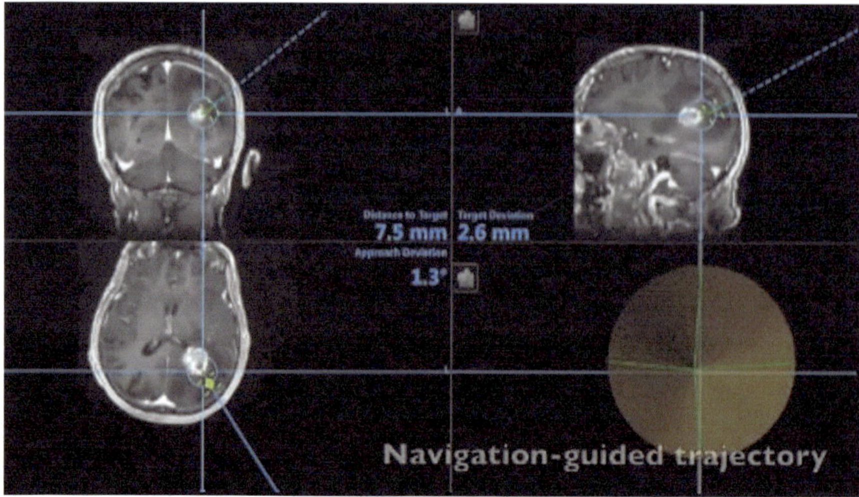


**Fig. 11.1** Navigation-guided trajectory. Frameless stereotactic navigation was utilized to plan and execute a surgical corridor based on assessing sagittal, coronal, and axial images. Identifying of appropriate sulcus for BrainPath retractor entry. (Bakhsheshian et al. [8]. The republishing license is re-attached for your records)

**Fig. 11.2** Identifying the appropriate sulcus is for BrainPath retractor entry

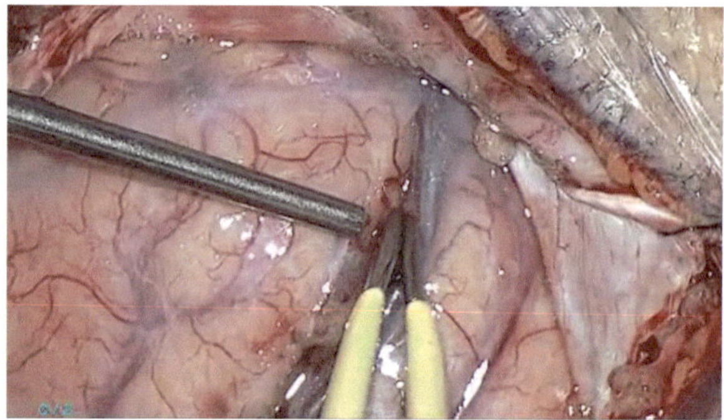

sulcus can be carefully dissected sharply under exoscopic visualization and magnification (Figs. 11.2 and 11.3) using a bimanual technique. A preselected tubular retractor length, based on the trajectory/approach distance, can then be passed to and docked on the superficial surface of the lesion with the aid of stereotactic navigation guidance. Once the superficial aspect of the lesion is reached, the tubular retractor can be fixated using a standard retractor system. The obturator can then be removed, and the exoscope can be used to visualize and resect the tumor at the distal end of the port (Fig. 11.4).

A pseudo en bloc resection can be performed, involving internal debulking with the use of a combination of tumor forceps, suction, tissue-resection device (e.g., cutting aspirator or ultrasonic aspirator), and/or bipolar cautery, followed by delivering the capsule of the tumor circumferentially in one piece. Tumor resection can

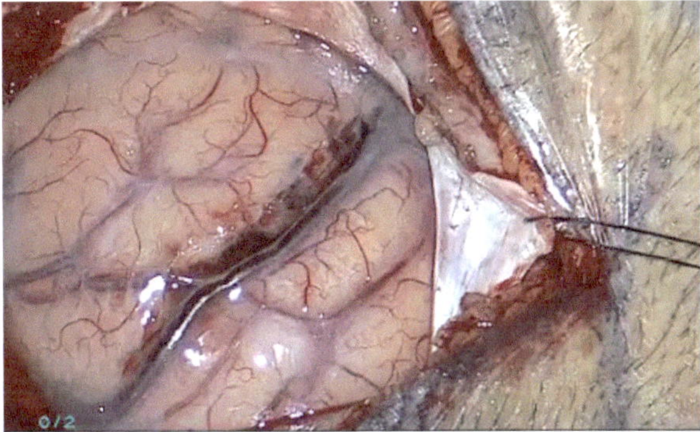

**Fig. 11.3** Sulcal opening used to introduce the tubular retractor

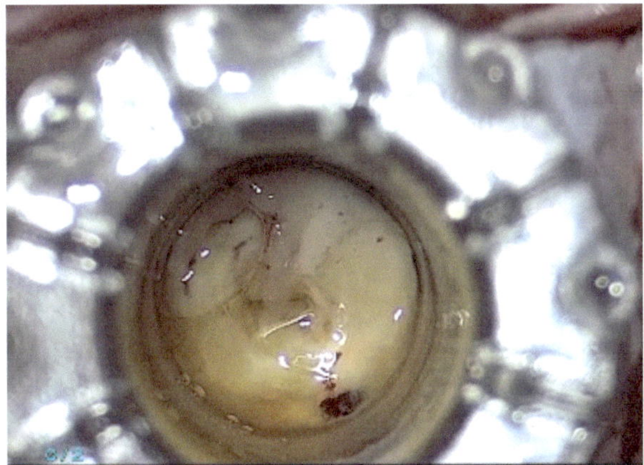

**Fig. 11.4** View of the metastatic lesion with the tubular retractor and exoscope

be performed using standard bimanual microsurgical methods, including piecemeal resection, a side-cutting aspirator, and/or ultrasonic aspirating instruments as needed [18, 19]. During internal debulking, it is important to confine the tumor cells to the tubular retractor to minimize potential dissemination of disease. In cases of larger tumors, the tubular retractor can be manipulated and toggled circumferentially to access the entire tumor. When lesions are adjacent to eloquent motor or speech regions, resection through a piecemeal fashion of tumors nearby eloquent regions may be preferred in an effort to avoid postoperative deficits and used in conjunction with subcortical motor mapping to determine distance to critical corticospinal tracts. In these cases, subtotal resection with the goal of optimizing an adaptive target for subsequent stereotactic radiosurgery may be the preferred option.

In general, hemostasis can be successfully acquired through standard microsurgical techniques, with bayoneted bipolar forceps and the application of standard hemostatic agents (Fig. 11.5). Following resection and achievement of hemostasis, the retractor can be withdrawn, and the dura, bone, and skin can be closed in a standard multilayer fashion. Patients should undergo postoperative stereotactic radiosurgery to the resection cavity within 3 weeks of the surgery.

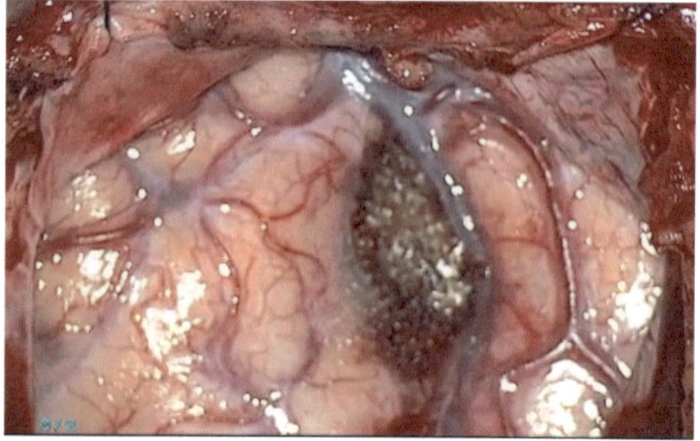

**Fig. 11.5** Sulcal entry point after the tubular retractor was withdrawn and hemostasis was achieved

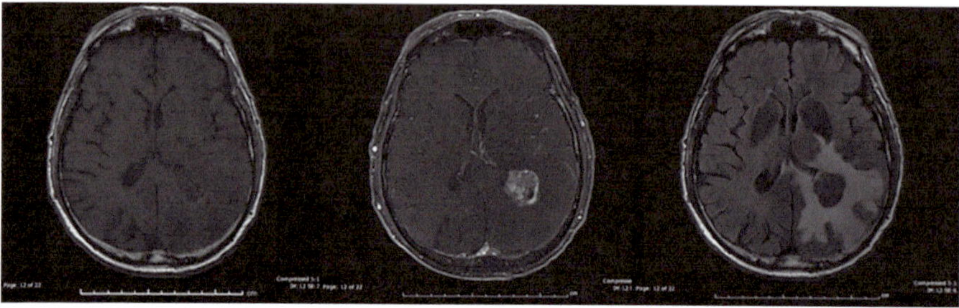

**Fig. 11.6** Example of preoperative imaging of deep-seated metastatic lesion. (Left) Preoperative T1-weighted MRI and (center) T1-weighted post-contrast MRI demonstrated 2.6 × 2.5 cm lobular heterogeneous enhancing lesion within the left parietal periatrial white matter, consistent with a metastatic lesion. (Right) FLAIR MRI demonstrated moderate to large amount of adjacent vasogenic edema and foci of hemorrhage within the lesion (observed on other sequences)

## Illustrative Case [8]

A 72-year-old man with a past medical history of stage IV colon adenocarcinoma presented with aphasia, right-sided apraxia, and visual field deficits. Magnetic resonance imaging (MRI) showed a single, heterogeneously enhancing 2 cm mass with a significant amount of surrounding vasogenic edema found within the left parietal periventricular white matter (Fig. 11.6) and extending anteriorly into the region of the internal capsule. Given the patient's neurologic symptoms, single nature of brain disease, location of lesion, and degree of surrounding edema, surgical resection via MIPS followed by adjuvant radiosurgery was recommended. Under navigational guidance (Fig. 11.1), a 3 cm craniotomy was performed in the left parieto-occipital region, and a 14 mm dural opening was made. A sulcus was identified for the entry point with navigation and dissected open (Figs. 11.2 and 11.3). A 50 mm BrainPath retractor was inserted into the dissected sulcus and cannulated to a depth of 45 mm using navigation guidance in parallel with the optic radiations and then secured. The obturator was then removed, and the exoscope was used to visualize and resect the

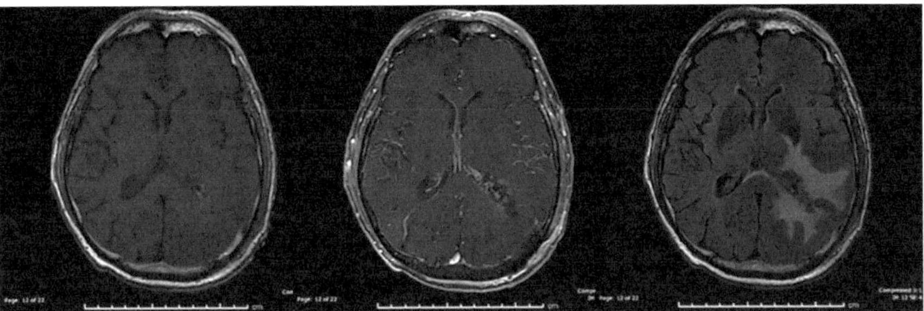

**Fig. 11.7** Example of postoperative imaging of deep-seated metastatic lesion. (Left) Immediate postoperative T1-weighted MRI and T1-weighted post-contrast MRI (center) demonstrated gross total resection of left parietal mass and decreased (right) signal on FLAIR

tumor and the distal end of the port (Fig. 11.4). The tumor was removed using a combination of suction, piecemeal resection, and side-cutting aspirator until an intraoperative GTR was achieved. There were no changes in somatosensory or motor evoked potential monitoring. Following meticulous hemostasis, the tube was gently withdrawn, and hemostasis was achieved along the tract using Surgicel (Fig. 11.5). Immediate postoperative MR imaging confirmed GTR (Fig. 11.7). The final pathology diagnosis was consistent with metastatic colon adenocarcinoma. There were no complications associated with the surgery, and the patient was discharged home on postoperative day 2. He subsequently received adjuvant radiosurgery to the resection cavity followed by chemotherapy and rapid tapering off corticosteroids. At 3-month follow-up, the patient's presenting neurologic symptoms had resolved. MRI at that time demonstrated no evidence of residual or recurrent tumor.

## Evidence

The resection of single, symptomatic brain metastases in conjunction with radiation-based treatments has already been shown to demonstrate an overall survival benefit in class I randomized clinical trial studies [4, 5]. Furthermore, acquiring gross total resection (GTR) of brain metastases has been shown to improve patient survival in retrospective comparative studies [20, 21]. Resections of metastatic lesions through a modern tubular port, even those prone to hemorrhage, do not appear to pose as a major obstacle for resection. The utilization of a navigable tubular retractor and exoscope appears to be a safe and feasible surgical option for trans-sulcal resection of carefully selected metastatic brain lesions.

There are a number of case series that have demonstrated the feasibility and safety in the use of MIPS with exoscopic visualization for deep-seated metastatic lesions [8–11].

Our institution led and published a multi-center retrospective study including 25 patients harboring metastatic brain tumors, where GTR was achieved in 80% of patient. In this series, 19 patients (76%) demonstrated neurologic improvement; 20% remained stable. Complications occurred in one patient (4.0%), which included postoperative hemiparesis and subsequent deep vein thrombosis. This patient had a 3.5 cm lesion (measured at widest diameter) with a firm capsule and core located in the deep left frontal lobe adjacent to the posterior internal capsule. During surgical resection of the medial portion of this lesion, reductions in right-sided motor evoked potentials were noted, and the resection was aborted (subtotal resection of brain metastases may be the surgical goal for selected deep-seated lesions located near eloquent regions). The patient had postoperative hemiparesis that gradually resolved. J.D. Day reported a single-surgeon experience with this approach in 20 metastatic brain tumors, where GTR was achieved in 19 (95%), postoperative hemorrhage occurred in 1 (5%) that did not require evacuation, no neurologic deficits, and perioperative mortality in 1 (5%) due to pulmonary complications in a patient with non-small cell lung carcinoma [9]. Gassie et al. investigated 15 deep-seated metastatic brain tumor cases and obtained GTR in 14 (93%) and observed no local complications [10]. Generally, this technique was not associated with a higher risk of complications, and most patients were able to undergo postoperative SRS.

To date, this technique has been performed with the aid of the microscope, endoscope, and exoscope using tubular retraction systems [16, 18, 22]. The use of an exoscope has a wider focal distance and volume of focus while providing high-quality views of the surgical field on a monitor [16, 17]. Thus, there has been a growing interest in investigating the use of the exoscope with modern tubular retraction systems for accessing subcortical brain lesions [16–18, 23, 24]. The use of an endoscope with modern tubular retractors has previously been shown to result in higher rates of subtotal resections [25, 26].

Deep-seated tumors typically require larger craniotomies and dural openings for access. Retraction during these cases may result in increased ischemic injury to adjacent normal tissue [27]. As a result, the surgical management of many deep-seated tumors has been limited by its associated complications and with the advent of radiosurgery as a viable treatment option. However, radiosurgery alone does not offer the benefits of relieving associated mass effect, debulking to increase effectiveness of adjuvant treatments, and tissue sampling for molecular analyses and targeted treatments.

Additional benefits with the current MIPS approach may also include shorter hospital length of stay. While a direct comparison between channel-based parafascicular and open traditional approaches cannot be drawn, median postoperative hospital stay appeared to be lower with the channel-based technique than prior reports (2 days vs. 6–7 days) [1, 28]. The hospital stay data can also be confounded by required additional diagnostic evaluations/consultations or length of inpatient rehabilitation.

## Additional Considerations

Deep-seated subcortical metastatic lesions represent a subset of the population of patients with metastatic tumors. There currently are no high-level comparative studies demonstrating their superiority over traditional approaches. However, the use of channel-based retraction is minimally invasive, which provides a safe alternative surgical approach.

Subtotal resection of brain metastases may be a cogent surgical goal for selected deep-seated lesions located near eloquent regions. Tumors in eloquent regions may require resection using a piecemeal or pseudo en bloc fashion, as an en bloc resection is not feasible in these regions. Previous investigations have suggested that piecemeal resection of single metastatic brain lesions may increase the risk for leptomeningeal disease and local recurrence when compared to en bloc resection [29, 30]. However, postoperative radiotherapy was not performed in those cases included in prior investigative studies, and it remains unclear if the benefit of en bloc resection would still be present with modern postoperative radiation treatment options.

A tumor's consistency (i.e., firmness) is an important factor to be aware of, as it may become a surgical obstacle. A softer tumor consistency will likely be more amenable for channel-based resection [8]. This is in line with reports that the soft consistency of intracerebral hematomas likely facilitates channel-based evacuation [23, 24]. Predicting the consistency of tumors, including adhesion to surrounding brain parenchyma, could provide valuable information for preoperative planning and predicting the extent of resection [31, 32]. At the very least, presurgical knowledge pertaining to the consistency of the lesion may help planning surface or deep docking into a tumor, as surface docking is mandated in very firm or calcified tumors.

## Conclusions

Brain metastases are the most common intracranial neoplasms, and their reported incidence continues to increase [1]. When used in combination with radiation-based treatments, safe maximal surgical resection has been advocated as a primary option for selected patients with brain metastasis [1, 6, 28]. Multiple case series have demonstrated that utilization of a navigable tubular retractor appears to be a safe and feasible surgical option for trans-sulcal, MIPS resection of carefully selected metastatic brain lesions. Additional benefits with the current approach may include shorter hospital length of stay, safer tissue acquisition, and optimization of target volume for subsequent stereotactic radiosurgery.

# References


1. D'Andrea G, Palombi L, Minniti G, Pesce A, Marchetti P. Brain metastases: surgical treatment and overall survival. World Neurosurg. 2017;97:169–77.
2. Andrews DW, Scott CB, Sperduto PW, Flanders AE, Gaspar LE, Schell MC, et al. Whole brain radiation therapy with or without stereotactic radiosurgery boost for patients with one to three brain metastases: phase III results of the RTOG 9508 randomised trial. Lancet. 2004;363(9422):1665–72.
3. Aoyama H, Shirato H, Tago M, Nakagawa K, Toyoda T, Hatano K, et al. Stereotactic radio-surgery plus whole-brain radiation therapy vs stereotactic radiosurgery alone for treatment of brain metastases: a randomized controlled trial. JAMA. 2006;295(21):2483–91.
4. Patchell RA, Tibbs PA, Walsh JW, Dempsey RJ, Maruyama Y, Kryscio RJ, et al. A ran-domized trial of surgery in the treatment of single metastases to the brain. N Engl J Med. 1990;322(8):494–500.
5. Vecht CJ, Haaxma-Reiche H, Noordijk EM, Padberg GW, Voormolen JH, Hoekstra FH, et al. Treatment of single brain metastasis: radiotherapy alone or combined with neurosurgery? Ann Neurol. 1993;33(6):583–90.
6. Kalkanis SN, Kondziolka D, Gaspar LE, Burri SH, Asher AL, Cobbs CS, et al. The role of sur-gical resection in the management of newly diagnosed brain metastases: a systematic review and evidence-based clinical practice guideline. J Neuro-Oncol. 2010;96(1):33–43.
7. Carpentier A, McNichols RJ, Stafford RJ, Itzcovitz J, Guichard JP, Reizine D, et al. Real-time magnetic resonance-guided laser thermal therapy for focal metastatic brain tumors. Neurosurgery. 2008;63(1 Suppl 1):ONS21–8; discussion ONS8–9.
8. Bakhsheshian J, Strickland BA, Jackson C, Chaichana KL, Young R, Pradilla G, et al. Multicenter investigation of channel-based subcortical trans-sulcal exoscopic resec-tion of metastatic brain tumors: a retrospective case series. Oper Neurosurg (Hagerstown). 2019;16(2):159–66.
9. Day JD. Transsulcal parafascicular surgery using BrainPath® for subcortical lesions. Neurosurgery. 2017;64(CN_suppl_1):151–6.
10. Gassie K, Alvarado-Estrada K, Bechtle P, Chaichana KL. Surgical management of deep-seated metastatic brain tumors using minimally invasive approaches. J Neurol Surg A Cent Eur Neurosurg. 2019;80(3):198–204.
11. Gassie K, Wijesekera O, Chaichana KL. Minimally invasive tubular retractor-assisted biopsy and resection of subcortical intra-axial gliomas and other neoplasms. J Neurosurg Sci. 2018;62(6):682–9.
12. Gaspar LE, Mehta MP, Patchell RA, Burri SH, Robinson PD, Morris RE, et al. The role of whole brain radiation therapy in the management of newly diagnosed brain metastases: a systematic review and evidence-based clinical practice guideline. J Neuro-Oncol. 2010;96(1):17–32.
13. Mehta MP, Paleologos NA, Mikkelsen T, Robinson PD, Ammirati M, Andrews DW, et al. The role of chemotherapy in the management of newly diagnosed brain metastases: a systematic review and evidence-based clinical practice guideline. J Neuro-Oncol. 2010;96(1):71–83.
14. Linskey ME, Andrews DW, Asher AL, Burri SH, Kondziolka D, Robinson PD, et al. The role of stereotactic radiosurgery in the management of patients with newly diagnosed brain metas-tases: a systematic review and evidence-based clinical practice guideline. J Neuro-Oncol. 2010;96(1):45–68.
15. Rahmathulla G, Recinos PF, Kamian K, Mohammadi AM, Ahluwalia MS, Barnett GH. MRI-guided laser interstitial thermal therapy in neuro-oncology: a review of its current clinical applications. Oncology. 2014;87(2):67–82.
16. Mamelak AN, Nobuto T, Berci G. Initial clinical experience with a high-definition exoscope system for microneurosurgery. Neurosurgery. 2010;67(2):476–83.
17. Mamelak AN, Danielpour M, Black KL, Hagike M, Berci G. A high-definition exoscope system for neurosurgery and other microsurgical disciplines: preliminary report. Surg Innov. 2008;15(1):38–46.

18. Eliyas JK, Glynn R, Kulwin CG, Rovin R, Young R, Alzate J, et al. Minimally invasive trans-sulcal resection of intraventricular and periventricular lesions through a tubular retractor system: multicentric experience and results. World Neurosurg. 2016;90:556–64.
19. McLaughlin N, Ditzel Filho LF, Prevedello DM, Kelly DF, Carrau RL, Kassam AB. Side-cutting aspiration device for endoscopic and microscopic tumor removal. J Neurol Surg B Skull Base. 2012;73(1):11–20.
20. Agboola O, Benoit B, Cross P, Da Silva V, Esche B, Lesiuk H, et al. Prognostic factors derived from recursive partition analysis (RPA) of Radiation Therapy Oncology Group (RTOG) brain metastases trials applied to surgically resected and irradiated brain metastatic cases. Int J Radiat Oncol Biol Phys. 1998;42(1):155–9.
21. Tendulkar RD, Liu SW, Barnett GH, Vogelbaum MA, Toms SA, Jin T, et al. RPA classification has prognostic significance for surgically resected single brain metastasis. Int J Radiat Oncol Biol Phys. 2006;66(3):810–7.
22. Greenfield JP, Cobb WS, Tsouris AJ, Schwartz TH. Stereotactic minimally invasive tubular retractor system for deep brain lesions. Neurosurgery. 2008;63(4 Suppl 2):334–9; discussion 9–40.
23. Labib MA, Shah M, Kassam AB, Young R, Zucker L, Maioriello A, et al. The safety and feasibility of image-guided BrainPath-mediated transsulcul hematoma evacuation: a multicenter study. Neurosurgery. 2017;80(4):515–24.
24. Bauer AM, Rasmussen PA, Bain MD. Initial single-center technical experience with the BrainPath system for acute intracerebral hemorrhage evacuation. Oper Neurosurg. 2017;13(1):69–76.
25. Kassam AB, Engh JA, Mintz AH, Prevedello DM. Completely endoscopic resection of intra-parenchymal brain tumors. J Neurosurg. 2009;110(1):116–23.
26. Hong CS, Prevedello DM, Elder JB. Comparison of endoscope- versus microscope-assisted resection of deep-seated intracranial lesions using a minimally invasive port retractor system. J Neurosurg. 2016;124(3):799–810.
27. Bander ED, Jones SH, Kovanlikaya I, Schwartz TH. Utility of tubular retractors to minimize surgical brain injury in the removal of deep intraparenchymal lesions: a quantitative analysis of FLAIR hyperintensity and apparent diffusion coefficient maps. J Neurosurg. 2016;124(4):1053–60.
28. Paek SH, Audu PB, Sperling MR, Cho J, Andrews DW. Reevaluation of surgery for the treatment of brain metastases: review of 208 patients with single or multiple brain metastases treated at one institution with modern neurosurgical techniques. Neurosurgery. 2005;56(5):1021–34; discussion -34.
29. Patel AJ, Suki D, Hatiboglu MA, Abouassi H, Shi W, Wildrick DM, et al. Factors influencing the risk of local recurrence after resection of a single brain metastasis. J Neurosurg. 2010;113(2):181–9.
30. Patel AJ, Suki D, Hatiboglu MA, Rao VY, Fox BD, Sawaya R. Impact of surgical methodology on the complication rate and functional outcome of patients with a single brain metastasis. J Neurosurg. 2015;122(5):1132–43.
31. Zada G, Yashar P, Robison A, Winer J, Khalessi A, Mack WJ, et al. A proposed grading system for standardizing tumor consistency of intracranial meningiomas. Neurosurg Focus. 2013;35(6):E1.
32. Yin Z, Hughes JD, Glaser KJ, Manduca A, Van Gompel J, Link MJ, et al. Slip interface imaging based on MR-elastography preoperatively predicts meningioma-brain adhesion. J Magn Reson Imaging. 2017;46(4):1007–16.

# Chapter 12
# Minimally Invasive Parafascicular Surgery (MIPS) for Primary and Metastatic Brain Neoplasms

J. D. Day

## Introduction

Subcortical neoplasms present a particularly challenging problem for surgical resection in terms of limiting disruption of cortical tissue and white matter. The lesions are by nature deep in the brain tissue, and therefore access is limited by the morbidity that is inherent in dissecting cortex and white matter to reach the lesion. Traditionally, a corticotomy with blunt white matter separation or division followed by placement of fixed blade retractors to access the lesion has been practiced. Dissecting through white matter with bipolar forceps is inherently disruptive to the tracts. Combined with retraction by fixed blade retractors that apply pressure, especially at the edge of the retractor blades, it is likely that significant damage to white matter can occur with this method. Further compounding the problem is the character of enhancing vision with the surgical microscope that has its own inherent limitations when viewing down a narrow corridor in terms of light delivery and depth of field. Focal depth is limited with the microscope. Light delivery down a narrow corridor is limited depending on the width and depth of the approach corridor. Given our current state of knowledge of brain connectivity, and technological developments in the areas of optics, computer power, image guidance, and miniaturized mechanical devices, a better strategy is mandated.

Different methods have been proposed to improve upon our ability to access such deep lesions while minimizing morbidity [1, 2]. The method that is discussed in this chapter utilizes a combination of imaging technology (e.g., diffusion tensor imaging), computerized image guidance, a tubular retraction device, a

J. D. Day (✉)
Department of Neurosurgery, University of Arkansas for Medical Sciences, Little Rock, AR, USA
e-mail: jdday@uams.edu

© Springer Nature Switzerland AG 2022
G. Zada et al. (eds.), *Subcortical Neurosurgery*,
https://doi.org/10.1007/978-3-030-95153-5_12

high-definition visualization platform, and a specially designed side-cutting aspiration resection device [3–5] to mitigate against excessive damage to white matter tracts while accessing subcortical lesions.

## Patient Selection

As with most every situation that neurosurgeons are called to intervene, patient selection for the particular method proposed is critical to a successful outcome. Even the most technically well-done operation can fail if the lesion is not amenable to the approach. This technique is certainly and particularly no exception to that rule. This surgical technique is appropriate for subcortical neoplasms, intracerebral hematomas [6], and selected intraventricular lesions. This discussion will focus on appropriate use for neoplasms.

Both primary and secondary subcortical neoplasms may be considered for resection with this technique. There are a number of considerations to take into account based upon preoperative imaging. Though lesions of any depth may be considered, a lesion that presents to the surface is not an ideal candidate for this technique unless a hybrid approach, incorporating both traditional microsurgery and a trans-sulcal parafascicular approach, is the operative plan. Many neoplasms that involve the cortical surface of course can be well handled through a small, targeted (i.e., image-guided) craniotomy and microsurgically removed. In general, lesions that are below the cortical surface are good candidates for the technique, especially if deeply located (Fig. 12.1). Tumors involving the basal ganglia and those that are periventricular or deep within lobar white matter are ideal (Fig. 12.2). Lesions in a cerebellar hemisphere may also be considered. Lesions that arise from, or extend to, the skull base are probably better treated via an alternative strategy.

## Preoperative Preparation and Planning

When considering utilization of this technique for subcortical tumors, complete imaging information is integral in formulating an operative strategy. Magnetic resonance imaging (MRI) must include diffusion-weighted imaging (DWI) and diffusion tensor imaging (DTI) with three-dimensional tractography studies to assist in surgical planning (Fig. 12.3). The essential importance of these studies cannot be overstated.

DWI studies help to determine the character of the neoplasm in terms of water content, which helps predict the density and firmness of the tumor (Fig. 12.4). This is particularly important in planning whether to penetrate the port into the tumor, a so-called depth cannulation, or to target the surface of the tumor, a so-called surface cannulation. The technical considerations of this will be discussed later in the discussion. In general, lesions that appear to be soft will be best approached by

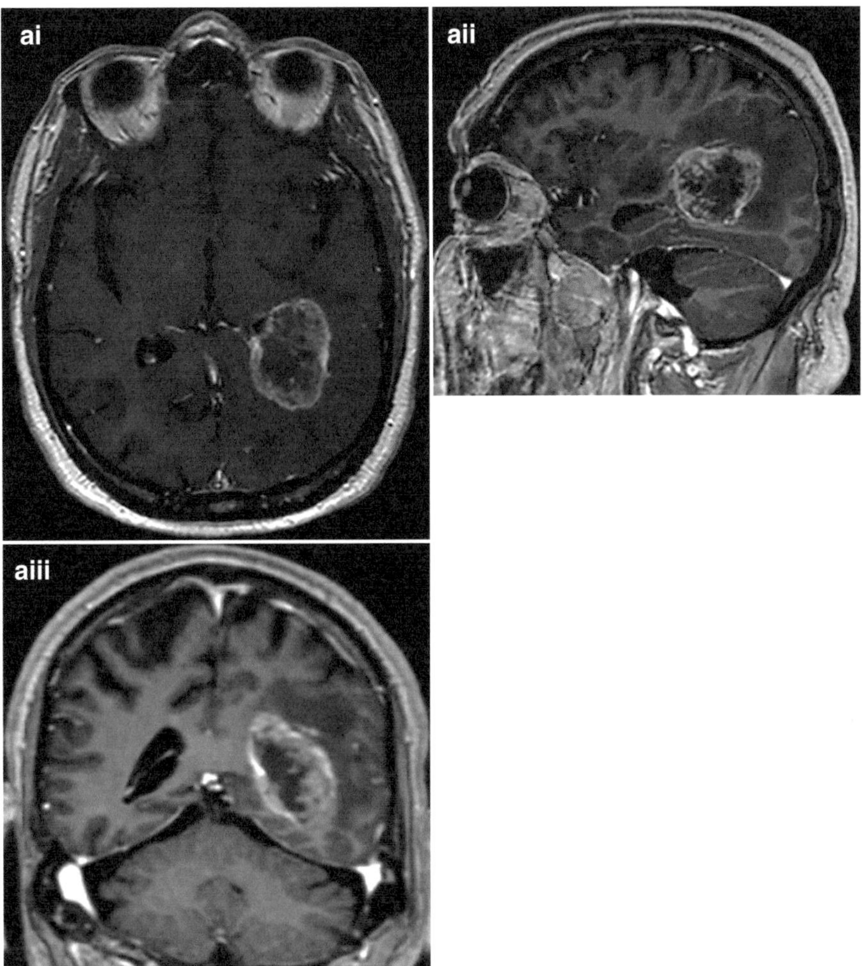

**Fig. 12.1** (**a**) Preoperative MRI T1 axial (i), sagittal (ii), and coronal (iii) views with contrast of a glioblastoma in a 63-year-old patient treated with the minimally invasive parafascicular surgery (MIPS) technique. (**b**) Postoperative MRI T1 axial (i), sagittal (ii), and coronal (iii) films demonstrating gross total resection. (**c**) Screenshot of axial slice of a three-dimensional tractography study on the patient prior to surgery. (**d**) (i) Preoperative MRI T1 with DTI mapping overlay demonstrating a left basal ganglia mass with displacement of the corticospinal tract. (ii, iii) Preoperative T2 axial and coronal views demonstrating significant peritumoral edema. (**e**) Postoperative MRI T1 axial (i), sagittal (ii), and coronal (iii) images demonstrating gross total resection

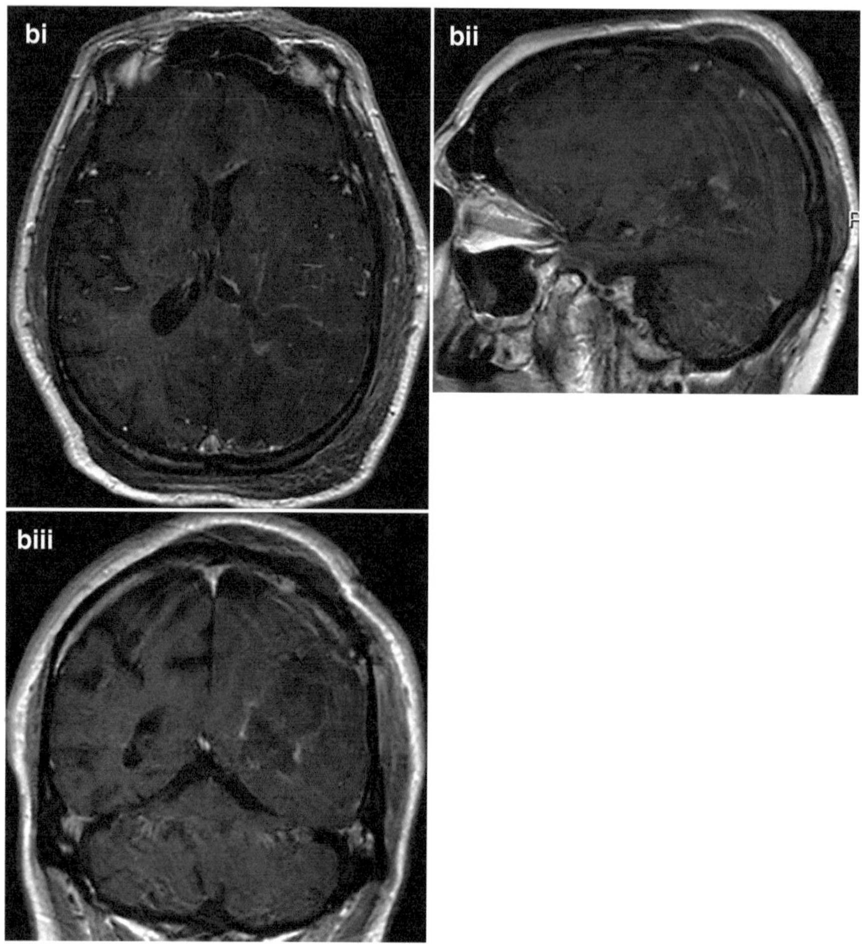

**Fig. 12.1** (continued)

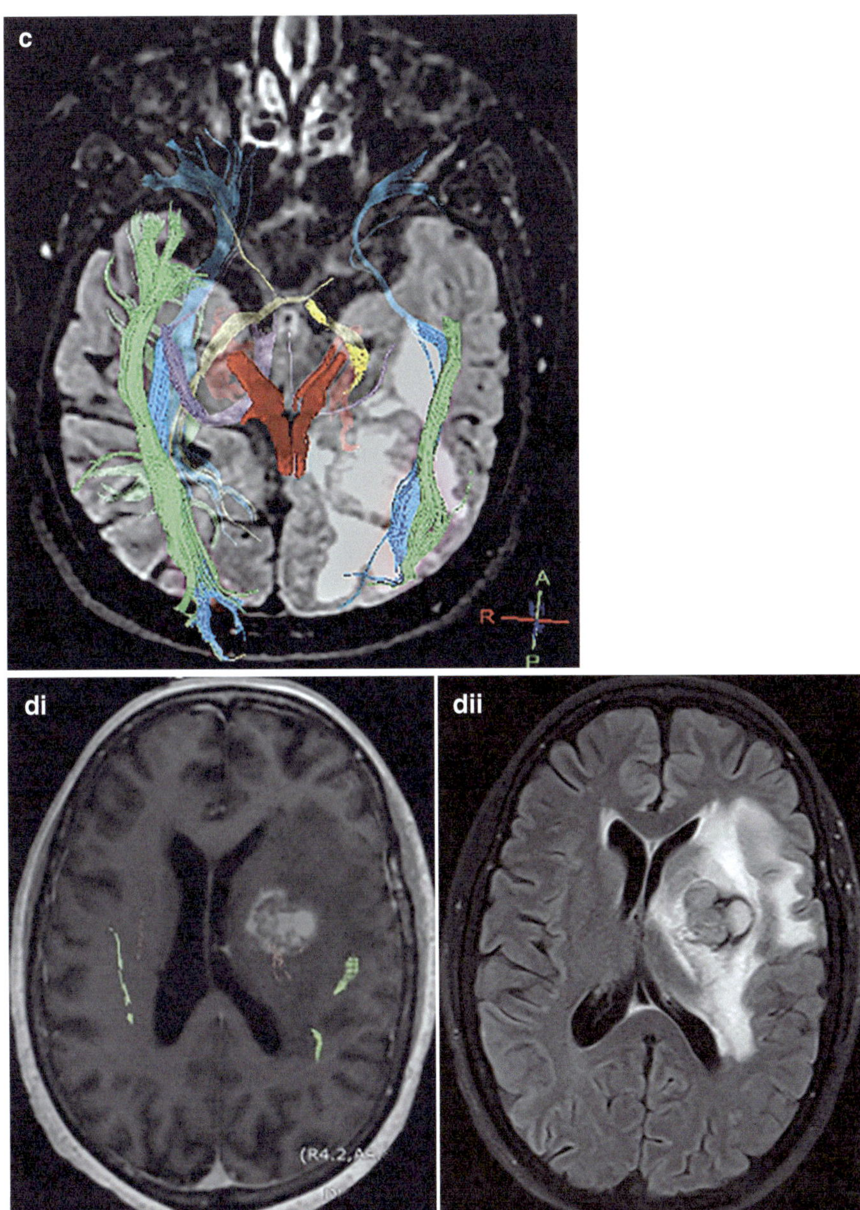

**Fig. 12.1** (continued)

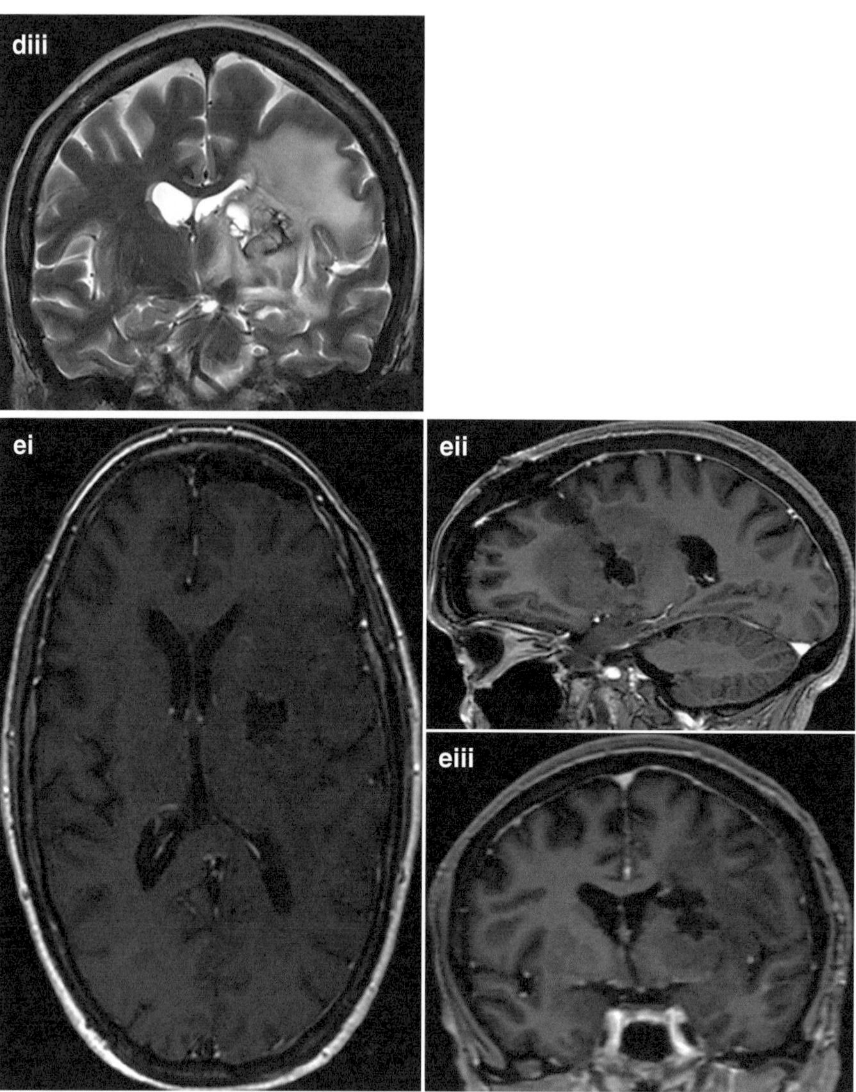

**Fig. 12.1** (continued)

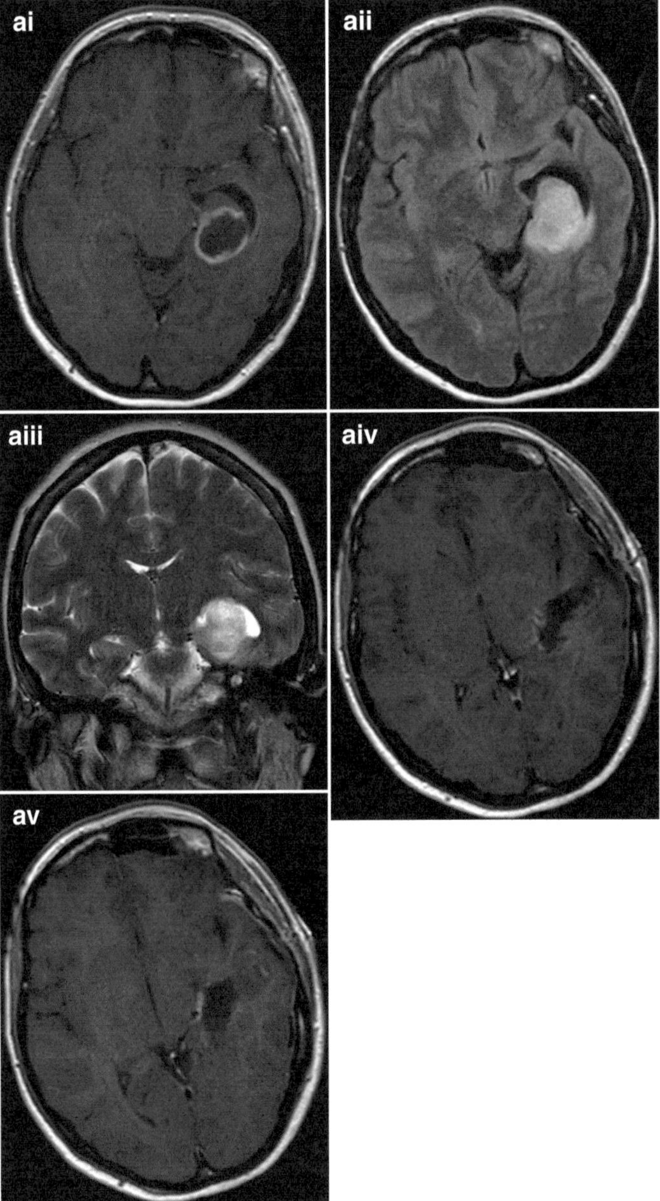

**Fig. 12.2** Examples of tumors amenable to a MIPS technique. (**a**) Preoperative MRI T1 with contrast axial (i), FLAIR axial (ii), and T2 coronal (iii) views of a left temporal glioblastoma in a 52-year-old woman. Postoperative T1 with contrast axial (iv, v) views showing approach tract via the superior temporal sulcus. (**b**) A 64-year-old woman with short-term memory loss with MRI T1 contrast axial (i), coronal (ii), and sagittal (iii) views showing a high-grade glioma. Postoperative T1 contrast axial (iv), coronal (v), and sagittal (vi) postoperative views showing the parieto-occipital approach trajectory. (**c**) Large right temporal mass in a 53-year-old man. Preoperative MRI T1 contrast axial (i), coronal (ii), and sagittal (iii) views prior to a posterior temporal MIPS approach. Axial (iv), coronal (v), and sagittal (vi) postoperative MRI T1 contrast imaging demonstrated gross total resection

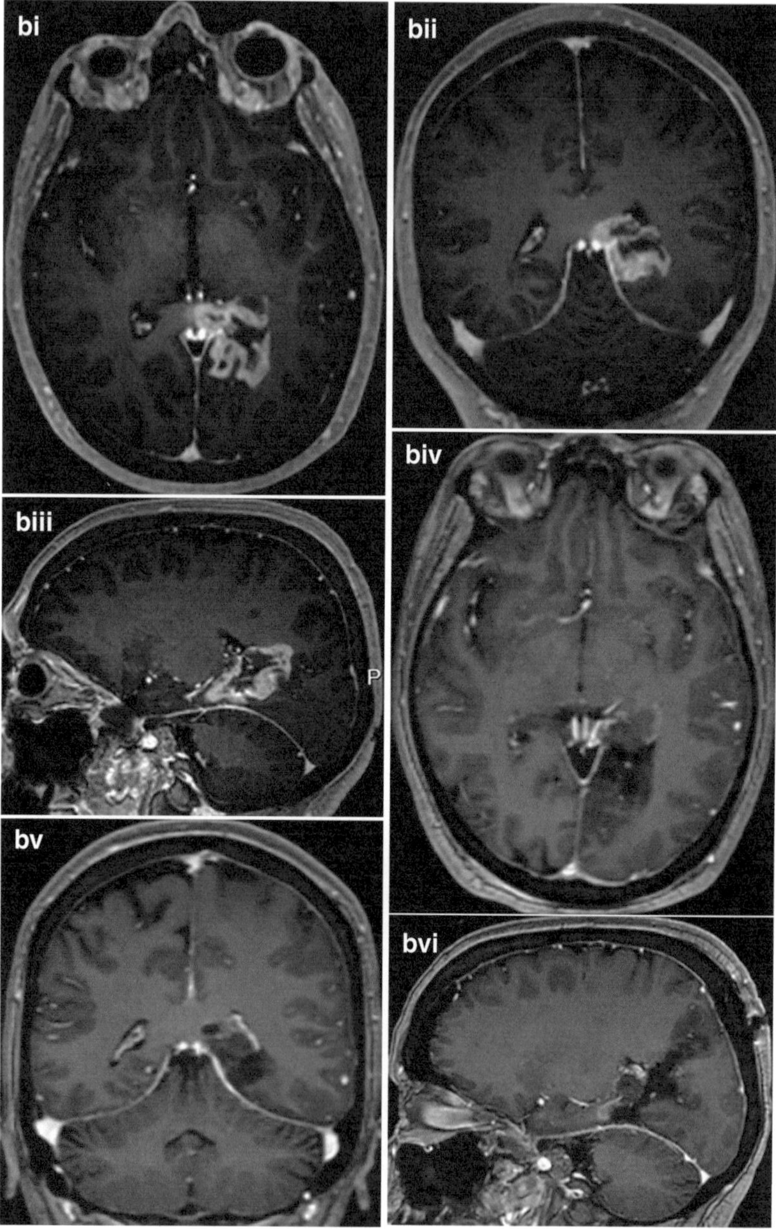

**Fig. 12.2** (continued)

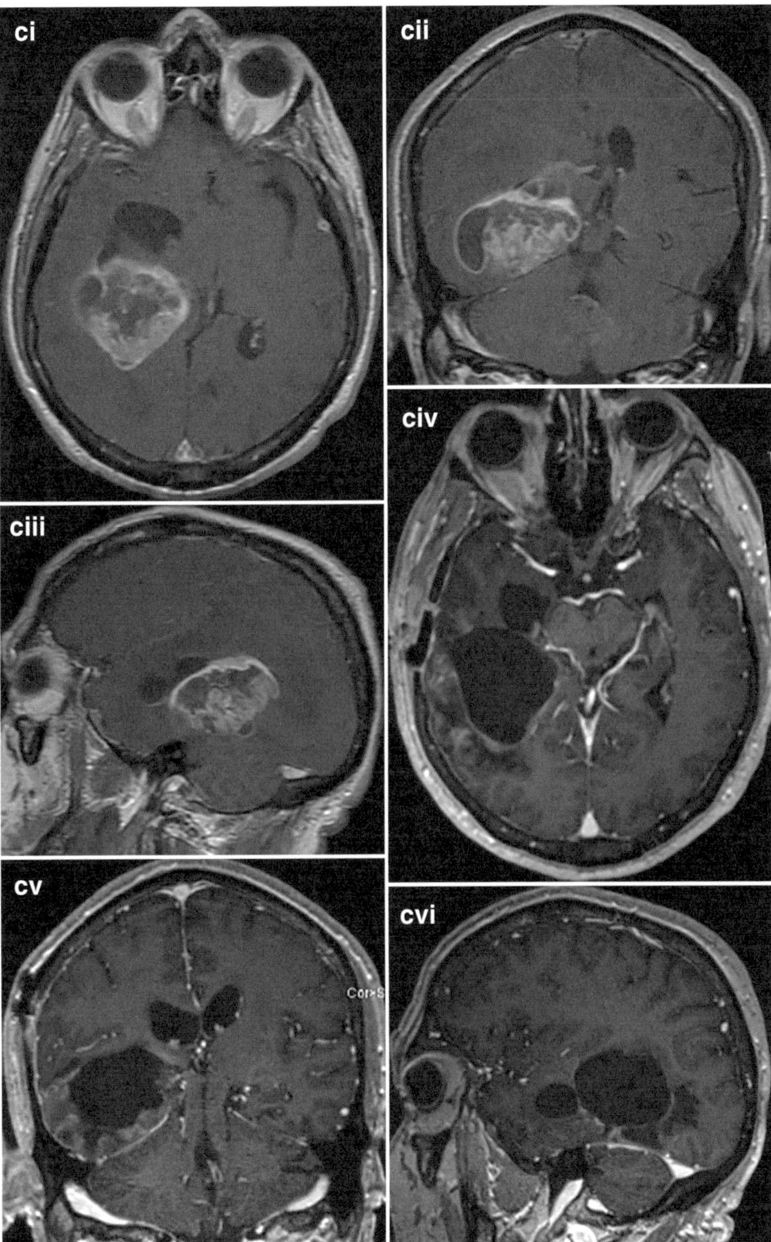

**Fig. 12.2** (continued)

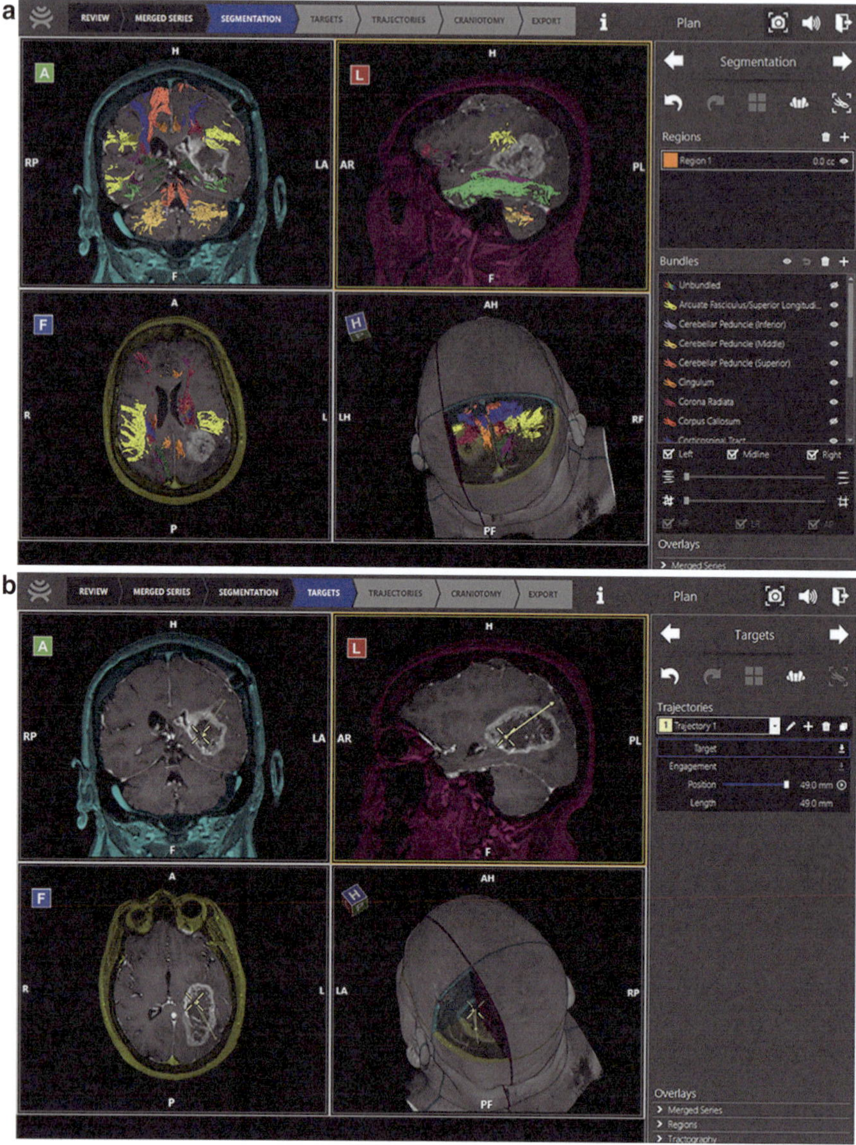



**Fig. 12.3** (**a**) Example case of a patient with a left parieto-occipital glioblastoma treated with MIPS utilizing the Synaptive Bright Matter software platform for preoperative evaluation and planning. Tractography is the first step in evaluating options for trajectory planning. (**b**) A trajectory to the lesion as parallel as possible to the displaced tracts is planned with a depth cannulation owing to the soft nature of the tumor determined on DWI. (**c**) The craniotomy planning feature of the software is utilized to help predict the appropriate craniotomy to effectively reach the entire lesion

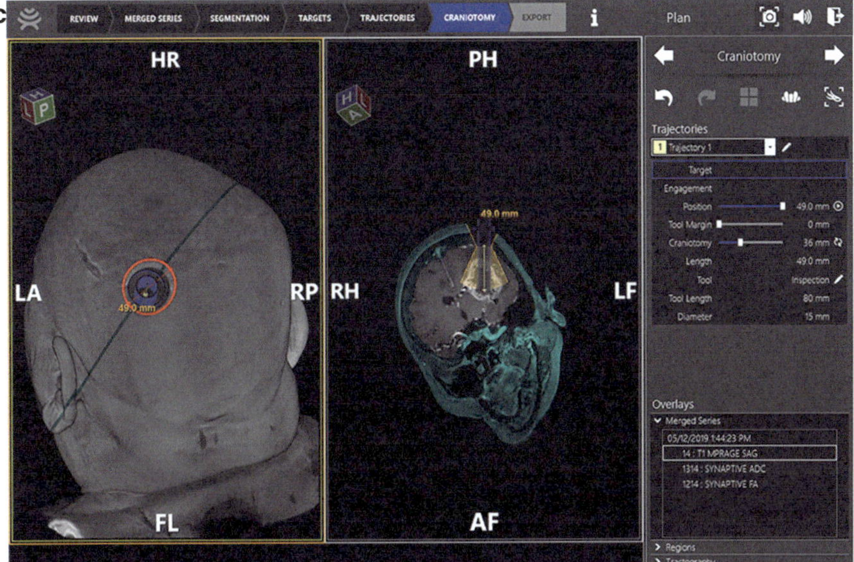



**Fig. 12.3**  (continued)

targeting a point in the depth of the tumor. More dense, firm lesions are planned so as to place the BrainPath retractor at the surface of the lesion.

Careful study of the MRI data is critical as part of this technique. The tubular port (e.g., BrainPath) is inserted in a trans-sulcal manner, and therefore this is an additional important planning aspect. A combination of the DTI data and the surface anatomy of the brain is considered in planning the approach (Fig. 12.5). A cannulation that is as parallel as possible to the direction of any major white matter fascicular bundle is optimal. Also of consideration is the shape of the lesion. As much as possible, the trajectory of approach should be planned along the long axis of a lesion. This is an important consideration as in most every case, a degree of toggling of the port is necessary to reach all portions of the tumor. Any limitation in toggling of the port must be considered and is included in at least some software packages for planning based upon the DTI data. A combination of these two factors, fascicular anatomy and tumor size and shape, is a primary consideration in surgical planning.

Patients may be operated either under general anesthesia or awake with conscious sedation. The selection of anesthetic method depends upon a number of factors, both patient and lesion location specific. Certainly, tumors in eloquent areas that lend themselves to physical examination and determination of function are generally operated in the author's practice under a protocol for awake craniotomy. An additional potential advantage of awake craniotomy is a faster recovery and discharge from the hospital. Therefore, it is often advantageous to employ an awake technique if the patient can tolerate the procedure. Factors that have been found to be a relative contraindication in the author's experience to an awake craniotomy are

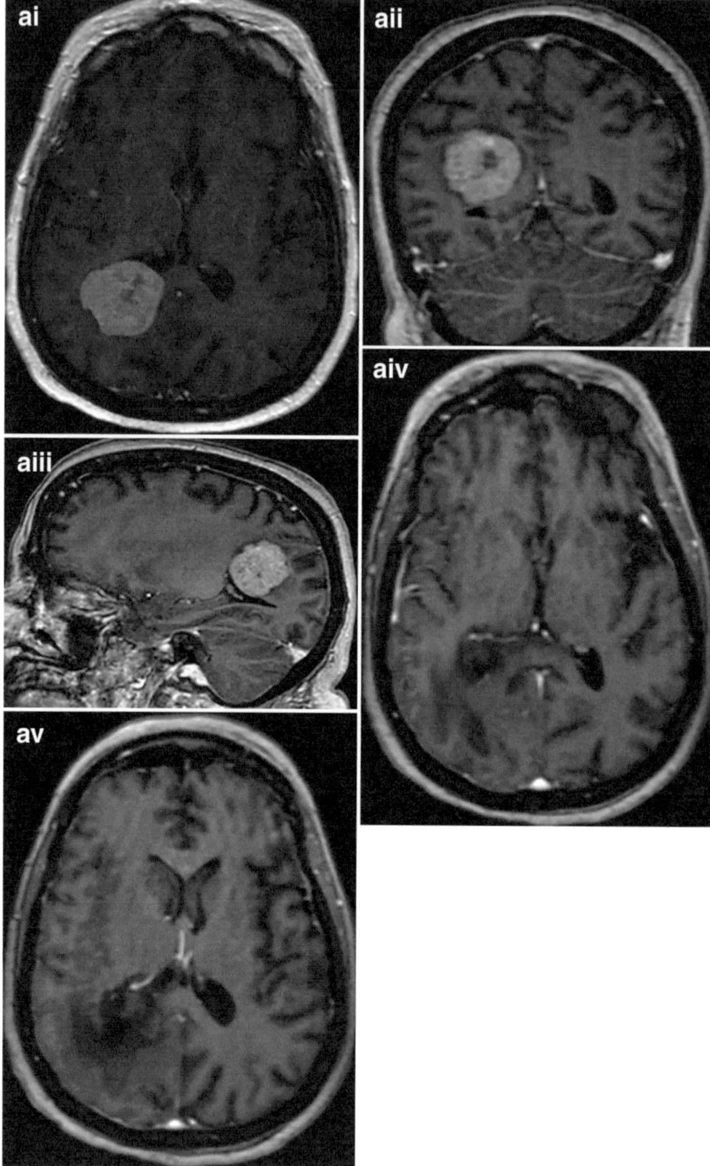

**Fig. 12.4** Evaluation of the characteristics of the tumor utilizing diffusion-weighted imaging is an important element of preoperative planning and helps to inform the decision regarding whether a surface or depth cannulation is most appropriate. (**a**) Preoperative MRI T1 contrast axial (i), coronal (ii), and sagittal (iii) images in a 34-year-old woman with metastatic lung cancer to the right parietal region. The diffusion-weighted image sequences, B0, B1000, ISO, DWI, and ADC, indicate that this is a solid tumor. The postoperative axial MRI T1 contrast images (iv, v) demonstrated a gross total resection of the tumor. (**b**) A 53-year-old woman presented with seizures, and the MRI T1 contrast axial (i, ii, iii) images demonstrated a large left frontal mass consistent with tumor. The B0, B1000, DWI, and ADC sequences indicated a high water content, soft tumor. Depth cannulation as part of a hybrid approach resulted in gross total resection (iv, v)

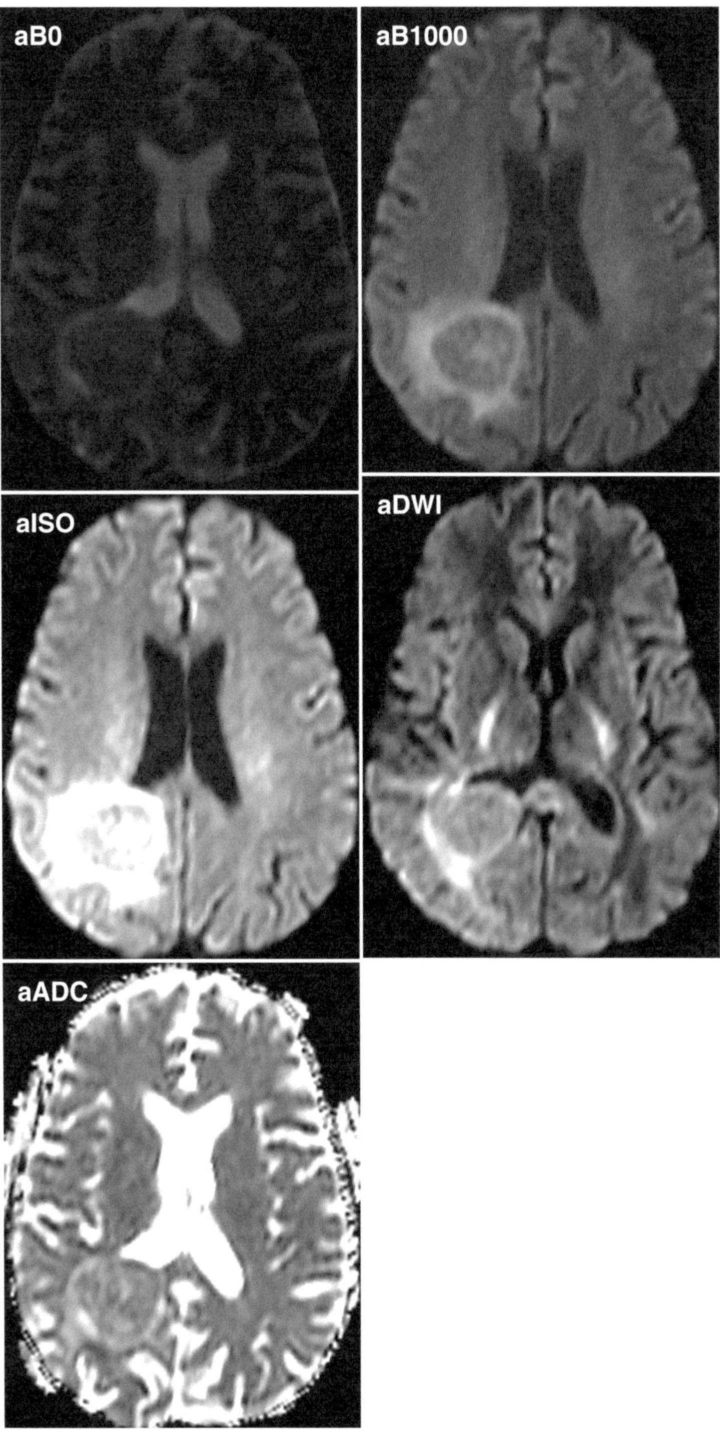



**Fig. 12.4** (continued)

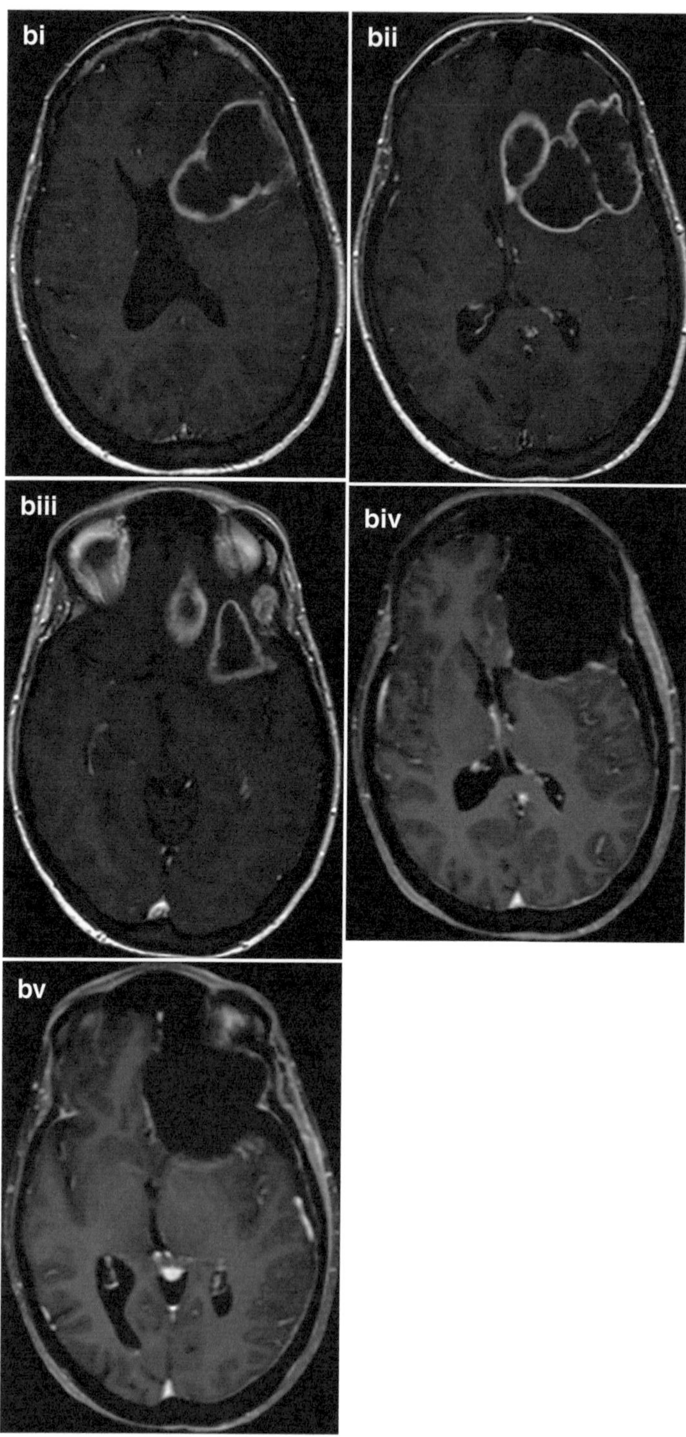

**Fig. 12.4** (continued)

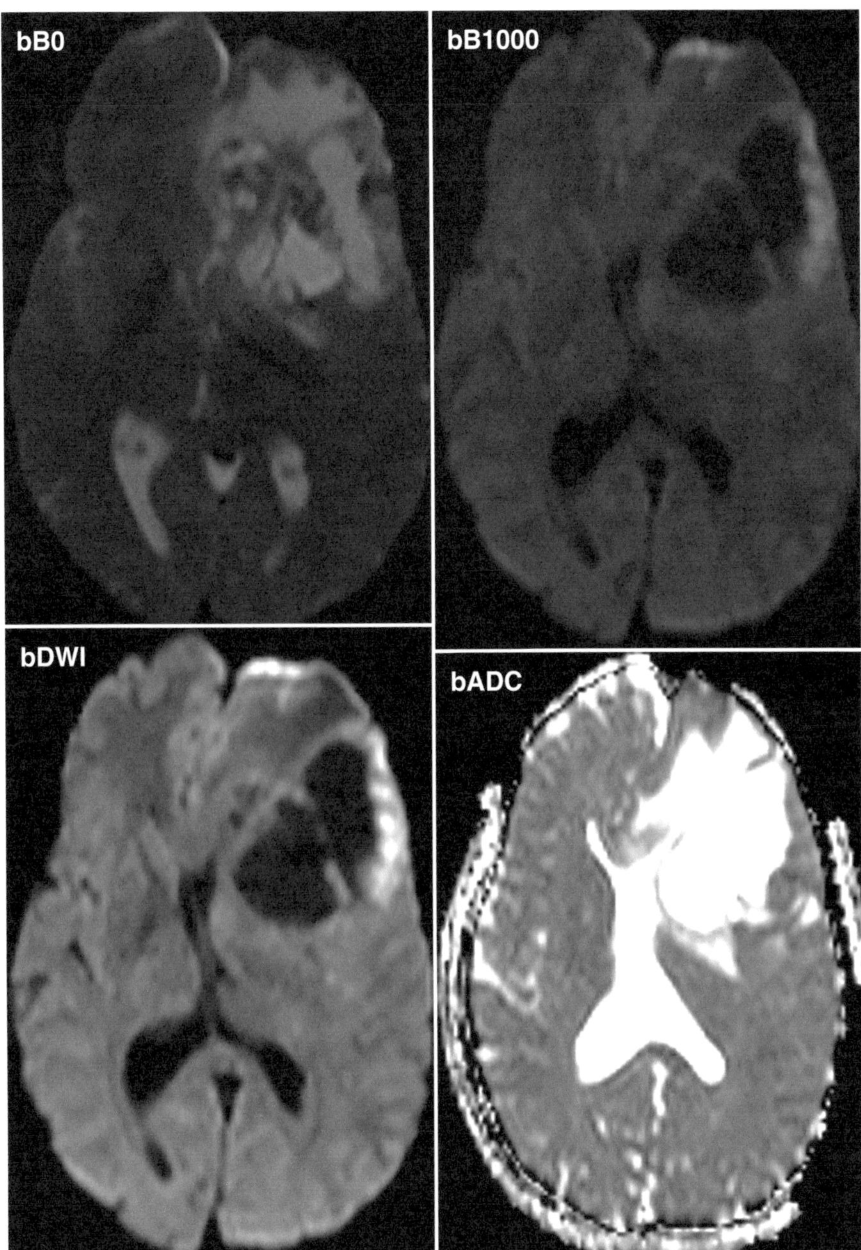


**Fig. 12.4** (continued)

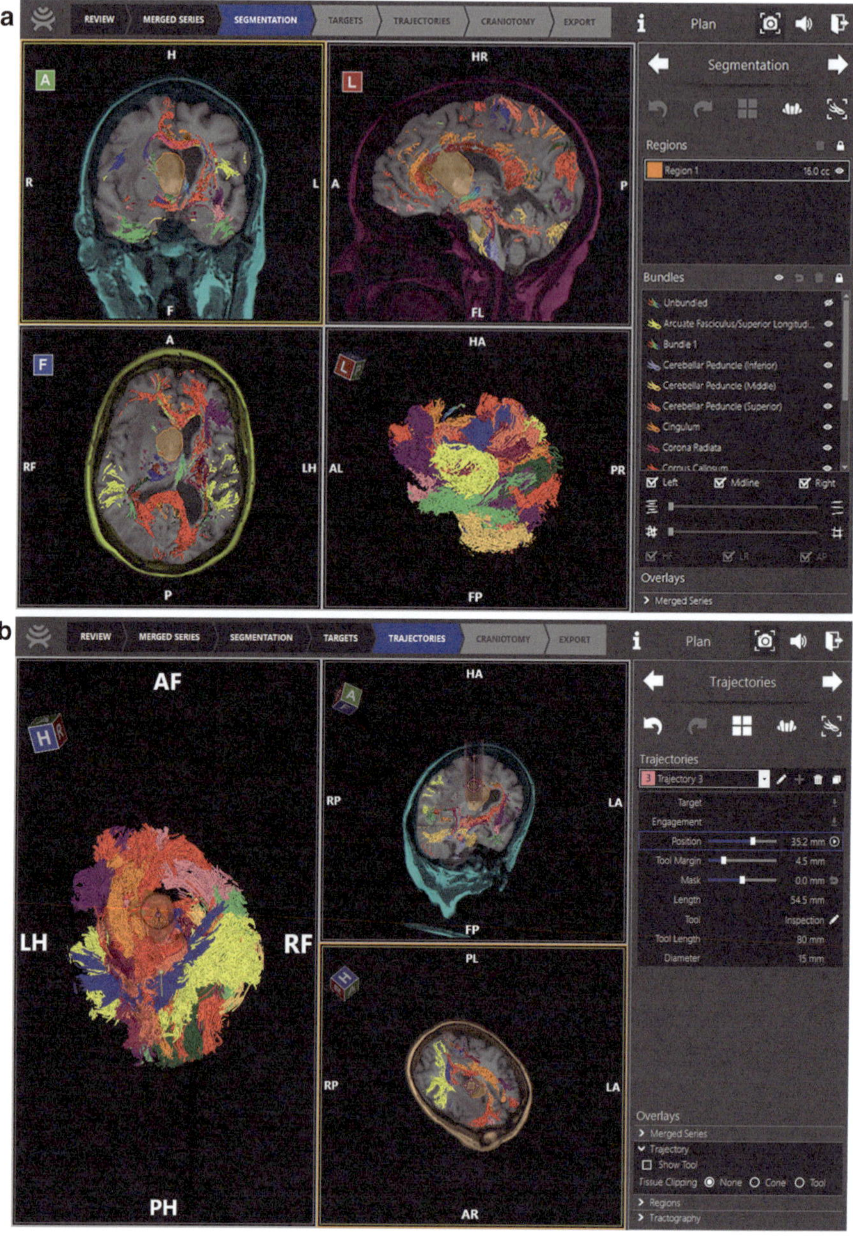

**Fig. 12.5** (**a**) The Bright Matter software system from Synaptive is demonstrated in the case of a periventricular glioma for planning of the MIPS approach by first considering the white matter anatomy and its deformation by the tumor. (**b**) An approach corridor is simulated as a subsequent step in the planning process, taking note of the white matter tracts that will interact with the cannulation of the port. (**c**) A final step in planning is determining the size and position of the craniotomy that will allow appropriate manipulation of the port to reach the entire extent of the lesion

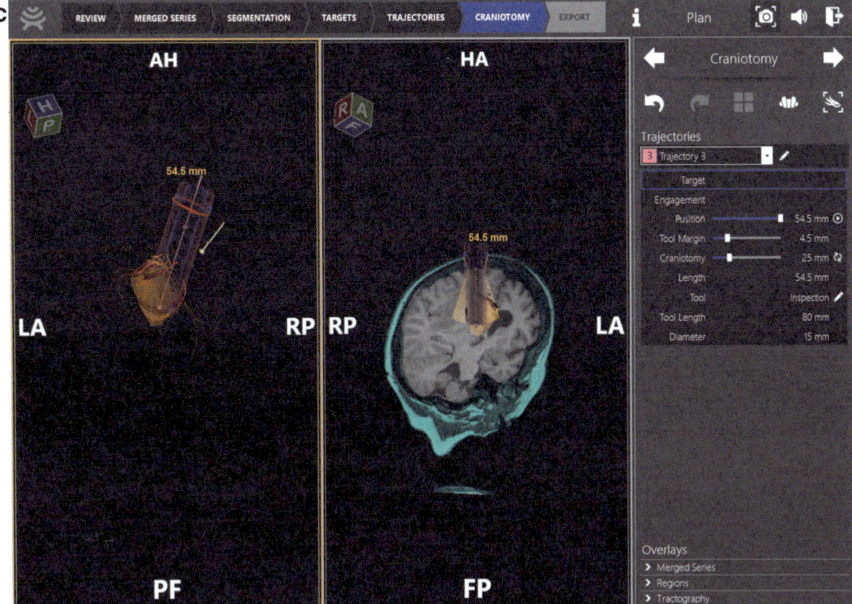


**Fig. 12.5**  (continued)

a history of drug use/abuse, alcohol abuse, psychiatric disorder, and general heightened anxiety. Some locations do not control neurologic functions that can be monitored through physical examination and therefore are typically done under general anesthesia to eliminate the general stress to the patient of an awake craniotomy, especially if any of the above contraindications are present.

## Surgical Technique

The patient is positioned according to the preoperative plan with respect to approach trajectory. This may call for positioning either supine, lateral, or park bench. Prone positioning may present particular problems owing to the image guidance platform requirements for registration. In the author's experience, the prone position presents particular challenges with this technique. The author's preferred alternative is a lateral or park bench position for posterior fossa or occipital lesions. In such cases, gravity is also a consideration in terms of how the brain will shift as tumor removal progresses. Accurately predicting how the brain will collapse on a resection cavity can mean the difference between a gross total and subtotal resection, especially in a soft tumor like some gliomas. Cavity collapse can result in a deep pocket of tumor that is missed and will require an early return to the operating room. A part of this element of preoperative consideration is deep versus surface cannulation with the

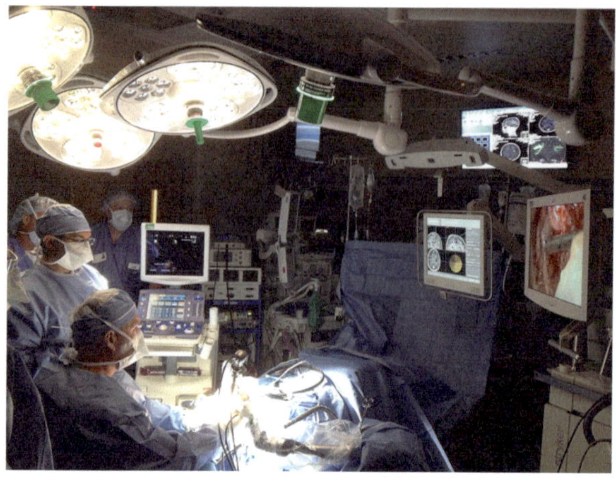

**Fig. 12.6** Optimal positioning of equipment and viewing screens is critical for surgeon comfort and ergonomics

port, depending on the predicted consistency of the neoplasm. Depth cannulation is generally the plan for soft neoplasms in the author's practice in order to resect deep portions of the tumor initially, attempting to avoid the effects of a collapsing resection cavity.

Once the patient is in position, the optimal positions of the various necessary equipment are arranged. Arrangement of the operating room is of particular importance for this technique (Fig. 12.6). Whatever the patient position, care is taken to place the viewing monitor and the image guidance monitor within direct view of the surgeon. It is not optimal, or comfortable, to have these monitors in a position that the surgeon has to turn his/her head while working. The monitors must be in the direct view of the operating surgeon. Also, of importance, optimal positioning of the exoscope (e.g., Storz Vitom) on the pneumatic arm (e.g., Mitaka arm) is of vital importance if utilizing this particular system. Particular care is taken to place the arm at an optimal position to hold the imaging device along the projected viewing angle and in a comfortable position for the surgeon. This is the case for any of the current systems in use.

With the patient positioned and the equipment arranged in the optimal position, the patient is registered in three-dimensional space with the image guidance system. A trajectory-centric system is preferred. The preplanned entry point is marked on the scalp, and it is important to test the preplanned trajectory to make sure it is attainable as the patient is positioned. After confirming that it is an attainable trajectory as the patient is positioned, the incision is planned. Typically, a slightly curved, "Lazy S" incision is optimal. The craniotomy required is approximately 2 cm in diameter; therefore, no more than a 4 cm incision is typically required. Depending upon the approach trajectory, the craniotomy may be necessarily shifted to accommodate the trajectory of the port. A minimum of hair removal is necessary, typically a thin strip along the line of incision.

The incision and craniotomy are made. It is best to retract the scalp with low-profile blunt scalp hooks to avoid a potential collision with the port and its holding mechanism. This can affect not only the ability to toggle the port as needed but also the depth the port can be placed. The dural opening is limited to just larger than the diameter of an average port such as the BrainPath device (13 mm). It may be advisable to utilize the ultrasound to confirm the position of the planned sulcus for entry prior to dural opening. The dural flaps are tacked up with suture. The exoscope is brought into place to view the cortical surface with magnification. The sulcal entry point is confirmed with the image guidance probe and adjusted as necessary. The arachnoid over the sulcus is opened using microsurgical technique. A wide opening of the arachnoid is not necessary; approximately 3–6 mm is sufficient for introduction of the port into the sulcus.

The port device is then advanced through the opening in the arachnoid into the sulcus and to the preplanned depth. The obturator tip is 10 mm beyond the rim of the retractor tube when using a port such as the BrainPath (Nico Corp., USA); therefore, the tube is advanced over the obturator to the preplanned depth and the obturator removed. In cases of depth cannulation, the port will be within the lesion. For surface cannulation cases, a cuff of white matter typically is retained over the lesion and is visible. This will be removed to expose the lesion.

The lesion is then resected utilizing a combination of suction, bipolar cautery, and a side-cutting aspirator such as the Myriad (Nico Corp., USA) device. Owing to the small diameter of the BrainPath port, other devices, such as an ultrasonic aspirator, are not small enough to utilize with this device. The optimal technique for resection is a "two-handed" technique whereby the surgeon uses the Myriad for suction and resection in one hand and the bipolar cautery for hemostasis and mobilization of tumor tissue simultaneously in the other. The Myriad device provides a small diameter suction tube with adjustable pressure in combination with a tissue cutting function that can be turned off and on. The small diameter of the device is key to allowing adequate visualization owing to the limited working diameter of the BrainPath device.

Once hemostasis is obtained, the BrainPath is withdrawn from the brain. A small piece of Gelfoam is then placed over the exposed brain and the dura closed with suture. The bone flap is replaced and secured with miniplates and screws. The scalp is then closed and a dressing applied.

The author's general practice is to admit the patient to our regular inpatient unit after post-anesthesia recovery. Patients are observed closely by the nursing staff with neurologic exam every 2 hours until 12–18 hours after surgery. Hospital length of stay varies between 1 and 3 days in general.

## Discussion

Accessing selected neoplastic subcortical lesions via a trans-sulcal parafascicular approach using a port retractor device is a viable and generally safe alternative to a traditional transcortical microsurgical approach. Essentially any primary or metastatic brain tumor in the subcortical space may be considered to utilize this strategy.

However, experience with the technique is necessary to make a sound judgment regarding the suitability of this approach for any particular case. This discussion will focus on particular surgical pearls that have been gained from the author's experience with various lesions.


## Primary Brain Tumors

Glial tumors located in a subcortical location are reasonable candidates for utilization of this strategy. High-grade tumors that are generally soft in consistency are well suited based upon the ability to resect the tumor essentially from the inside-out. Abnormal tumor tissue that is readily discernible from surrounding white matter can be well resected with suction or the Myriad® device. Adjustments in viewing angle and toggling the BrainPath® appropriately to resect the tumor in all quadrants can result in a gross total resection of the enhancing portion of the lesion. The ability to obtain a gross total resection is dependent upon the location, size, and experience with this technique.

In general, the author's strategy is to perform a depth cannulation if the DWI information indicates that the tumor will be sufficiently soft. The reasons for this are multiple. First, resecting the deep portion first allows for a soft tumor to collapse into the cavity created, thus delivering itself in large part into the cavity much like what is experienced in evacuation through the port in an intracerebral hematoma case. It is important to identify any predetermined anatomical landmarks in the depth prior to retracting the port more superficially. As the port is gradually retracted, it is toggled appropriately to resect tumor until normal-appearing white matter is encountered at all margins of the cavity. As always, the author advocates a two-handed technique whereby the side-cutting aspirator is held in the non-dominant hand and used to suction and resect tumor while the dominant hand utilizes the bipolar cautery forceps to continually manage hemostasis and to mobilize tumor tissue toward the resection device. This technique provides an efficient way to resect tumor while maintaining a hemostatic field.

In many specialized centers, the importance of tumor genetics has taken on a central role in treatment decisions for glial tumors. This technique has been incorporated and expanded in the author's institution as a part of the movement toward personalized medicine treatment of brain tumors. Targeted tumor collection is made efficient with this technique to sample particular areas of interest that may better define therapeutic targets on a molecular genetic basis, in particular the periventricular progenitor zone.

A hybrid approach is incorporated in selected cases to provide certain advantages of both port-based resection and traditional open microsurgery. In such cases, typical is a tumor that extends from the periventricular area out to the cortical surface. In these cases, the deep portion of the tumor is planned for resection via a port technique, passing through the tumor, in order to sample and resect the hypothesized progenitor zone. Subcortical stimulation is used when appropriate to help preserve motor function. This zone is that which is expected to harbor the least amount of genetic heterogeneity, thus potentially offering the most accurate determination of potential therapeutic targets. In performing such a hybrid approach, the surface involvement of the tumor is taken into account necessarily, and therefore the craniotomy is appropriately sized. Once the deep portion is resected, the sulcal borders of the tumor at the surface are utilized to complete the resection with a traditional microsurgical approach. Utilization of 5-ALA is also routine in our practice and can be viewed both microsurgically and through the port (Fig. 12.7).

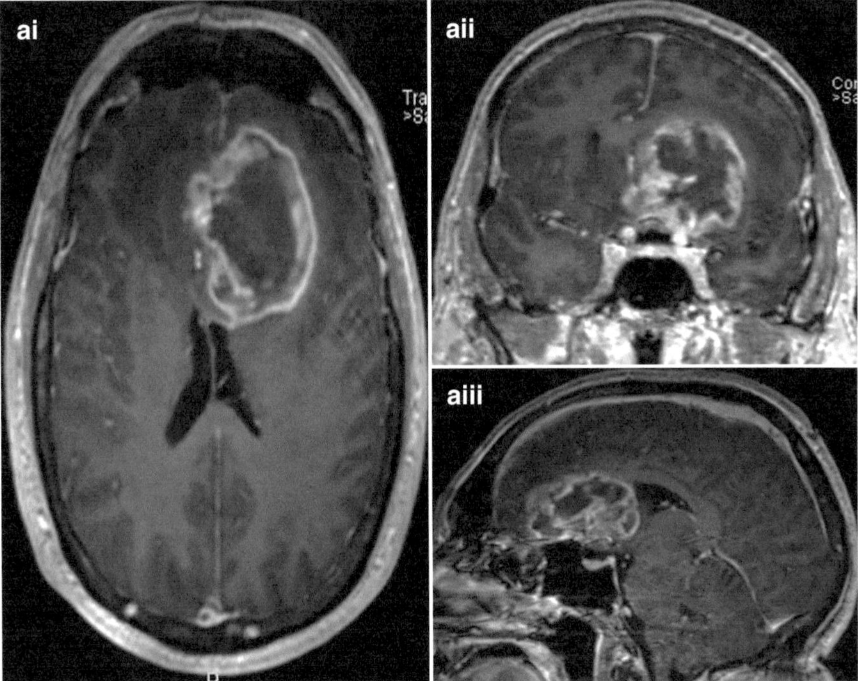


**Fig. 12.7** (**a**) A 57-year-old man presented with mass effect symptoms and imaging suggestive of a high-grade glioma (MRI T1 with contrast axial (i), coronal (ii), and sagittal (iii)). (**b**) The operative plan was developed based upon tractography, utilizing a frontal trajectory (i, ii, iii). The patient was administered 5-ALA which is visible through the port with the appropriate 450 nM filter. (**c**) Postoperative MRI T1 contrast axial (i), coronal (ii), and sagittal (iii) images demonstrated a gross total resection

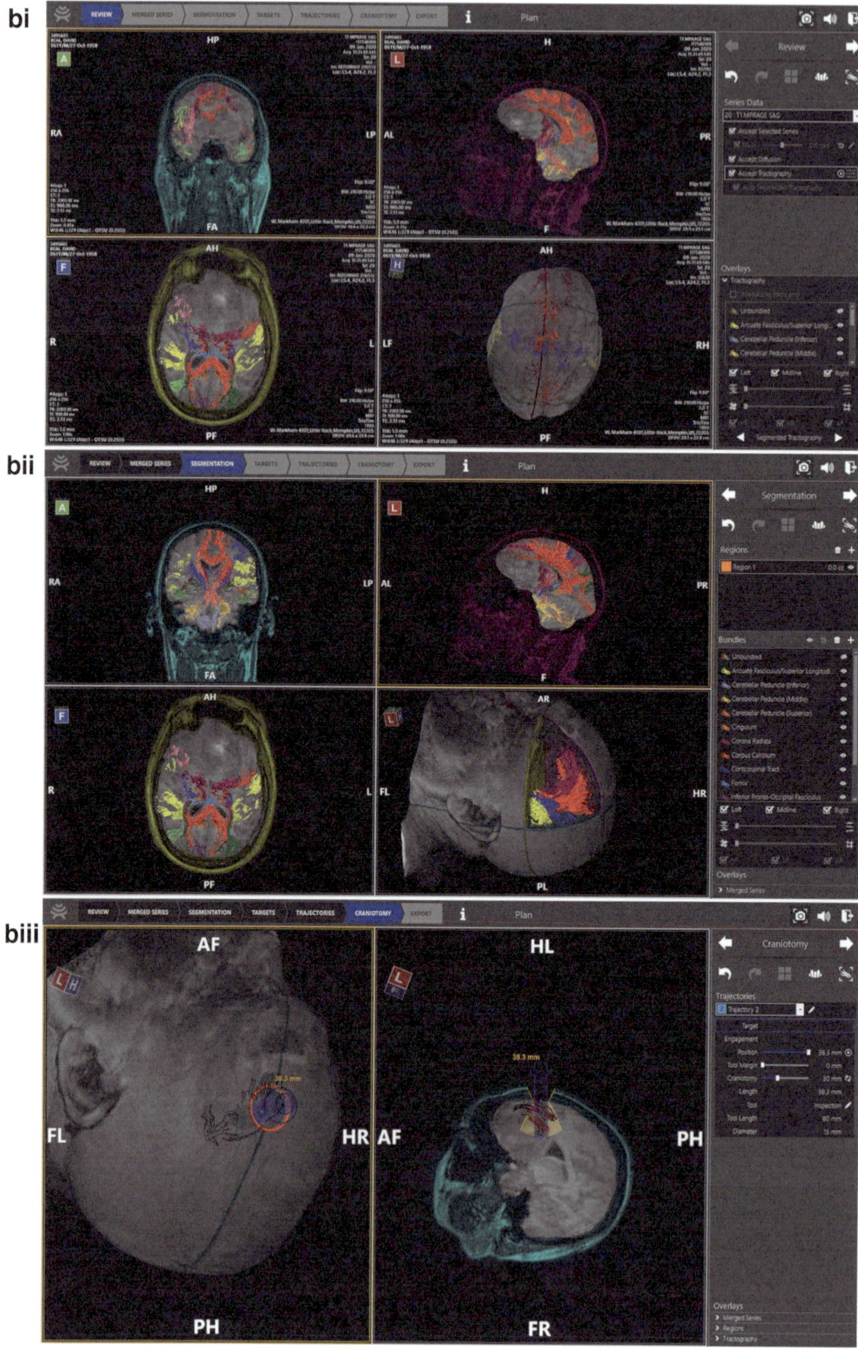

**Fig. 12.7** (continued)

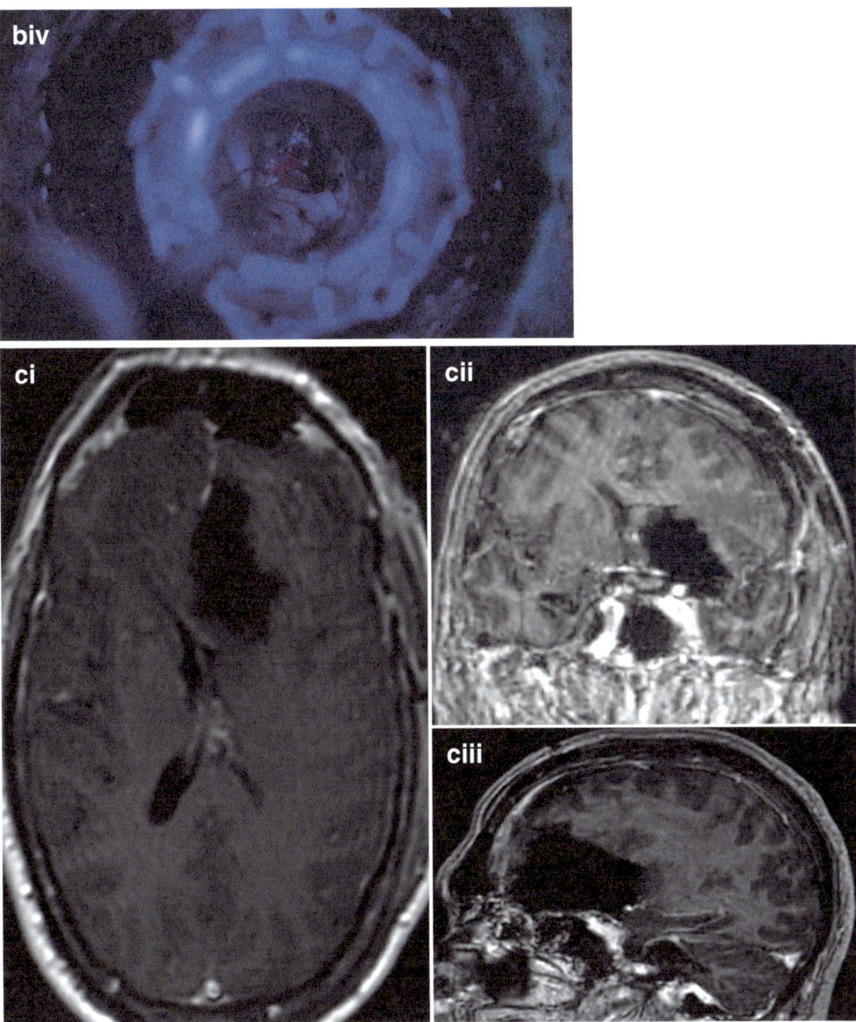

**Fig. 12.7** (continued)

## *Metastatic Tumors*

Aside from location, a particularly important element of preoperative evaluation in cases of metastatic tumors is an analysis of the DWI. Predicting the character of the tumor tissue with respect to its firmness based upon water content is helpful in terms of selecting the depth of cannulation with a port such as the BrainPath®. As in high-grade primary lesions, a soft lesion is amenable to a so-called depth cannulation, targeting the tube depth to a point within the tumor. This results in a resection strategy characterized by an inside-out resection, stopping at the white matter borders of the lesion. Metastatic tumors with a high degree of central tumor necrosis are amenable to this strategy. However, this is not an appropriate strategy with this method in the case of a firm tumor.

In the case of a firm tumor, a so-called "surface cannulation" is appropriate, targeting the capsule of the mass and not penetrating the tumor tissue. Many metastatic lesions are firm enough that they will not be penetrable with a port. Whether the lesion is large or small, a firm tumor may be displaced by the port if firm and a depth cannulation is attempted. This is a result of the tumor "rolling" out of the field of view by displacement during cannulation. Awareness of this particular potential pitfall will help mitigate the possibility of difficulty localizing the mass. Experience also helps in predicting how a lesion may roll out of the pathway of the port. Also helpful in such situations is utilizing ultrasound down the port to visualize the tumor.

Resection of metastatic tumors through the port is very much like doing so with a microsurgical technique. The firm nature of most metastatic tumors lends itself to following the margins of the lesion around the tumor and resecting with a side-cutting aspirator device. This is an outside-to-inside technique in contrast to resecting soft tumors via a depth cannulation. In general, the author's experience demonstrates that a gross total resection of deep subcortical metastatic tumors, while minimizing tissue disruption, is possible with this technique and has become the preferred method in practice. Surgical resection is typically followed up with adjuvant stereotactic radiosurgery.

## *Intraventricular Lesions*

Intraventricular lesions can be well suited to this technique. Operative planning must take into consideration how the port will access the ventricle. In most tumor cases, the tumor extends to the ventricular lumen from the wall of the ventricle. In such cases, the ventricle is essentially entered through the tumor as part of the resection. Good examples of this are ependymomas (Fig. 12.8) and subependymal giant cell astrocytomas. In other cases, such as a central neurocytoma, for example, the origin of the tumor is deep, and the path the port will take into the ventricular lumen must be taken into account. With insufficient ventricular caliber and a particular trajectory, it is possible that the port could shear off structures in the wall of the ventricle, such as the caudate head. Visualization of the ventricular anatomy is at least equivalent to that obtained endoscopically. A particular advantage in visualization with the exoscope through the port is if any significant bleeding is encountered. The ability to isolate and coagulate the bleeding point is superior in this technique versus the endoscopic technique when blood in cerebrospinal fluid can greatly obscure vision. The port technique allows operating in a dry field and is more efficient to resect a tumor of any significant size.

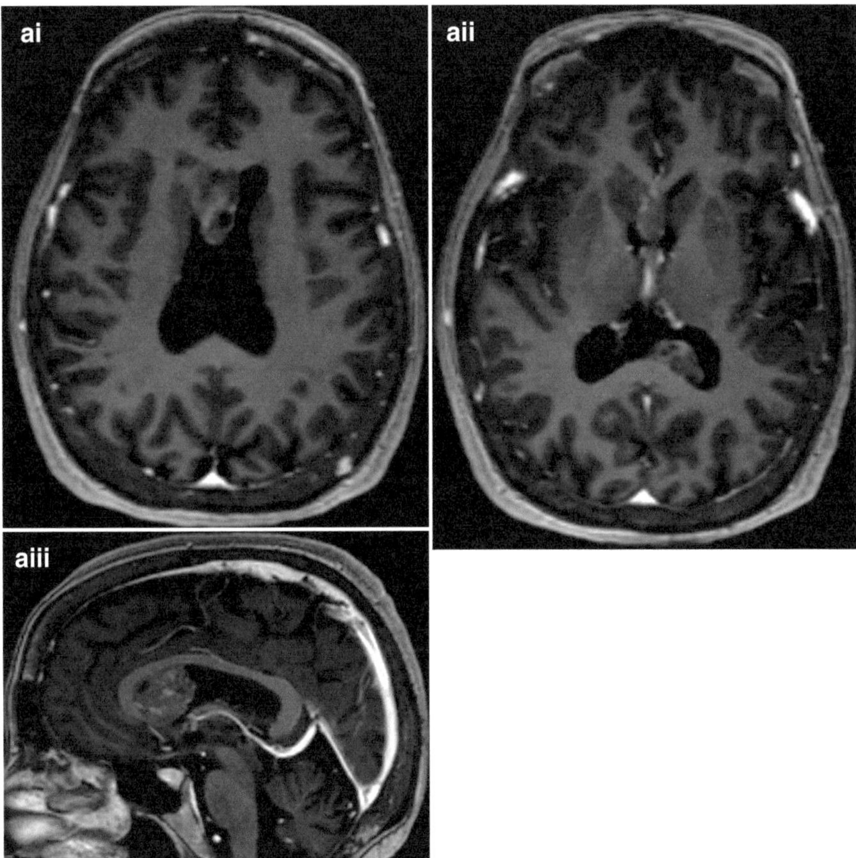


**Fig. 12.8** Intraventricular lesions can be addressed with the MIPS technique when proper considerations are taken into account. (**a**) This patient had two foci of metastatic ependymoma and was responsive to prior treatment with a good Karnofsky performance score. Two procedures were performed to resect the lesions in the right frontal horn and the left atrium as seen on the T1 contrast axial (i, ii) and sagittal (iii) images. (**b**) Postoperative MRI T1 contrast axial (i) and sagittal (ii, iii, iv) images demonstrated gross total resection of the lesions

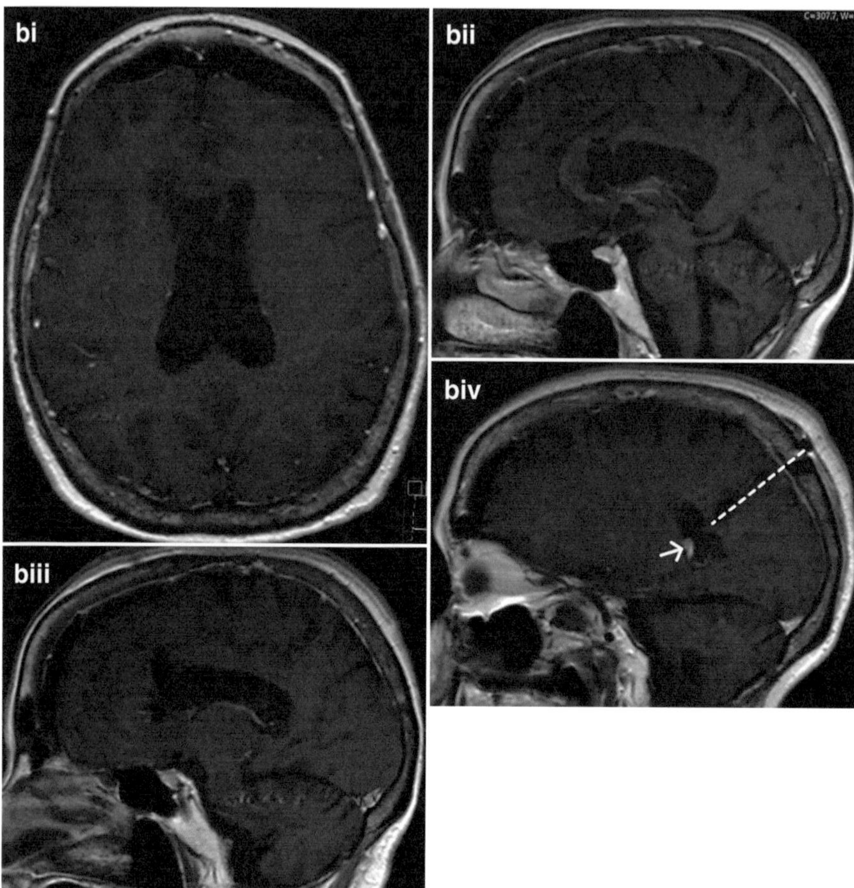

**Fig. 12.8** (continued)

## Conclusion

The current armamentarium of minimally invasive techniques in cranial surgery includes a number of strategies that take advantage of our current state of technology in advanced imaging, high-definition viewing platforms, and innovative instrumentation. The BrainPath® device for access to subcortical lesions is being adopted across multiple centers as an attractive alternative to traditional microsurgical transcortical techniques. Accumulated experience with this technique will lead to further refinements in defining the indications for this approach, as well as improvements in instrumentation and operative technique.

# References


1. Ogura K, Tachibana E, Aoshima C, Sumitomo M. New microsurgical technique for intraparenchymal lesions of the brain: transcylinder approach. Acta Neurochir. 2006;148(7):779–85; discussion 85.
2. Nagatini K, Takeuchi S, Feng D, Mori K, Day JD. High-definition exoscope system for microneurosurgery: use of an exoscope combination with tubular retraction and frameless neuronavigation for microsurgical resection of deep brain lesions. No Shinkei Geka. 2015;43(7):611–7. https://doi.org/10.11477/mf.1436203086. Japanese. PMID: 26136325.
3. Day JD. Transsulcal parafascicular surgery using BrainPath® for subcortical lesions. Neurosurgery. 2017;64(CN Suppl 1):151–6. https://doi.org/10.1093/neuros/nyx324.
4. Dlouhy BJ, Dahdaleh NS, Greenlee JD. Emerging technology in intracranial neuroendoscopy: application of the NICO Myriad. Neurosurg Focus. 2011;30(4):E6.
5. McLaughlin N, Ditzel Filho LF, Prevedello DM, Kelly DF, Carrau RL, Kassam AB. Side-cutting aspiration device for endoscopic and microscopic tumor removal. J Neurol Surg Part B Skull Base. 2012;73(1):11–20.
6. Labib MA, Shah M, Kassam AB, Young R, Zucker L, Maioriello A, et al. The safety and feasibility of image-guided BrianPath-mediated transsulcal hematoma evacuation: a multicenter study. Neurosurgery. 2017:1–10. https://doi.org/10.1227/NEU.0000000000001316.

# Chapter 13
# Trans-sulcal, Channel-Based Parafascicular Biopsy Techniques

Evan D. Bander and Rohan Ramakrishna

## Introduction

Advancing tools in genetic analysis, epigenetics, and proteomics have revealed the wide genetic heterogeneity of tumors. Simple histopathology and microscopic diagnoses are no longer sufficient to classify tumors in neuro-oncology. The new World Health Organization (WHO) grading of central nervous system tumors has acknowledged this by making molecular markers a critical element of an integrated diagnosis. These molecular markers can be essential indicators of prognosis [1–5] and response to treatment/chemotherapy [6, 7] and represent targets for innovative new therapies.

With these scientific advances comes the need to tailor our clinical management. The need for larger quantities of tissue for advanced analysis and biobanking is now of paramount importance to help guide patient therapies. Obtaining minimal tissue for the purpose of only histologic diagnosis is no longer sufficient. With the growing need for tissue, tools such as tubular/channel-based retractors have become operative adjuncts in biopsies to maximize access and visualization of deep-seated lesions while minimizing collateral tissue damage compared to fixed blade retractors [8, 9]. Tubular retractors have been recognized for use in the resection of deep intracranial tumors and for evacuation of subcortical hematomas and neoplastic lesions of the

E. D. Bander
New York-Presbyterian Hospital, Weill Cornell Medicine, Department of Neurosurgery, New York, NY, USA
e-mail: evb2005@nyp.org

R. Ramakrishna (✉)
New York-Presbyterian Hospital, Weill Cornell Medicine, Department of Neurological Surgery, New York, NY, USA
e-mail: ror9068@med.cornell.edu

© Springer Nature Switzerland AG 2022
G. Zada et al. (eds.), *Subcortical Neurosurgery*,
https://doi.org/10.1007/978-3-030-95153-5_13

brainstem, basal ganglia, and ventricles [10–33]. Now their use has also been refined to obtain biopsy samples via small craniotomies and a trans-sulcal course for the tubular retractor.

## Traditional/Alternative Approaches

Before turning to the use of channel-based biopsies, we first must consider the alternatives. Traditionally, deep-seated unresectable tumors or those in highly eloquent locations had been sampled using navigated stereotactic frame-based or frameless needle biopsies [34–39]. These needle biopsies provide small volume specimens and sample tissue from limited locations along the same trajectory. Multiple specimens can be taken from the same or different locations in the tumor; however, each pass of the needle incurs a further risk of hematoma. Diagnostic success with this technique varies widely, but success rates can be as low as 60–70% in some cases [40–44]. Non-diagnostic samples can occur at high rates (13%, Table 13.1), sometimes requiring repeat operations to obtain a diagnosis [9]. Furthermore, there is a non-trivial rate of misdiagnosis or under-grading of tumors, which has been reported to occur in 9.2–28.0% of neoplastic lesions, respectively [43, 45]. Finally, for high-grade lesions, retrieved tissue may often be necrotic, limiting the diagnostic utility.

Given that stereotactic biopsies are minimally invasive and blind procedures, visualization of hemostasis cannot be achieved. As such, hematomas related to the procedure often cannot be diagnosed and treated until after the operation. Standard of care varies between institutions, but in a survey of surgeons, Warnick et al. found that ~59% of respondents obtain post-operative CT on all stereotactic biopsy patients [46]. The rate of immediate post-operative hematoma in the literature varies between 2% and 8% [9, 46–49]. Many of these post-operative hematomas remain

**Table 13.1** Comparison of stereotactic and tubular biopsy outcomes

| | Stereotactic biopsy ($n = 146$) | Transtubular biopsy ($n = 18$) | |
|---|---|---|---|
| | Mean (SD) or freq (%) | Mean (SD) or freq (%) | $p$-value[a] |
| *Biopsy/pathology outcomes* | | | |
| Non-diagnostic sample obtained | 19 (13.0%) | 0 (0%) | 0.1346 |
| Permanent section volume (cm$^3$) | 0.3 (0.9) | 1.26 (1.1) | **<0.0001** |
| *Patient outcomes* | | | |
| Post-biopsy hemorrhage | 3 (2.1%)[b] | 1 (5.6%)[#] | 0.3691 |
| Re-operation necessary for diagnosis | 6 (4.1%) | 0 (0%) | 1.000 |

Adapted from Bander et al. [9]
[a]All categorical variables were analyzed using Fisher's exact test. All continuous variables were analyzed using the Wilcoxon rank sum test
[b]All post-biopsy hemorrhages remained clinically silent and none required clinical intervention

clinically silent, but rarely these can require surgical intervention and cause neurologic morbidity.

Open craniotomy for biopsy of a mass is also a practical alternative to stereotactic and tubular biopsy techniques. This approach allows for a significant volume of tissue for sampling, debulking of tumor, and direct visualization of hemostasis. It also allows for approaches to regions of the brain not easily accessible to channel-based methods (subtemporal, midbrain, pineal, lesions arising from the skull base, etc.).

## Channel-Based Benefits and Patient Selection

The passage of a tubular retractor parallel to white matter tracts theoretically minimizes the damage and transection of these subcortical fascicles. Meanwhile, the single passage of a tubular retractor offers the ability to sample tumor at multiple points along the retractor's path through the tumor while also allowing for intra-operative hemostasis to be obtained under direct visualization. Tubular/channel-based biopsy can be offered for deep lesions that are "unresectable," in that the risks of near total resection outweigh the potential oncologic benefits. Subcortical, insular, corpus callosum, thalamic, periventricular, and/or bilateral masses ("butterfly lesions"), for which more extensive resections would result in post-operative neurologic deficits, are considered good candidates for transtubular biopsy (Fig. 13.1). Compared to stereotactic needle biopsy, the tubular retractor system allows the surgeon to transition their surgical goals with ease intra-operatively, all while maintaining a minimally invasive approach. The tubular approach provides for significant tissue for frozen diagnosis, and in the case of lesions where pathology suggests that a debulking may be clinically beneficial, the channel-based system can allow for subsequent minimally invasive debulking of the tumor within the limits of preserving neurologic function.

We suggest that transtubular biopsies be considered with any subcortical lesion. In particular, diffuse tumors with little to no contrast enhancement may uniquely benefit from the extensive tissue generated from this technique. These latter cases are most prone to misdiagnosis or under-grading and therefore mostly likely to benefit from larger tissue volumes. Evidence suggests that pathologic diagnosis from stereotactic biopsy of low-grade gliomas agrees with open resection pathologic type and grade in only 36% of cases and can result in over-grading of tumors in 11% and under-grading in 28% of cases [43]. For these same reasons, patients with recurrent gliomas are an ideal and important patient population to consider for channel-based biopsy. While these patients already have a diagnosis, the tumors are highly heterogeneous [50], at risk for sampling bias, and the tumor genetics can be important in determining late-stage treatment decisions. Moreover, these tumors evolve over time so the tumor genetics at initial presentation may not be representative at recurrence. These patients historically have been offered stereotactic needle

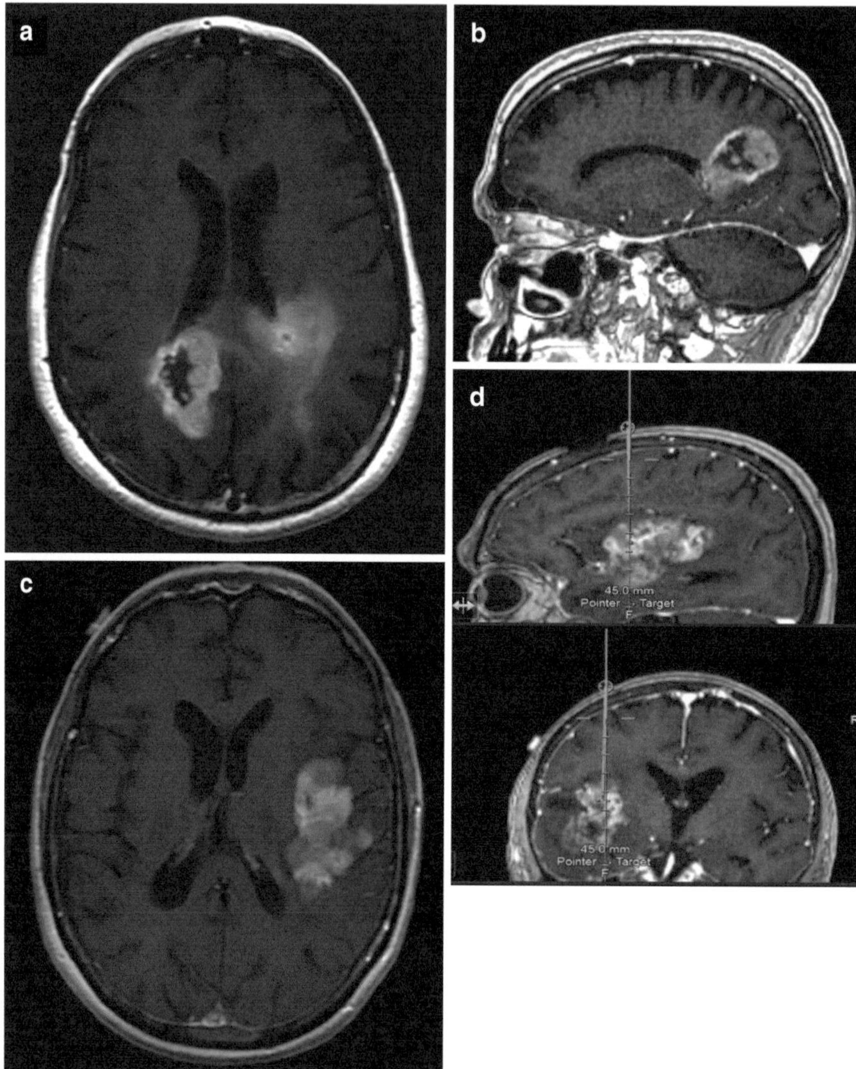

**Fig. 13.1** Examples of appropriate tumors and trajectories for channel-based biopsy. (**a**, **b**) Axial and sagittal T1 + contrast MR images of bilateral enhancing mass of splenium of corpus callosum, biopsied through a tubular retractor. (**c**) Recurrent left-sided, dominant insular, enhancing tumor with prior diagnosis of anaplastic astrocytoma. (**d**) Intra-operative navigation demonstrating channel-based trajectory for biopsy. Pathology consistent with glioblastoma. (**e**, **f**) Examples of pre-operative trajectory plans made using Brainlab software for channel-based biopsies

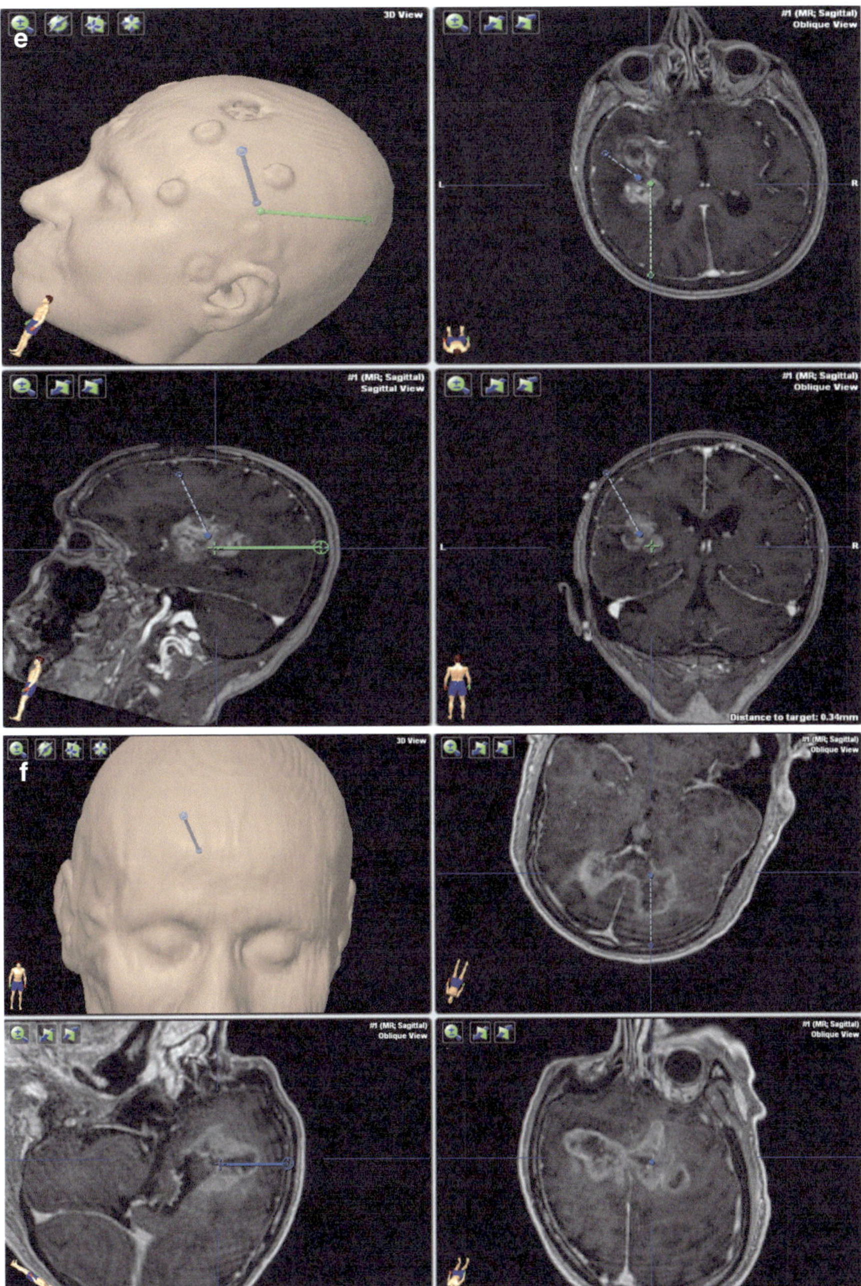

**Fig. 13.1** (continued)

biopsy, but given the potential for inadequate sampling and insufficient material for genetic testing, tubular biopsy is a viable alternative to provide more tissue to the pathologist.

Tubular retractors offer their greatest benefit when accessing a deep lesion with a significant volume of intervening normal tissue between the cortex. Masses that have deep components but come close to the cortical surface and/or could be easily reached by a small craniotomy and corticectomy without the need for deep dissection through normal tissue are better offered open procedures. However, if deep lesions approach the cortex in eloquent areas, an alternative approach could be the introduction of a tubular retractor via a more distant sulcus in non-eloquent brain. The trajectory of the tubular retractor in these cases would need to be determined by the fiber tracts surrounding the tumor in these cases. Stereotactic needle or open biopsies are favored in brainstem or cerebellar lesions. These tissues contain a high density of white matter tracts that are not easily separated by a retractor. Furthermore, tumors arising from the skull base are often most easily accessed via open craniotomy, and channel-based approaches offer little benefit.

Few studies have assessed the diagnostic accuracy and complication rate of tubular biopsy. Channel-based techniques were initially viewed as a rescue, minimally invasive approach for non-diagnostic stereotactic biopsies [51]. However, this approach is beginning to gain attention as a primary biopsy method. In a study of 18 consecutive channel-based biopsies, 100% of surgeries resulted in a pathologic diagnosis [9] (Table 13.1). Furthermore, channel-based biopsies allow for a significantly larger (~4x) volume of specimen for permanent pathology compared to stereotactic approaches. No study has yet determined if the larger volume of tissue obtained results in more diagnostic/genetic/research testing, but the theoretic advantage remains. Complications from these procedures also remain a concern as there is little data for comparison. The rate of hemorrhage, despite the ability to obtain hemostasis, remains present (~5%). To better define the role and limitations of channel-based biopsy, further work must be done.

## Surgical Technique

General principles of trans-sulcal channel-based surgery have been extensively discussed elsewhere [10–13, 26, 27]. The goal of a channel-based biopsy is to avoid the major pitfalls of under-grading and misdiagnosis that plague other minimally invasive biopsy techniques such as stereotactic biopsy. As with other techniques, the target of the biopsy should be planned to sample an area that recapitulates the most aggressive features of that tumor. Pre-operative imaging is vital in this regard. Identifying a region with increased permeability (i.e., contrast enhancement) and/or the region with a high level of perfusion/metabolic activity on PET or MR perfusion imaging can help minimize the risk of under-grading and misdiagnosis [52–54]. Diffusion tensor imaging (DTI) can also be used to determine a path that runs parallel to and minimizes the retractor crossing major white matter fascicles. With a stereotactic biopsy, each separate target, depth, or region of interest requires a separate pass of the biopsy needle, and each pass of the needle carries a risk of causing complications. However, using a channel-based method, the cannula is inserted along the long axis of the tumor, and samples can be taken from multiple depths along the retractor's trajectory without repeated passes of the retractor. Tubular retractor length can be chosen based on the distance to the chosen target. The diameter of the retractor can be chosen by surgeon preference. An 11-mm-diameter channel allows for minimal footprint, while also suitable access for suctioning and use of a small pituitary forceps for sampling and bipolar cautery for hemostasis. Operative instrumentation used in endoscopic endonasal surgery can be quite useful for working at depths in the tubular retractor.

Once the trajectory has been chosen using the pre-operative imaging, a small craniotomy can be made over the chosen sulcal entry point. Using the intra-operative navigation system, the retractor with an introducer/obturator in place can be guided along the planned trajectory. Depending on the retractor system, the introducer may extend different lengths beyond the channel retractor itself, and this must be kept in mind when passing the system to the appropriate depth. The retractor should be passed to the maximal depth of the planned biopsy, and the introducer is then removed from the retractor. If there is concern based on imaging that the lesion may be fibrous, dense, or firm, the retractor can be passed to the surface of the lesion and biopsy be taken from the lesion's surface. An operating microscope or an exoscope can be used for visualization at the depth of the retractor. Samples can then be taken with pituitary forceps and sent for frozen pathology. After taking a sample, any hemostatic agent and bipolar cautery can be used to obtain hemostasis. The tubular retractor can then be slowly removed to allow for further sampling of tumor at shorter depths along the planned trajectory. Obtaining hemostasis after each sample is paramount and a significant advantage of this biopsy technique. After removal of the retractor, ultrasound can be used to confirm no immediate hematoma has resulted from the biopsy, prior to closure of the dura and replacement of the bone plate. Figure 13.2 demonstrates the steps of the procedure.

Post-operative management may vary per institution, but patients can be monitored in the recovery room and then overnight in either an intensive care unit or step-down unit. Imaging can be reserved for patients with neurologic deficit given the intra-operative visualization of hemostasis.

## Future Advances

The current use of channel-based approaches to biopsy remains understudied. While channel-based approaches are becoming increasingly popular, studies comparing complication rates, diagnostic success rates, and rate of tissue utilization all remain unclear. This technique offers theoretical advantages over traditional open and stereotactic biopsy techniques in appropriately chosen patients, but large-scale, randomized, or prospective trials could better define these advantages. Furthermore,

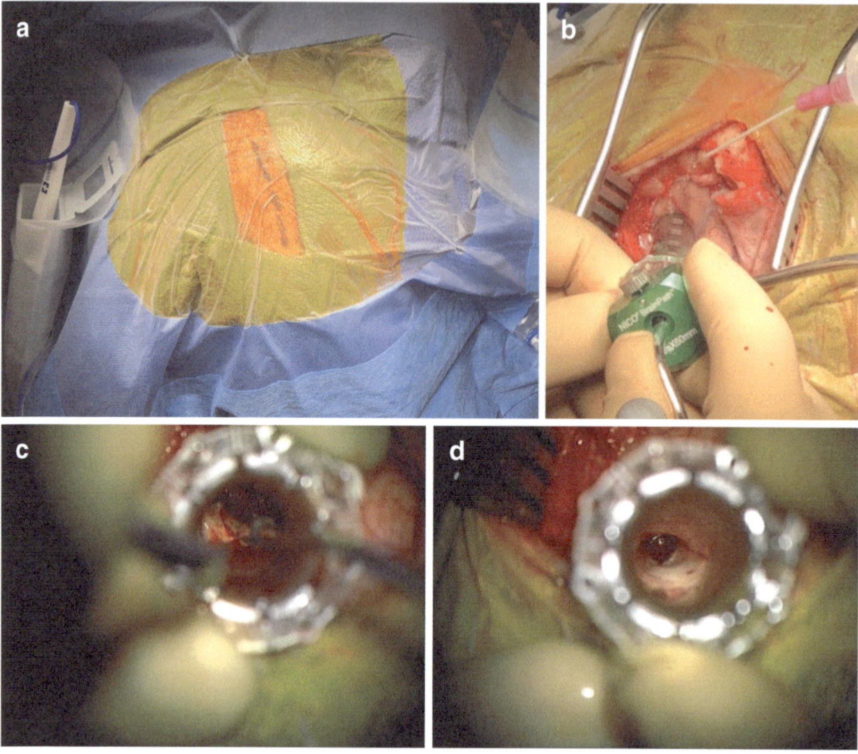

**Fig. 13.2** Procedural steps of channel-based biopsy. (**a**) Localized, small incision and craniotomy are planned. (**b**) Trans-sulcal introduction of the tubular retractor using image guidance. (**c**) Two-handed biopsy using suction and pituitary forceps. (**d**) Removal of retractor under direct visualization with attention paid to hemorrhage or potential biopsy at other depths

while early evidence demonstrates a relatively similar safety profile to stereotactic biopsy, this requires further confirmation.

The potential benefits of combining channel-based biopsy techniques with advances in intra-operative identification of tumor tissue are clear. Fluorescent agents such as fluorescein or 5-aminolevulinic acid can allow for intra-operative confirmation of diagnostic specimens with a high positive predictive value [55, 56]. Raman spectroscopy, which can identify the presence of tumor cells in a specimen with a high sensitivity, represents yet another intra-operative adjunct to increase the likelihood of obtaining diagnostic specimens [57–60]. The use of these technologies could balance the need for obtaining larger volumes of tissue, by accurately predicting the presence of diagnostic tissue in the specimen.

Ultimately, while obtaining larger volumes of tumor tissue has become a prime goal for genetic and epigenetic testing, evidence remains lacking that this data can shift the curve on patient survival and outcomes. Currently, early evidence, including the SHIVA trial, has not supported molecularly targeted treatments, or precision medicine, improving outcomes [61]. As such, in order to continue qualifying the goal of obtaining large tissue samples for these molecular tests, we must show that the patient will clinically benefit from this data.

# References


1. Jones C, Perryman L, Hargrave D. Paediatric and adult malignant glioma: close relatives or distant cousins? Nat Rev Clin Oncol. 2012;9(7):400–13.
2. Patel AP, Tirosh I, Trombetta JJ, Shalek AK, Gillespie SM, Wakimoto H, et al. Single-cell RNA-seq highlights intratumoral heterogeneity in primary glioblastoma. Science. 2014;344(6190):1396–401.
3. Pfister S, Remke M, Benner A, Mendrzyk F, Toedt G, Felsberg J, et al. Outcome prediction in pediatric medulloblastoma based on DNA copy-number aberrations of chromosomes 6q and 17q and the MYC and MYCN loci. J Clin Oncol Off J Am Soc Clin Oncol. 2009;27(10):1627–36.
4. Schwalbe EC, Lindsey JC, Nakjang S, Crosier S, Smith AJ, Hicks D, et al. Novel molecular subgroups for clinical classification and outcome prediction in childhood medulloblastoma: a cohort study. Lancet Oncol. 2017;18(7):958–71.
5. Parsons DW, Jones S, Zhang X, Lin JC-H, Leary RJ, Angenendt P, et al. An integrated genomic analysis of human glioblastoma multiforme. Science. 2008;321(5897):1807–12.
6. Rivera AL, Pelloski CE, Gilbert MR, Colman H, De La Cruz C, Sulman EP, et al. MGMT promoter methylation is predictive of response to radiotherapy and prognostic in the absence of adjuvant alkylating chemotherapy for glioblastoma. Neuro-Oncol. 2010;12(2):116–21.
7. Cancer Genome Atlas Research Network, Brat DJ, Verhaak RGW, Aldape KD, Yung WKA, Salama SR, et al. Comprehensive, integrative genomic analysis of diffuse lower-grade gliomas. N Engl J Med. 2015;372(26):2481–98.
8. Bander ED, Jones SH, Kovanlikaya I, Schwartz TH. Utility of tubular retractors to minimize surgical brain injury in the removal of deep intraparenchymal lesions: a quantitative analysis of FLAIR hyperintensity and apparent diffusion coefficient maps. J Neurosurg. 2015;2:1–8.
9. Bander ED, Jones SH, Pisapia D, Magge R, Fine H, Schwartz TH, et al. Tubular brain tumor biopsy improves diagnostic yield for subcortical lesions. J Neuro-Oncol. 2019;141:121–9.
10. Greenfield JP, Cobb WS, Tsouris AJ, Schwartz TH. Stereotactic minimally invasive tubular retractor system for deep brain lesions. Neurosurgery. 2008;63(4 Suppl 2):334–9; discussion 339–340.
11. Kelly PJ, Goerss SJ, Kall BA. The stereotaxic retractor in computer-assisted stereotaxic microsurgery. Technical note. J Neurosurg. 1988;69(2):301–6.
12. Day JD. Transsulcal parafascicular surgery using BrainPath® for subcortical lesions. Neurosurgery. 2017;64(CN_suppl_1):151–6.
13. Akai T, Shiraga S, Sasagawa Y, Okamoto K, Tachibana O, Lizuka H. Intra-parenchymal tumor biopsy using neuroendoscopy with navigation. Minim Invasive Neurosurg MIN. 2008;51(2):83–6.
14. Almenawer SA, Crevier L, Murty N, Kassam A, Reddy K. Minimal access to deep intracranial lesions using a serial dilatation technique: case-series and review of brain tubular retractor systems. Neurosurg Rev. 2013;36(2):321–30.
15. Fahim DK, Relyea K, Nayar VV, Fox BD, Whitehead WE, Curry DJ, et al. Transtubular microendoscopic approach for resection of a choroidal arteriovenous malformation. J Neurosurg Pediatr. 2009;3(2):101–4.
16. Herrera SR, Shin JH, Chan M, Kouloumberis P, Goellner E, Slavin KV. Use of transparent plastic tubular retractor in surgery for deep brain lesions: a case series. Surg Technol Int. 2010;19:47–50.

17. Jho H-D, Alfieri A. Endoscopic removal of third ventricular tumors: a technical note. Minim Invasive Neurosurg MIN. 2002;45(2):114–9.
18. Jo K-W, Shin HJ, Nam D-H, Lee J-I, Park K, Kim JH, et al. Efficacy of endoport-guided endoscopic resection for deep-seated brain lesions. Neurosurg Rev. 2011;34(4):457–63.
19. Kassam AB, Engh JA, Mintz AH, Prevedello DM. Completely endoscopic resection of intraparenchymal brain tumors. J Neurosurg. 2009;110(1):116–23.
20. Kelly PJ. Future perspectives in stereotactic neurosurgery: stereotactic microsurgical removal of deep brain tumors. J Neurosurg Sci. 1989;33(1):149–54.
21. Moshel YA, Link MJ, Kelly PJ. Stereotactic volumetric resection of thalamic pilocytic astrocytomas. Neurosurgery. 2007;61(1):66–75; discussion 75.
22. Nishihara T, Nagata K, Tanaka S, Suzuki Y, Izumi M, Mochizuki Y, et al. Newly developed endoscopic instruments for the removal of intracerebral hematoma. Neurocrit Care. 2005;2(1):67–74.
23. Otsuki T, Jokura H, Yoshimoto T. Stereotactic guiding tube for open-system endoscopy: a new approach for the stereotactic endoscopic resection of intra-axial brain tumors. Neurosurgery. 1990;27(2):326–30.
24. Patil A-A. Stereotactic excision of deep brain lesions using probe guided brain retractor. Acta Neurochir. 1987;87(3–4):150–2.
25. Raza SM, Recinos PF, Avendano J, Adams H, Jallo GI, Quinones-Hinojosa A. Minimally invasive trans-portal resection of deep intracranial lesions. Minim Invasive Neurosurg MIN. 2011;54(1):5–11.
26. Recinos PF, Raza SM, Jallo GI, Recinos VR. Use of a minimally invasive tubular retraction system for deep-seated tumors in pediatric patients. J Neurosurg Pediatr. 2011;7(5):516–21.
27. Ross DA. A simple stereotactic retractor for use with the Leksell stereotactic system. Neurosurgery. 1993;32(3):475–6; discussion 476.
28. Constantini S, Mohanty A, Zymberg S, Cavalheiro S, Mallucci C, Hellwig D, et al. Safety and diagnostic accuracy of neuroendoscopic biopsies: an international multicenter study. J Neurosurg Pediatr. 2013;11(6):704–9.
29. Chrastina J, Novak Z, Riha I, Hermanova M, Feitova V. Diagnostic value of brain tumor neuroendoscopic biopsy and correlation with open tumor resection. J Neurol Surg Part A Cent Eur Neurosurg. 2014;75(2):110–5.
30. Ichinose T, Goto T, Morisako H, Takami T, Ohata K. Microroll retractor for surgical resection of brainstem cavernomas. World Neurosurg. 2010;73(5):520–2.
31. Ratre S, Yadav YR, Parihar VS, Kher Y. Microendoscopic removal of deep-seated brain tumors using tubular retraction system. J Neurol Surg Part A Cent Eur Neurosurg. 2016;77(4):312–20.
32. Jo K-I, Chung SB, Jo K-W, Kong D-S, Seol H-J, Shin H-J. Microsurgical resection of deep-seated lesions using transparent tubular retractor: pediatric case series. Childs Nerv Syst. 2011;27(11):1989–94.
33. Eichberg DG, Buttrick SS, Sharaf JM, Snelling BM, Shah AH, Ivan ME, et al. Use of tubular retractor for resection of colloid cysts: single surgeon experience and review of the literature. Oper Neurosurg [Internet]. [cited 2018 Dec 16]; Available from: https://academic.oup.com/ons/advance-article/doi/10.1093/ons/opy249/5092712.
34. Rahman M, Murad GJA, Mocco J. Early history of the stereotactic apparatus in neurosurgery. Neurosurg Focus. 2009;27(3):E12.
35. Krieger MD, Chandrasoma PT, Zee C-S, Apuzzo MLJ. Role of stereotactic biopsy in the diagnosis and management of brain tumors. Semin Surg Oncol. 1998;14(1):13–25.
36. Kickingereder P, Willeit P, Simon T, Ruge MI. Diagnostic value and safety of stereotactic biopsy for brainstem tumors: a systematic review and meta-analysis of 1480 cases. Neurosurgery. 2013;72(6):873–81; discussion 882; quiz 882.
37. Reithmeier T, Lopez WO, Doostkam S, Machein MR, Pinsker MO, Trippel M, et al. Intraindividual comparison of histopathological diagnosis obtained by stereotactic serial biopsy to open surgical resection specimen in patients with intracranial tumours. Clin Neurol Neurosurg. 2013;115(10):1955–60.

38. Hall WA. The safety and efficacy of stereotactic biopsy for intracranial lesions. Cancer. 1998;82(9):1749–55.
39. Dammers R, Haitsma IK, Schouten JW, Kros JM, Avezaat CJJ, Vincent AJPE. Safety and efficacy of frameless and frame-based intracranial biopsy techniques. Acta Neurochir. 2008;150(1):23–9.
40. Khatab S, Spliet W, Woerdeman PA. Frameless image-guided stereotactic brain biopsies: emphasis on diagnostic yield. Acta Neurochir. 2014;156(8):1441–50.
41. Castle M, Nájera E, Samprón N, Bollar A, Urreta I, Urculo E. Frameless stereotactic biopsy: diagnostic yield and complications. Neurocir Astur Spain. 2014;25(2):56–61.
42. Woodworth G, McGirt MJ, Samdani A, Garonzik I, Olivi A, Weingart JD. Accuracy of frameless and frame-based image-guided stereotactic brain biopsy in the diagnosis of glioma: comparison of biopsy and open resection specimen. Neurol Res. 2005;27(4):358–62.
43. Muragaki Y, Chernov M, Maruyama T, Ochiai T, Taira T, Kubo O, et al. Low-grade glioma on stereotactic biopsy: how often is the diagnosis accurate? Minim Invasive Neurosurg MIN. 2008;51(5):275–9.
44. Jackson RJ, Fuller GN, Abi-Said D, Lang FF, Gokaslan ZL, Shi WM, et al. Limitations of stereotactic biopsy in the initial management of gliomas. Neuro-Oncol. 2001;3(3):193–200.
45. Slowiński J, Harabin-Slowińska M, Mrówka R. Smear technique in the intra-operative brain tumor diagnosis: its advantages and limitations. Neurol Res. 1999;21(1):121–4.
46. Warnick RE, Longmore LM, Paul CA, Bode LA. Postoperative management of patients after stereotactic biopsy: results of a survey of the AANS/CNS section on tumors and a single institution study. J Neuro-Oncol. 2003;62(3):289–96.
47. Field M, Witham TF, Flickinger JC, Kondziolka D, Lunsford LD. Comprehensive assessment of hemorrhage risks and outcomes after stereotactic brain biopsy. J Neurosurg. 2001;94(4):545–51.
48. Bernstein M, Parrent AG. Complications of CT-guided stereotactic biopsy of intra-axial brain lesions. J Neurosurg. 1994;81(2):165–8.
49. Shakal AAS, Mokbel EAH. Hemorrhage after stereotactic biopsy from intra-axial brain lesions: incidence and avoidance. J Neurol Surg Part A Cent Eur Neurosurg. 2014;75(3):177–82.
50. Sottoriva A, Spiteri I, Piccirillo SGM, Touloumis A, Collins VP, Marioni JC, et al. Intratumor heterogeneity in human glioblastoma reflects cancer evolutionary dynamics. Proc Natl Acad Sci. 2013;110(10):4009–14.
51. Chen Y-N, Omay SB, Shetty SR, Liang B, Almeida JP, Ruiz-Treviño AS, et al. Transtubular excisional biopsy as a rescue for a non-diagnostic stereotactic needle biopsy-case report and literature review. Acta Neurochir (Wien). 2017;159(9):1589–95.
52. Moussazadeh N, Tsiouris AJ, Ramakrishna R. Advanced imaging for biopsy guidance in primary brain tumors. Cureus [Internet]. [cited 2018 Aug 27];8(2). Available from: https://www.ncbi.nlm.nih.gov/pmc/articles/PMC4803649/.
53. Chiang GC, Kovanlikaya I, Choi C, Ramakrishna R, Magge R, Shungu DC. Magnetic resonance spectroscopy, positron emission tomography and radiogenomics—relevance to glioma. Front Neurol [Internet]. 2018 [cited 2018 Mar 1];9. Available from: https://www.frontiersin.org/articles/10.3389/fneur.2018.00033/full.
54. Salama GR, Heier LA, Patel P, Ramakrishna R, Magge R, Tsiouris AJ. Diffusion weighted/tensor imaging, functional mri and perfusion weighted imaging in glioblastoma—foundations and future. Front Neurol [Internet]. 2018 [cited 2018 Mar 1];8. Available from: https://www.frontiersin.org/articles/10.3389/fneur.2017.00660/full.
55. Rey-Dios R, Hattab EM, Cohen-Gadol AA. Use of intraoperative fluorescein sodium fluorescence to improve the accuracy of tissue diagnosis during stereotactic needle biopsy of high-grade gliomas. Acta Neurochir. 2014;156(6):1071–5.
56. Widhalm G, Minchev G, Woehrer A, Preusser M, Kiesel B, Furtner J, et al. Strong 5-aminolevulinic acid-induced fluorescence is a novel intraoperative marker for representative tissue samples in stereotactic brain tumor biopsies. Neurosurg Rev. 2012;35(3):381–91.

57. Koljenović S, Choo-Smith L-P, Bakker Schut TC, Kros JM, van den Berge HJ, Puppels GJ. Discriminating vital tumor from necrotic tissue in human glioblastoma tissue samples by Raman spectroscopy. Lab Investig. 2002;82(10):1265–77.
58. Kalkanis SN, Kast RE, Rosenblum ML, Mikkelsen T, Yurgelevic SM, Nelson KM, et al. Raman spectroscopy to distinguish grey matter, necrosis, and glioblastoma multiforme in frozen tissue sections. J Neuro-Oncol. 2014;116(3):477–85.
59. Jermyn M, Mok K, Mercier J, Desroches J, Pichette J, Saint-Arnaud K, et al. Intraoperative brain cancer detection with Raman spectroscopy in humans. Sci Transl Med. 2015;7(274):274ra19.
60. Desroches J, Jermyn M, Pinto M, Picot F, Tremblay M-A, Obaid S, et al. A new method using Raman spectroscopy for in vivo targeted brain cancer tissue biopsy. Sci Rep. 2018;8(1):1–10.
61. Tourneau CL, Delord J-P, Gonçalves A, Gavoille C, Dubot C, Isambert N, et al. Molecularly targeted therapy based on tumour molecular profiling versus conventional therapy for advanced cancer (SHIVA): a multicentre, open-label, proof-of-concept, randomised, controlled phase 2 trial. Lancet Oncol. 2015;16(13):1324–34.

# Chapter 14
# Trans-sulcal, Channel-Based Parafascicular Surgery for Colloid Cysts

Lina Marenco-Hillembrand and Kaisorn L. Chaichana

## Introduction

Colloid cysts are rare, slow-growing intracranial tumors that represent <1% of all intracranial malignancies [1]. These lesions classically occur within the third ventricle and can block the foramina of Monro, causing isolated hydrocephalus of the lateral ventricles [2]. Surgery for these lesions is technically demanding and can be associated with significant morbidity and mortality because of the challenges in access, visualization, ability to achieve hemostasis, and potential for morbidity of surrounding structures [3–5]. Conventional microsurgical approaches for accessing and resecting colloid cysts within the intraventricular space involve a large craniotomy, extensive white matter dissection, and use of several fixed retractor blades to provide an adequate corridor for resection [6]. More recently, with the development of specialized tubular or channel-based retractors, resection can be achieved through these protected corridors with smaller openings, less white matter dissection, and minimal collateral damage [7–9]. In this chapter, we will discuss the techniques of a trans-sulcal, channel-based approach for the surgical resection of colloid cysts.

## Ventricular Anatomy

The ventricles consist of the lateral (right and left), third, and fourth ventricles [10]. The anatomy of the ventricles can be difficult to understand because of the complexity of anatomical structures in close proximity to each of the ventricles that are variable in the axial, coronal, and sagittal planes [10].

L. Marenco-Hillembrand · K. L. Chaichana (✉)
Department of Neurosurgery, Mayo Clinic Florida, Jacksonville, FL, USA
e-mail: marenco.lina@mayo.edu; chaichana.kaisorn@mayo.edu



G. Zada et al. (eds.), *Subcortical Neurosurgery*,
https://doi.org/10.1007/978-3-030-95153-5_14

The lateral ventricles are bilateral cavities that consist of a frontal horn, body, atrium and occipital horn, and temporal horn [10]. The frontal horn of the lateral ventricle extends from the genu of the corpus callosum to the foramen of Monro, where at the anterior surface resides the forceps minor of the genu of the corpus callosum, the superior surface is the body of the corpus callosum, the lateral surface is the head of the caudate nucleus, the medial surface is the septum pellucidum, and the inferior surface is the rostrum of the corpus callosum [10]. The body of the lateral ventricle extends from the foramen of Monro to the point where the corpus callosum attaches to the fornix posteriorly to the septum pellucidum, where the superior surface is the body of the corpus callosum, the lateral surface is the body of the caudate, the medial surface is the septum pellucidum, the medial inferior surface is the fornix, and the lateral inferior surface is the thalamus [10]. The atrium and occipital horn resemble a triangle with the apex oriented posteriorly, where the anterior surface are the fornix medially and the thalamus laterally, the superior surface is the corpus callosum, the lateral surface are the tapetum of the corpus callosum and tail of the caudate nucleus, the medial surface are the calcar avis and the bulb of the corpus callosum, and the inferior surface is the collateral triangle [10]. The temporal horn extends from the amygdala to the anterior wall of the atrium, where its anterior surface is the amygdala; the superior surface are the amygdala, head of the hippocampus, sublenticular portion of the internal capsule, and tail of the caudate nucleus; the lateral surface are the optic radiations (which also extend into the superior surface) and tapetum of the corpus callosum; the medial surface is the choroidal fissure; and the inferior surface are the hippocampus medially and the collateral eminence laterally [10].

The third ventricle is a midline cavity that communicates with the lateral ventricles through the bilateral foramen of Monro and with the fourth ventricle through the cerebral aqueduct [10]. Colloid cysts most commonly occur in the rostral third ventricle near the foramen of Monro [1]. The anterior surface of the third ventricle consists of the lamina terminalis; the superior surface has four layers and consists of the fornices and hippocampal commissure, the superior membrane of the tela choroidea, a vascular layer with the two internal cerebral veins and branches of the medial posterior choroidal arteries, and the inferior membrane of the tela choroidea; the lateral surface is the hypothalamic sulcus; the posterior surface are the superior pineal recess, habenular commissure, pineal recess, and posterior commissure; and the inferior surface are the optic recess, infundibular recess, tuber cinereum, mammillary bodies, and posterior perforated substance [10]. The fourth ventricle is a midline cavity located between the brainstem and cerebellum and connects to the third ventricle through the cerebral aqueduct and to the cisterna magna through the foramina of Magendie and Luschka [10]. The superior surface consists of the superior medullary velum between the superior cerebellar peduncles, the inferior surface are the tela choroidea and the inferior medullary velum, the anterior surface or the floor are the pons and medulla, and the posterior surface or roof is the cerebellum [10].

## Approaches to the Ventricular System

The ventricles can be accessed safely through the different corridors that can be divided into skull base and trans-calvarial approaches. The lateral ventricles are accessed primarily through trans-calvarial approaches, which can further be divided into intra- and extra-axial routes. This intra-axial or trans-cortical route to the lateral ventricles is typically preferred when the ventricles are large in caliber [11]. The advantages of this approach are that it minimizes manipulation of the anterior cerebral arteries, corpus callosum, and cingulate gyri, but the disadvantages are there is a potential for increased risk of seizures and damage to the superficial cortex and white matter [12]. For lesions involving the frontal horn or body of the lateral ventricle, an intra-axial route involves the frontal lobe at Kocher's point [11, 13]. This frontal lobe location is typically in the mid-pupillary line in the sagittal plane and 4–6 centimeters in front of the coronal suture [11, 13]. This point allows avoidance of the superior longitudinal fasciculus laterally, the sagittal striatum medially, and the corticospinal tracts posteriorly [11, 13]. For lesions involving the atrium and occipital horn, an intra-axial route involves a superior parietal lobule approach in the mid-pupillary line [11]. This parietal lobe location avoids the somatosensory and motor cortex anteriorly, the visual cortex posteriorly, and the superior longitudinal fasciculus laterally [11]. For lesions involving the temporal horn, an intra-axial route involves a direct lateral approach, with an understanding that visual field fibers reside along the lateral walls of the temporal horns of the lateral ventricle, as well as potentially in the superior longitudinal fasciculus and inferior longitudinal fasciculus more posteriorly [11].

An alternative approach to the lateral ventricles for the frontal horn, body, atrium, and occipital horn is a trans-calvarial approach through primarily an extra-axial route [12, 13]. This extra-axial, as compared to intra-axial, route involves an interhemispheric approach, where the anterior-posterior entry is dependent on which portion of the lateral ventricle is targeted [12, 13]. A more frontal interhemispheric approach is preferred for the frontal horn and body, while a parietal interhemispheric approach is preferred for the occipital horn and atrium [12, 13]. This extra-axial, interhemispheric route is typically preferred when the ventricles are small in caliber [12, 13]. The advantages of this approach are that it avoids cortical and subcortical entry and violation, thus minimizing the potential for seizures, but the disadvantages are potential injury to the cingulate gyrus, anterior cerebral arteries, and corpus callosum, as well as increased time of dissection [12, 13]. In this approach, the trajectory is between the hemispheres until the corpus callosum is identified. The corpus callosum is sectioned and the lateral ventricles are entered [12, 13]. The sectioning of the corpus callosum is typically limited to 2–3 cm, and entry in the anterior third of the corpus callosum is preferred to minimize potential disconnection problems that are more common posteriorly [12, 13].

The third ventricle can be entered in both skull base and trans-calvarial approaches along its anterior, posterior, inferior, and superior surfaces [12, 13]. The anterior access to the third ventricle is through the lamina terminalis through a skull base, subfrontal, extra-axial approach [12, 13]. The inferior access is through the interpeduncular cistern through a skull base, extra-axial, endoscopic transsphenoidal transsellar approach [12, 13]. The posterior access is through the pineal region typically through a trans-cranial, extra-axial, supracerebellar infratentorial or occipital transtentorial approaches [12, 13]. The superior access is through the lateral ventricles through a trans-calvarial approach as detailed in the above [12, 13]. This can be done through either an intra-axial, trans-cortical or extra-axial, interhemispheric, transcallosal route [12, 13]. Once the lateral ventricles are entered, the choroidal fissure along the roof of the third ventricle can be opened to enter the cavity of the third ventricle [12, 13]. The choroidal fissure should be opened on the forniceal side of the fissure medial to the internal cerebral veins in order to avoid the veins on the thalamic side of the fissure [12, 13].

The fourth ventricle is accessed through a trans-calvarial approach with either an extra-axial or intra-axial route [12, 13]. The advantage of the extra-axial route is that it avoids manipulation of the cerebellar vermis and hemispheres to minimize postoperative ataxia, but the disadvantages are potential injury to branches of the posterior inferior cerebellar arteries [12, 13]. The most commonly used approach is an extra-axial, telovelar approach [12, 13]. In this approach, a midline suboccipital craniotomy is done, and the cerebellomedullary fissure is opened to exposure the tela choroidea and inferior medullary velum to expose the floor of the fourth ventricle from the obex to the aqueduct [12, 13]. Alternatively, the fourth ventricle can be accessed through an intra-axial approach, where a midline suboccipital craniotomy is done followed by splitting the inferior vermis to enter the fourth ventricle [12, 13]. The splitting of the inferior vermis should be limited to the bottom half as involvement of the superior vermis can potentially lead to cerebellar mutism [12, 13].

## Open Microsurgery: Extra-axial Versus Intra-axial Approaches to the Ventricles

The general neurosurgical tenet is to minimize collateral damage. For intra-axial surgery, this typically involves taking advantage of the extra-axial space to minimize distance to the intraparenchymal lesion [14]. For access to the lateral ventricles and to the superior roof of the third ventricle, many neurosurgeons prefer an interhemispheric transcallosal approach to the lateral ventricle and opening of the choroidal fissure to access the third ventricle if needed [12, 13]. This approach minimizes the amount of brain substance that has to be violated and limits the potential parenchymal injury and therefore is associated with less risk of postoperative seizures [12, 13]. However, this approach puts several potential vascular structures at risk including the sagittal sinus and the anterior cerebral artery and its branches, as well as the cingulate gyrus and corpus callosum [12, 13]. Similarly, the extra-axial approaches to the third ventricle including the subfrontal trans-lamina terminalis and endonasal transsphenoidal transsellar approaches as well the telovelar approach to the fourth ventricle are preferred because they avoid traversing brain parenchyma [12, 13].

The trans-cortical approach was generally avoided in the past because of potential parenchymal injury since this approach involves a large craniotomy, large corticectomy through the gyrus, extensive white matter resection, and placement of bladed retractors before entering the ventricle [14]. The morbidity associated with cortical and subcortical violations can be relatively significant and may explain the increased risk of seizures, venous strokes, and/or encephalomalacia [14]. The cortical approach, regardless of method, is often preferred for cases of hydrocephalus since the enlarged ventricles provide not only a protected corridor for ventricular surgery but decreased distance of brain that needs to be violated to enter the ventricle [14].

The risks and complications of the trans-cortical approach can be minimized [14]. Minimally invasive approaches can have similar, if not improved, risk profiles to extra-axial approaches [6–9]. This is because modern channel-based retractors may be used to reduce potential surgical risks [6–9]. These retractors can displace rather than sever white matter tracts to allow parafascicular access to the ventricle, thus minimizing subcortical injury [6–9]. Additionally, these retractors provide circumferential equivalent retraction forces to minimize shear forces on the white matter [6–9]. Furthermore, these channeled retractors provide a protected corridor for access and resection [6–9]. In addition, a trans-sulcal approach can be used in combination with the channel-based retractor [6–9]. The use of trans-sulcal approaches utilizes the sulcus instead of the gyrus, which minimizes the working distance to the ventricle and the cortex that needs to be violated [6–9]. Therefore, the modern transcortical, trans-sulcal parafascicular approach can minimize potential cortical and subcortical injury while not subjecting critical vascular structures to risk and can be safely utilized for third ventricular access [6–9, 12, 13].

## Patient Selection and Indications for Surgical Removal of Colloid Cysts

Surgical management of colloid cysts is indicated in the presence of symptoms associated with increased intracranial pressure (headaches, visual changes, reduced level of consciousness) or progression on neurological imaging (including hydrocephalus) [1]. The main goal of surgery is to remove the cystic contents as well as the capsule in order to prevent recurrence [15, 16]. The techniques that are currently available for the surgical management of colloid cysts include stereotactic aspiration, endoscopy, and microsurgery [17]. Stereotactic aspiration is largely reserved for patients who are unsuitable for a craniotomy due to medical comorbidities [18]. Open microsurgery remains the gold standard for the treatment of colloid cyst of the third ventricle. However, this technique involves the transgression of neural tissue which can lead to complications including postoperative seizures and requires prolonged brain retraction leading to increased edema and higher rates of postoperative neurological deficits [17, 19]. In order to minimize the damage to eloquent brain parenchyma that is experienced with open approaches and the use of flat blade retractors, minimally invasive surgery such as neuroendoscopy or the trans-sulcal insertion of port systems has become widely utilized within the last couple of decades [19, 20]. Despite neuroendoscopy being advocated as superior to microsurgery, the drawbacks associated with this technique include the lack of stereoscopic vision and difficulty in conducting a bimanual technique; it is also not optimal for large cysts and overall is associated with lower extents of resection and higher recurrence rates due to incomplete removal of the capsule [21]. In contrast, minimally invasive parafascicular surgery (MIPS) reduces the likelihood of brain injury during resection by using naturally occurring corridors to access the ventricles while simultaneously minimizing damage to the underlying association fibers [19].

## Retractors Used for the Resection of Colloid Cysts

Retractors are critical for trans-cortical approaches to the ventricles regardless if they are trans-sulcal or trans-gyral [6–9]. The cortex and white matter need to be retracted in order to gain access to the ventricle, allow for illumination, provide a view for microscopic magnification, and prevent inadvertent tissue injury during lesion resection [6–9]. The retractors that are available come in two varieties – bladed retractors and channel-based retractors. There are a variety of bladed retractor systems including Leyla, Fukushima, Greenberg, and Budde' systems, among others. In these retractor systems, a retractor blade made of silicone or metal is inserted into the brain and retracted with a fixed arm. For ventricular access, one, two, three, or four retractors are placed into the brain to retract the cortex and subcortical white matter. The advantages of the bladed retractor system are that they can provide a large corridor for microscopic visualization and surgical resection, ease of use, and familiarity to neurosurgeons. The disadvantages are that they provide inequivalent forces which can cause white matter shearing, they do not provide a protected corridor where brain tissue can be damaged with repeated entry into the surgical site, and prolonged pressure can lead to tissue ischemia, venous congestion, and eventual encephalomalacia [6].

Channel-based retractors provided a channel in which the ventricle can be accessed and the lesion can be resected [3–5, 7–9, 22–27]. The most commonly used channel-based retractors are the peel-away catheters (Fig. 14.1), ovular-shaped retractor (Vycor ViewSite™), and circular sheath (Nico BrainPath™) (Fig. 14.2) retractors [3–5, 7–9, 22–27]. This concept of a retractor system for intracranial pathology began with Dr. Patrick Kelly in the 1980s where he used metal-based, channel retractors to access deep-seated intraparenchymal lesions that where stereotactically mapped [26–28]. Peel-away catheters allow for endoscopic-assisted

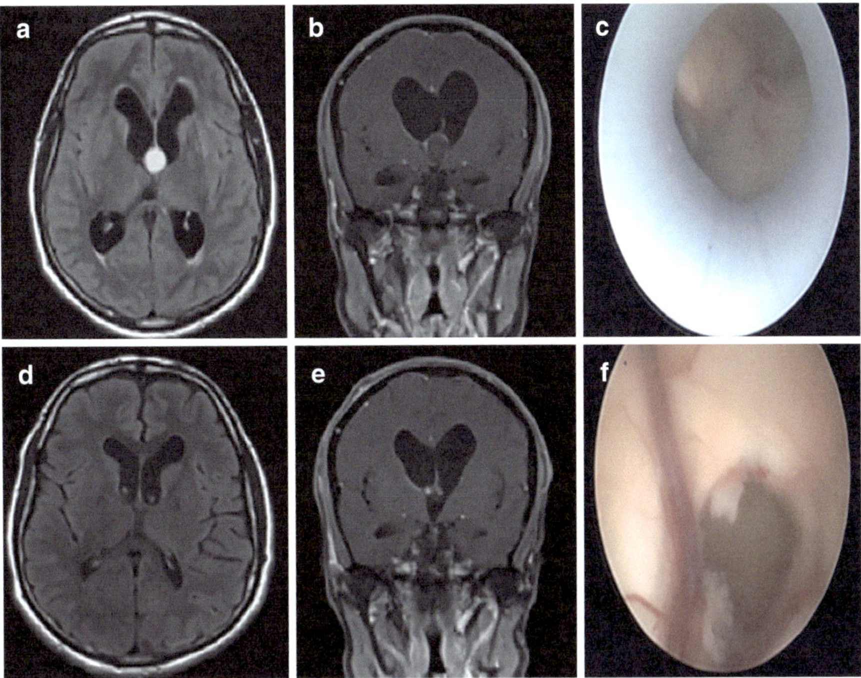

**Fig. 14.1** Trans-sulcal approach to the right lateral ventricle with a peel-away, channel-based retractor. A peel-away channel-based retractor was used to access a colloid cyst for endoscopic-guided resection. (**a**, **b**) preoperative MRI demonstrating a colloid cyst and obstructive hydrocephalus; (**c**) peel-away catheter with view through the endoscope of the right lateral ventricle; (**d**, **e**) postoperative MRI demonstrating gross total resection of the colloid cyst; (**f**) view through the endoscope after gross total resection

surgery through working-channel endoscopes and vary in diameter from 8 French to 16 French. Surgery through the peel-away catheter leaves the smallest footprint on the brain of the retractors because of its small dimensions, but surgery is limited to endoscopic working channels. This usually translates into lack of bimanual techniques and difficulty with simultaneous resection and hemostasis. The ovular-shaped retractor is oval-shaped, is transparent, and comes in different diameters (12–28 mm) and lengths (30–70 mm) [4, 5]. This retractor provides a larger working corridor for microscopic or exoscopic visualization and bimanual techniques, but its oval shape limits its use to trans-gyral instead of trans-sulcal approaches [4, 5]. The circular sheath is circle-shaped, is transparent, can be navigationally guided, and also comes in different diameters (11.5–13.5 mm) and lengths (50–95 mm) [3, 8, 9, 22, 24]. The circular sheath, like the ovular retractor, provides a sufficient corridor for both microscopic or exoscopic visualization and bimanual techniques, but it can be used with both trans-sulcal and trans-gyral approaches, and its smaller diameter puts less white matter tracts at risk [3, 8, 9, 22, 24]. The smaller corridor, however, can be challenging for resection and hemostasis as compared to the larger

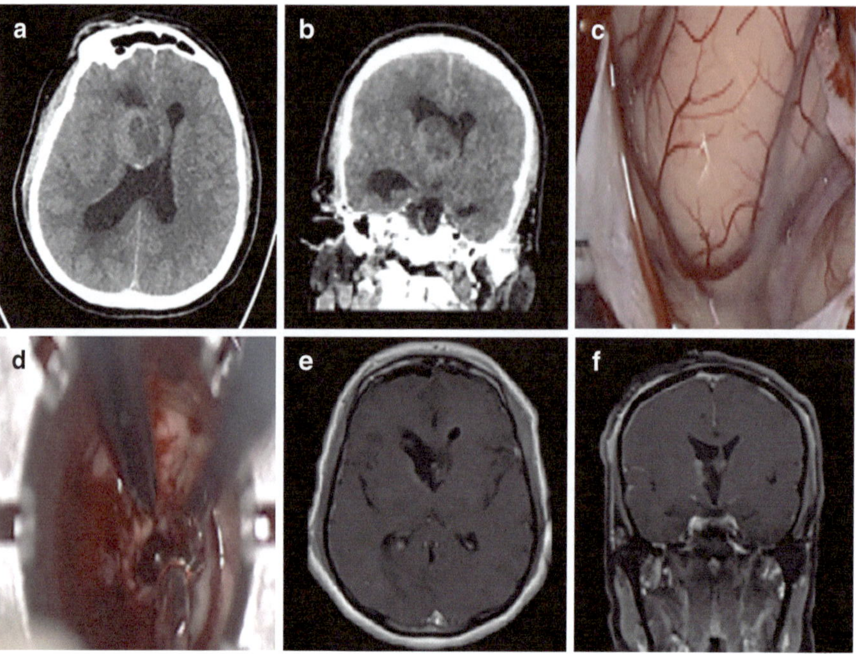

**Fig. 14.2** Trans-sulcal approach to the right lateral ventricle with a circular-shaped, channel-based retractor for the resection a large colloid cyst. A circular-shaped retractor (BrainPath™) was used to access the colloid cyst under microscopic guided resection. (**a–c**) Preoperative MRI demonstrating a large, ring-enhancing, T1/T2 hyperintense lesion within the third ventricle and obstructive hydrocephalus. (**d–f**) Postoperative MRI showing gross total resection of the lesion and resolution of the hydrocephalus

ovular-shaped retractors [3, 8, 9, 22, 24]. Regardless of channel-based retractor type, they are advantageous for trans-calvarial, intra-axial approaches because they provide equivalent circumferential retraction forces to minimize shearing of the white matter tracts, create a protected corridor to minimize collateral damage during the resection, and can be used to access deep lesions [3, 8, 9, 22, 24]. The disadvantages of these channel-based retractors, however, are the corridor is smaller, achieving hemostasis may be more challenging, and a limited number of instruments can be utilized and exclude ultrasonic aspirators [3, 8, 9, 22, 24].

## Surgical Technique

Prior to surgery, the patient undergoes high-resolution magnetic resonance imaging (MRI) with thin-cut (1.5 mm) T2-weighted images to delineate the sulcal anatomy. If there is concern of eloquent white matter tract involvement, then diffusion tensor imaging (DTI) is also done to help delineate the white matter tracts. In general, the sulcus that is in a non-eloquent area of the brain (i.e., avoidance of motor or somatosensory cortex) would be targeted. Sometimes, this is not possible given the location of the lesion. This chosen sulcus should be non-eloquent and provide the shortest corridor between the bottom of the sulcus and the ventricle. Using navigation guidance, a linear skin incision approximately 3–4 cm is made over the chosen sulcus. A 3 cm craniotomy is done with the sulcus in the center of the craniotomy flap. The dura is opened in a cruciate fashion. Under exoscope visualization, the sulcus is opened sharply to mobilize the sulcal arteries and veins and opened to the bottom of the sulcus. Under navigation guidance, the channel-based retractor is passed into the ventricle, and the obturator will be withdrawn. The retractor is then locked in place with the retractor system. For small ventricles, ultrasound can help with surgical trajectory.

Resection within the ventricle is then done meticulously and precisely. The corridor within the channel-based retractor is much smaller than the corridor created by a bladed retractor system. In the bladed retractor system, the blades can be manipulated to generate larger spaces with more force, while the channel-based retractor is fixed. However, the access provided by the channel-based retractor should be sufficient for a wide range of lesion sizes if the surgery is done carefully. When working within the ventricle, it is important to understand that bleeding can escape within the ventricular system and not be visualized. Moreover, it is important to remember that the ventricles are surrounded by critical neurovascular structures. Hemostasis should be obtained before cyst debulking to minimize intraventricular bleeding. Resection should also be methodical and systematic to avoid multiple sites of bleeding that would be difficult to address. Cyst decompression is performed first so the cyst capsule can be identified and excised safely. The use of a side-cutting aspiration device (Nico Myriad™) can facilitate cyst debulking as other devices such as an ultrasonic aspirator will not fit down the channel. The channel-based retractor can also be toggled to facilitate resecting larger lesions. After the resection, if there is concern of potential for unilateral obstruction, a septum pellucidotomy is done, and an extraventricular drain (EVD) is left. The dura, bone, and skin are closed in standard fashion.

## Case Examples

### *Case #1: Peel-Away Channel-Based Retractor Resection of a Medium-Sized Colloid Cyst*

A 32-year-old male with no significant past medical history presented with progressive headaches and intermittent nausea and vomiting. Head CT and MRI demonstrated a ring-enhancing lesion at the foramen of Monro with obstructive hydrocephalus (Fig. 14.1). He underwent a right frontal burr hole at Kocher's point, sulcal opening under microscopic guidance, and placement of a 14-French peel-away catheter into the ventricle. The peel-away catheter was used as a channel for endoscopic-guided resection (Storz Lotta™) of the mass. A septum pellucidotomy was also done prophylactically in case the foramen became obstructed. An extra-ventricular drain was kept for 1 day. The patient was discharged on postoperative day 2 to home with an intact neurological exam and resolution of his headache and fatigue. Final pathology was a colloid cyst. He was 24 months from surgery without evidence of recurrence, and the ventricles have decreased in caliber.

## Case #2: Oval-Shaped, Channel-Based Retractor Resection of a Medium-Sized Colloid Cyst

A 34-year-old right-handed female presented with a long-standing history of headaches associated with nausea, vomiting, and visual changes. A previous MRI revealed a T1 hyperintense, T2 hypointense lesion at the foramen of Monro, consistent with a colloid cyst. On follow-up imaging, there was a progressive enlargement in the size of the lesion as well as obstructive hydrocephalus. She initially opted for endoscopic removal of the cyst, but the procedure was aborted due to inadequate visualization. Subsequently, she underwent a right frontal craniotomy for the removal of the cyst. Kocher's point was located using neuro-navigation, the previous incision was identified and extended anteriorly as well as inferiorly, and the craniotomy was performed to encompass the EVD. An oval-shaped, channel-based retractor (Vycor ViewSite™) was inserted adjacent to the EVD under navigation guidance for microscopic resection of the mass. The superficial aspect of the right frontal horn was entered, and the catheter was followed down to identify the foramen of Monro. The cyst was identified and debulked, achieving gross total resection. The EVD was removed on postoperative day 2, and the patient was discharged on postoperative day 3 with an intact neurological examination. The final pathology was consistent with a colloid cyst. She is 3 months out from surgery; her headaches have resolved and show no evidence of recurrence.

## Case #3: Circular-Shaped, Channel-Based Retractor Resection of a Large Colloid Cyst

A 26-year-old right-handed male with developmental delay presented due to progressive headaches accompanied by nausea and vomiting. A CT scan was performed and revealed a large third ventricular mass. A subsequent MRI showed a large, ring-enhancing, T1/T2 hyperintense, third ventricular brain lesion measuring 5 cm in diameter with uncompensated obstructive hydrocephalus, consistent with a large colloid cyst (Fig. 14.2). Urgent surgical resection was indicated to obtain relief of the mass effect. The patient underwent a right frontal trans-sulcal approach for a colloid cyst. Kocher's point was identified on the right side, an anterior trajectory to the frontal horn was chosen, and a burr hole was drilled at the future position of the EVD. A 50 mm circular sheath (Nico BrainPath™) was passed under navigation guidance through the superior frontal sulcus into the anterior part of the frontal horn and cannulated superficially into the outer part of the ventricle. The colloid cyst was identified and cauterized. Following cauterization, the cyst was internally debulked using suction with the NICO Myriad, after which the cyst walls were coagulated. On the contralateral side, the tumor was debulked until the contralateral lateral wall was identified. An EVD was passed through the BrainPath device and placed into the lateral ventricle. Following surgery, the patient was transferred to the neuro-ICU for observation and then to the general floor. The drain was removed on postoperative day 5. The patient was discharged to rehab 1 month after the surgery. Final pathology was positive for a colloid cyst. At 2-month follow-up, the patient is doing well, his headaches have ceased, and he denies any new cognitive or neurological deficits after surgery. Follow-up imaging shows gross total resection of the cyst and resolution of the hydrocephalus.

## Conclusions

Traditional microsurgical techniques used to access colloid cysts involve large craniotomies, extensive white matter dissection, and bladed retractor systems, which can introduce significant morbidity just with access alone. In recent years, the use of channel-based retractor systems, which include peel-away catheters, ovular retractors, and circular sheaths, has allowed entrance to the ventricles through minimally invasive approaches reducing collateral injury. These channel-based retractors allow for binocular vision and bimanual handling of tissues and provide access via the trans-sulcal instead of the trans-gyral space to minimize cortical injury and approach the ventricles in a parafascicular manner.

## References


1. Beaumont TL, Limbrick DD Jr, Rich KM, Wippold FJ 2nd, Dacey RG Jr. Natural history of colloid cysts of the third ventricle. J Neurosurg. 2016;125(6):1420–30.
2. Louis DN, Ohgaki H, Wiestler OD, et al. The 2007 WHO classification of tumours of the central nervous system. Acta Neuropathol. 2007;114(2):97–109.
3. Eliyas JK, Glynn R, Kulwin CG, et al. Minimally invasive transsulcal resection of intraventricular and periventricular lesions through a tubular retractor system: multicentric experience and results. World Neurosurg. 2016;90:556–64.
4. Raza SM, Recinos PF, Avendano J, Adams H, Jallo GI, Quinones-Hinojosa A. Minimally invasive trans-portal resection of deep intracranial lesions. Minim Invasive Neurosurg. 2011;54(1):5–11.
5. Recinos PF, Raza SM, Jallo GI, Recinos VR. Use of a minimally invasive tubular retraction system for deep-seated tumors in pediatric patients. J Neurosurg Pediatr. 2011;7(5):516–21.
6. Chaichana KL, Vivas-Buitrago T, Jackson C, et al. The radiographic effects of surgical approach and use of retractors on the brain after anterior cranial fossa meningioma resection. World Neurosurg. 2018;112:e505–13.

7. Gassie K, Wijesekera O, Chaichana KL. Minimally invasive tubular retractor-assisted biopsy and resection of subcortical intra-axial gliomas and other neoplasms. J Neurosurg Sci. 2018;62(6):682–9.

8. Iyer R, Chaichana KL. Minimally invasive resection of deep-seated high-grade gliomas using tubular retractors and exoscopic visualization. J Neurol Surg A Cent Eur Neurosurg. 2018;79(4):330–6.

9. Jackson C, Gallia GL, Chaichana KL. Minimally invasive biopsies of deep-seated brain lesions using tubular retractors under exoscopic visualization. J Neurol Surg A Cent Eur Neurosurg. 2017;78(6):588–94.

10. Rhoton AL Jr. The lateral and third ventricles. Neurosurgery. 2002;51(4 Suppl):S207–71.

11. Gungor A, Baydin S, Middlebrooks EH, Tanriover N, Isler C, Rhoton AL Jr. The white matter tracts of the cerebrum in ventricular surgery and hydrocephalus. J Neurosurg. 2017;126(3):945–71.

12. Anderson RC, Ghatan S, Feldstein NA. Surgical approaches to tumors of the lateral ventricle. Neurosurg Clin N Am. 2003;14(4):509–25.

13. Rhoton AL Jr. The cerebrum. Anatomy. Neurosurgery. 2007;61(1 Suppl):37–118; discussion 118–119.

14. Campero A, Ajler P, Emmerich J, Goldschmidt E, Martins C, Rhoton A. Brain sulci and gyri: a practical anatomical review. J Clin Neurosci. 2014;21(12):2219–25.

15. Vorbau C, Baldauf J, Oertel J, Gaab MR, Schroeder HWS. Long-term results after endoscopic resection of colloid cysts. World Neurosurg. 2019;122:e176–85.

16. Boogaarts HD, Decq P, Grotenhuis JA, et al. Long-term results of the neuroendoscopic management of colloid cysts of the third ventricle: a series of 90 cases. Neurosurgery. 2011;68(1):179–87.

17. Eichberg DG, Buttrick SS, Sharaf JM, et al. Use of tubular retractor for resection of colloid cysts: single surgeon experience and review of the literature. Oper Neurosurg (Hagerstown, Md). 2019;16(5):571–9.

18. Rajshekhar V. Rate of recurrence following stereotactic aspiration of colloid cysts of the third ventricle. Stereotact Funct Neurosurg. 2012;90(1):37–44.

19. Lin M, Bakhsheshian J, Strickland B, et al. Navigable channel-based trans-sulcal resection of third ventricular colloid cysts: a multicenter retrospective case series and review of the literature. World Neurosurg. 2020;133:e702–10.

20. Azab WA, Najibullah M, Yosef W. Endoscopic colloid cyst excision: surgical techniques and nuances. Acta Neurochir. 2017;159(6):1053–8.

21. Sheikh AB, Mendelson ZS, Liu JK. Endoscopic versus microsurgical resection of colloid cysts: a systematic review and meta-analysis of 1,278 patients. World Neurosurg. 2014;82(6):1187–97.

22. Bakhsheshian J, Strickland BA, Jackson C, et al. Multicenter investigation of channel-based subcortical trans-sulcal exoscopic resection of metastatic brain tumors: a retrospective case series. Oper Neurosurg (Hagerstown). 2019;16:159–66.

23. Bander ED, Jones SH, Kovanlikaya I, Schwartz TH. Utility of tubular retractors to minimize surgical brain injury in the removal of deep intraparenchymal lesions: a quantitative analysis of FLAIR hyperintensity and apparent diffusion coefficient maps. J Neurosurg. 2016;124(4):1053–60.

24. Day JD. Transsulcal parafascicular surgery using BrainPath® for subcortical lesions. Neurosurgery. 2017;64(CN_suppl_1):151–6.

25. Kelly PJ. Stereotactic biopsy and resection of thalamic astrocytomas. Neurosurgery. 1989;25(2):185–94; discussion 194–185.

26. Kelly PJ, Goerss SJ, Kall BA. The stereotaxic retractor in computer-assisted stereotaxic microsurgery. Technical note. J Neurosurg. 1988;69(2):301–6.

27. Kelly PJ, Kall BA, Goerss SJ. Computer-interactive stereotactic resection of deep-seated and centrally located intraaxial brain lesions. Appl Neurophysiol. 1987;50(1–6):107–13.

28. Kelly PJ. Future perspectives in stereotactic neurosurgery: stereotactic microsurgical removal of deep brain tumors. J Neurosurg Sci. 1989;33(1):149–54.

# Chapter 15
# Trans-sulcal, Channel-Based Parafascicular Surgery for Intracerebral Hematoma

Rima Sestokas Rindler and Gustavo Pradilla

## Introduction

Primary, spontaneous intracerebral hemorrhage (ICH) is a significant cause of morbidity and mortality worldwide [1, 2]. There has been a tremendous effort over the last few decades to employ surgical hematoma evacuation to improve the functional outcome of patients that survive their stroke event [3]. Each clinical trial to date has offered some modification to the previous one in the hopes of discovering "the optimal way." Despite our excellent collective ability to attain near-complete hematoma evacuation with current techniques, there is no clear established impact on overall long-term patient outcome [4–6]. Approach-related morbidity has been invoked as a potential culprit, specifically with regard to disruption of cerebral cortex and white matter tracts. As a result, current-day efforts are focused on refining how the lesion is accessed while adhering to two principles: maximal hematoma evacuation while maintaining minimal disruption of normal brain tissue. Novel or enhanced technologies from the last decade have allowed surgeons to trial different approaches to hematoma evacuation while staying true to these principles.

These efforts have culminated in the development of the trans-sulcal, channel-based parafascicular surgery as one such approach. Each component of the technique has been carefully selected for certain perceived advantages of achieving the surgical goals. The basis for the approach is to provide adequate access to and visualization of deep subcortical hematomas (exoscope-assisted port-based channel), minimize cortical disruption (trans-sulcal entry), and maintain the integrity of white matter tracts through a corridor that runs parallel to the tracts (parafascicular).

R. S. Rindler
The Mayo Clinic, Department of Neurosurgery, Rochester, MN, USA

G. Pradilla (✉)
Neurological Surgery, Emory University School of Medicine, Atlanta, GA, USA
e-mail: gpradil@emory.edu

© Springer Nature Switzerland AG 2022
G. Zada et al. (eds.), *Subcortical Neurosurgery*,
https://doi.org/10.1007/978-3-030-95153-5_15

Advanced technologies in operative instrumentation, optical and biomechanical sciences, and neuroimaging provide critical support for successfully executing this approach. In this chapter, we will detail the historical context and rationale for each component of the approach and describe the current state of technological innovation.

# The Principles for Surgical Evacuation of Intracerebral Hematoma

## Patient and Pathology Selection

The impact of surgical evacuation of primary, spontaneous ICH on improving patient long-term functional outcome is still up for debate [4, 7]. Several factors must be considered in the decision to evacuate an ICH, including its location and size, as well as the clinical status of the patient. The vast majority of spontaneous intracerebral hemorrhages occur in either the deep gray matter or the subcortical white matter of the cerebral hemispheres. There is little evidence, including in the most recent trials, that any form of evacuation of deep gray matter hemorrhages has any impact on overall outcome, but that lobar hemorrhages (e.g., frontal, temporal, occipital, parietal) may experience some benefit. There is evidence that blood and blood breakdown products are cytotoxic and might lead to secondary neurological injury that impedes or worsens patient recovery if left to reabsorb naturally [8]. The size of presenting hematomas also matters. Size can range from a tiny blush to an almost holo-hemispheric hemorrhage. In our institution, a potentially "operative" hematoma is considered to be $\geq 30$ cm$^3$, especially if associated with significant midline shift or clinical herniation syndromes. Finally, the current and pre-ictus clinical status of the patient becomes important: surgical intervention is pursued for non-elderly patients with a good baseline medical and functional status (modified Rankin Scale score 0 or 1), in a normal coagulation state, with a non-moribund neurological exam (Glasgow Coma Scale, GCS score $\geq 5$). Some argue that hematoma evacuation, if complete, can relieve elevated intracranial pressure and local mass effect on the brain, thereby also potentially avoiding the need for a decompressive hemicraniectomy and its associated risks. Given the clinical equipoise still present in many of these situations, it is ultimately at the treating neurosurgeon's discretion, in discussion with the patient and/or the patient's family, whether to proceed with ICH evacuation.

Our institution has employed the channel-based parafascicular approach to deep and lobar ICHs in patients with selected criteria above, as described in a prospective, multicenter, observational study by Labib et al. [9]. The approach to the clot is based on the integrity and location of the white matter tracts adjacent to the hematoma, The early collective experience in 39 patients from 11 centers achieved statistically significant improvements in postoperative GCS, with a clot evacuation of ≥90% in 72% of patients. The Cleveland Clinic series evaluated 18 patients with similar results, including improvement of the median GCS from 10 preoperatively to 14 postoperatively [10]. Our institutional experience of 17 patients suggests equivalent safety profile and a slight functional benefit to minimally invasive surgery over medical management [11]. From these experiences, a multicenter randomized controlled trial (Early MiNimally-invasive Removal of IntraCerebral Hemorrhage, ENRICH) was designed to specifically address the question of whether minimal cortical and subcortical disruption for hematoma evacuation improves outcomes (www.enrichtrial.com, NCT02880878). The trial remains ongoing anticipated through 2021.

## *Principle I: Maximal Hematoma Evacuation*

Hematoma evacuation is maximized in order to prevent secondary cytotoxic brain injury caused by the presence of the blood breakdown products or hypoxic brain injury caused by decreased perfusion from local mass effect. Complete hematoma evacuation requires sufficient tools for access and visibility. Intracerebral hematomas generally maintain a circular or oval shape and typically involve a single brain region or compartment. Past strategies have involved planning the surgical trajectory along the long axis of the lesion (STITCH I and II) in an open, non-port-based technique [6, 12]. The proximal-most face of the clot is first encountered and is then "chased" to its base. As the clot is debulked from the center, the surrounding rind of clot can be collapsed into the field, much like a tumor resection. This technique is most easily applied for superficial clots that reach the cortical surface, but more challenging for deeper clots. Port-based methods and visual intraoperative technologies have thus been applied to such cases to overcome these issues [9]. Port-based approaches maintain an unobstructed surgical corridor without excessive retraction or shearing of the surrounding brain. In contrast to standard microsurgical approaches, the primary target for port-based navigation is at the distal base of the clot. The resection then proceeds in a distal to proximal fashion. The clot in the direct field of view is evacuated, and clot from the surrounding rind falls into view. The tube can be adjusted 10–15 degrees in a radial fashion for added visibility. Addition of an exoscope or microscope is requisite to enhanced lighting and magnification of the surgical field. Advantages of the exoscope include uniform illumination and magnification of the entire surgical field, including proximal and deep targets; creation of a wide focal field that can be projected onto a high-definition screen viewed by the surgeon and team; and long focal length (15–31 mm) and working distance (20–65 cm) [13]. All of these factors enhance visibility of the hematoma target.

## *Principle II: Maintaining the Integrity of Cerebral Cortex and Subcortical White Matter Tracts*

The second principle for successful hematoma evacuation is minimizing disruption to normal brain tissue along the planned surgical trajectory to the hematoma and the tissue at risk immediately adjacent to the hematoma. These principles can be upheld again with port-based technologies and through careful planning of the surgical trajectory. In a port-based technique, a single and no more than two trajectories are attempted toward the target. Once docked, the tube acts as a physical barrier for healthy brain against the instruments as they are passed to and from the target. Even more importantly, however, the choice of cortical entry point and trajectory is critical for protecting undisturbed white matter tracts and avoiding iatrogenic neurological deficits. A trans-sulcal entry point through a non-eloquent area is optimal in order to prevent injury to the cortical mantle or cerebral vasculature. The planned trajectory should be parafascicular, or parallel to the major white matter tracts, especially if they are not injured by the primary hemorrhagic event.

For proper execution of these principles, it is necessary to (1) visualize the tracts and (2) note the relationship of the tracts to the hematoma, particularly the location and extent of destruction. High-quality neuroimaging is critical for this purpose in the form of high-resolution, three-dimensional, volumetric MRI with whole brain tractography [diffuse tensor imaging (DTI)]. DTI characterizes the anisotropic, or asymmetric, diffusion of water molecules along white matter tracts to identify the density and location of these tracts within the brain [14, 15]. Differences in this anisotropy between each imaged voxel are used to create a 2D grayscale map that is then reconstructed in a 3D color-coded fashion [16]. In this way, the most salient white matter tracts can be visualized in relation to the hemorrhage and planned operative trajectory and avoided. Of particular importance are the projection fibers of the optic radiations and pyramidal/corticospinal tracts and the unilateral association fibers of the arcuate fasciculus (AF), superior longitudinal fasciculus (SLF), inferior longitudinal fasciculus (ILF), uncinate fasciculus (UF), inferior fronto-occipital fasciculus (IFO), and cingulate fasciculus (CF). The chosen path from the cortical surface to the hematoma should traverse parallel to these fibers as much as possible. An anterior, frontal approach is best utilized for anterior basal ganglia hemorrhages, taking advantage of the corridor between the SLF and CF. For posterior hematomas, the parieto-occipital sulcus is the entry point to the lesion, posterior to the primary sensory cortex fibers. A directly lateral approach to deeper lesions is ideally avoided, as this would transgress tracts in a perpendicular fashion, but may be appropriate for lesions that come directly to the cortical surface [17].

Obtaining such high-quality imaging with DTI does come with challenges. In pathologies such as ICH, peri-hematomal edema or primary tract violation may decrease tract anisotropy and introduce artifact that leads to poor visualization of preserved tracts. Additionally, DTI post-processing requires time and neuroradiological expertise, which could impact valuable time to treatment. Finally, intraoperative shifts in brain parenchyma could also affect the accuracy of DTI neuronavigation during the operation [18].

Once a trajectory is planned, the surgical technique and tools are critical to maintaining the integrity of the surrounding brain during access and hematoma removal. For this reason, port or channel-based instruments are valuable for gaining access to deep lesions, as they typically cause temporary and circumferential stretching rather than tissue destruction along the path. Hematoma removal should employ non-ablative, non-thermal techniques unless absolutely necessary.

## Surgical Technique

To adhere to the principles outlined above, our group has adopted specific techniques, tools, and workflow to efficiently plan and safely execute evacuation of acute ICH [17].

Preoperative Planning

We utilize the Synaptive neuronavigation system (Synaptive Medical, Toronto, Canada) for preoperative planning purposes to visualize the target and subcortical tracts and plan the operative corridor (Fig. 15.1). The system imports and overlays standard MRI sequences (T1, T2, and DTI) to automatically incorporate and display whole brain tractography (Modus Plan™, Bright Matter™; Fig. 15.2). We use the system for trajectory planning and have found that the overlay of white matter tracts with respect to location of the hematoma is especially useful. As we simulate our planned surgical corridor, we are able to identify any traversing fiber tracts that are at risk of damage and adjust the plan accordingly. We then utilize the neuronavigation system in real time to guide the BrainPath unit along our planned trajectory to the lesion (Figs. 15.1 and 15.2). Other neuronavigation systems are also well suited for this purpose.

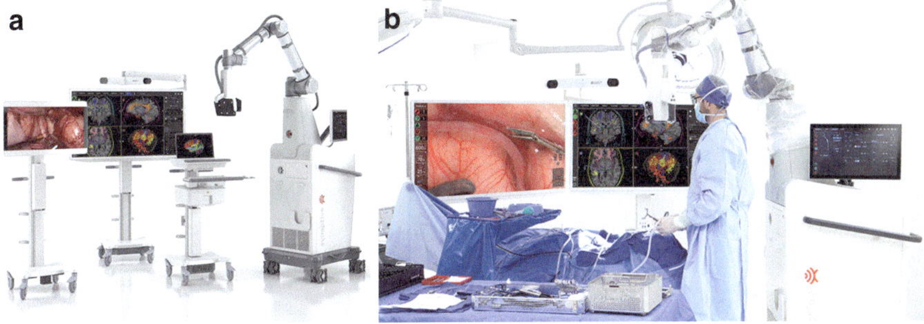

**Fig. 15.1** The Synaptive Integrated Suite. (**a**) From left to right, intraoperative exoscope monitor, neuronavigation screen with BrightMatter Guide, Modus Plan workstation, Modus robotic exoscope. (**b**) The Synaptive Integrated Suite intraoperative setup

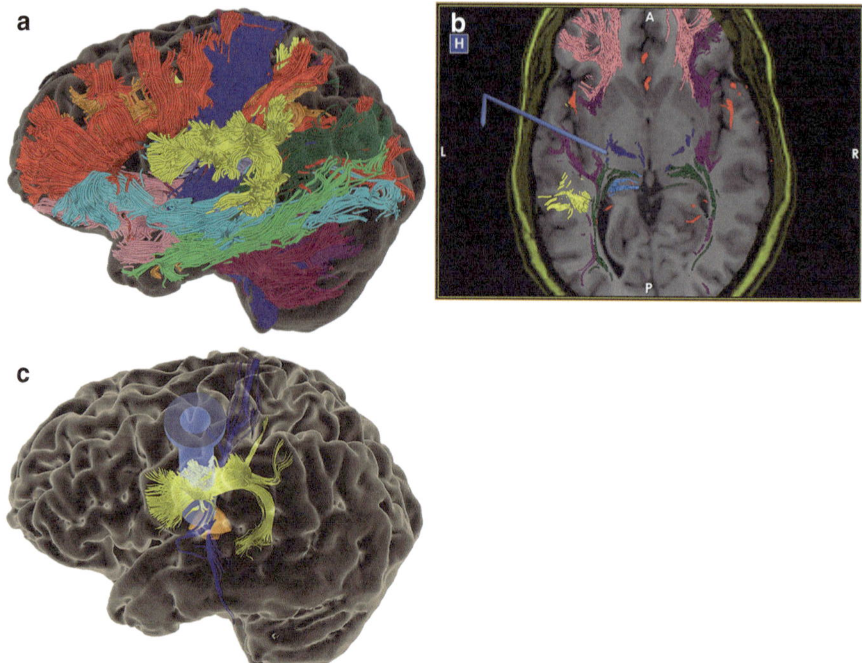

**Fig. 15.2** Magnetic resonance imaging of the brain with overlayed diffusion tensor imaging of white matter tracts overlayed into cortical and subcortical brain matter using Synaptive Modus Plan (**a**), intraoperative neuronavigation using BrightMatter with a neuronavigation probe in blue (**b**), and port-based entry (**c**)

## Operative Equipment

We use the BrainPath® system (NICO Corporation, Indianapolis, IN) as our port-based channel (Fig. 15.3) [19]. This was designed specifically for trans-sulcal access to deep-seated lesions with a special focus on minimizing injury to adjacent tissue. The system is comprised of a hollow, metallic obturator that inserts into a clear, plastic cylindrical sheath. The obturator accommodates a stereotactic pointer through its center that assists with intraoperative navigation during initial placement of the port. The obturator, sheath, and navigation probe are assembled and advanced as a unit to the intracranial target. The obturator has a blunt, cone-shaped tip that extends either 8 mm or 15 mm beyond the edge of the sheath. The tip of the obturator is 2 mm and dilates to a 13.5 mm diameter. It comes in a variety of lengths (50, 60, 75, 95 mm). The sheath is made of frosted plastic to minimize glare to the surgeon. The working diameter of the port is 12 mm that allows for bimanual microsurgical technique.

Visualization for microsurgical dissection is maintained with a mounted exoscope (Vitom HD exoscope, Optronics, Goleta, CA; VisionSense, VisionSense,

**Fig. 15.3**  NICO BrainPath channel-based intracranial access equipment. (**a**) Assembly of inner cannula and plastic obturator sheath in various widths and lengths. (**b**) BrainPath inner cannula tip size relative to a dime. (**c**) BrainPath inner cannula insertion into brain parenchyma via corticectomy, magnified view from exoscope

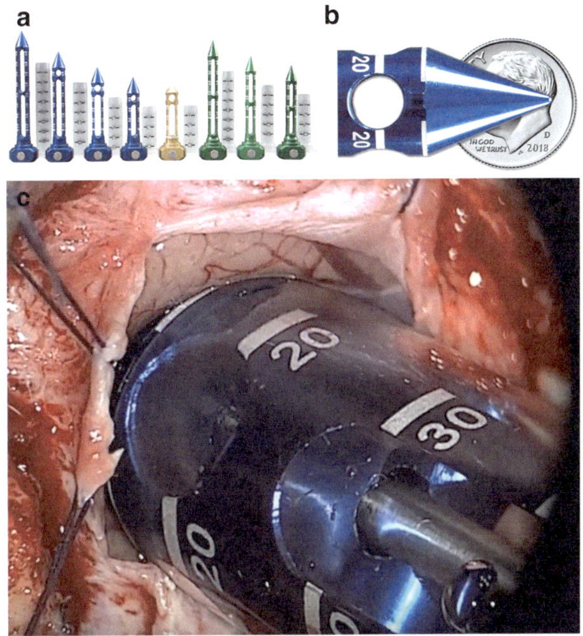

Philadelphia, PA; BrightMatter Vision, Synaptive Medical, Toronto, Canada). The manual mount employs gas-powered push-button mechanism for zero-gravity mobilization (i.e., Point Setter, Mitaka Kohki Co, Tokyo, Japan) (Fig. 15.4). Alternatively, a robotic-mounted exoscope automatically realigns to the neuronavigation probe to maintain coaxial visibility with the sheath (ModusV™, Synaptive Medical, Toronto, Canada; Fig. 15.1). Clot removal is performed with a motor-driven, suction-debriding device, in addition to regular suction tips, for clot removal (NICO Myriad NOVUS®, NICO Corporation, Indianapolis, IN; Fig. 15.5). Additional lighting is available with certain suction-aspiration handpieces that enhances intraoperative visibility (NICO Myriad-LX Light Source ®, NICO Corporation, Indianapolis, IN). A comprehensive list of additional tools and equipment necessary to execute the procedure is included in Fig. 15.6 as our group has previously published [13].

Perioperative Care

The patient is stabilized from a cardiopulmonary standpoint prior to transfer to the operating room. This may require endotracheal intubation, supplementary oxygenation, or vasoactive agents to maintain a systolic blood pressure <160 mmHg. As patients presenting with acute ICH often are hypertensive at baseline, it is important to avoid hypotension and precipitate watershed ischemia while controlling

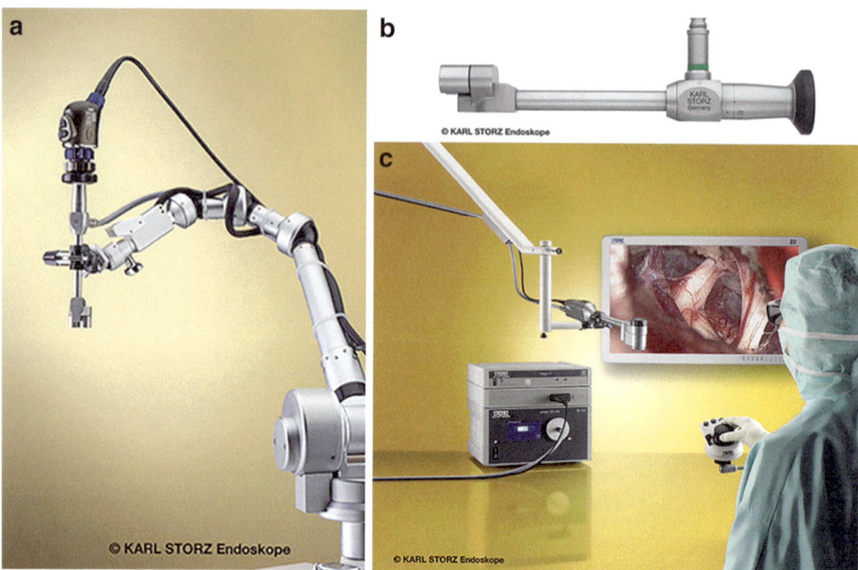

**Fig. 15.4** 2D exoscope (**a**, **b**; VITOM HD 0-degree Endoskope KARL STORZ Endoscopy-America, Inc.) mounted on a pneumatic, zero-gravity Point Setter arm (**a** Mitaka Kohki Company). VITOM 3D 4 K exoscope (**c**), mounted on a VERSACRANE holding arm connected to a 3D monitor, IMAGE1S Connect camera control unit (top), IMAGE1S D3-Link (middle), Xenon Light Source (bottom). Surgeon holding the IMAGE1 Pilot

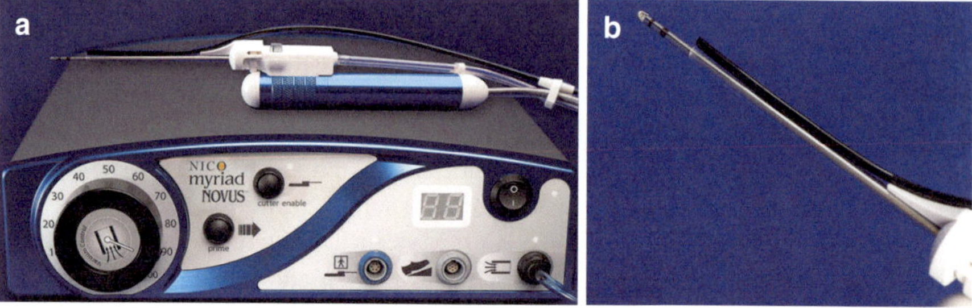

**Fig. 15.5** NICO Myriad equipment for mechanical suction-aspiration of intraparenchymal hematoma (**a**). NICO Myriad NOVUS LX with light source to improve visibility within the BrainPath sheath. (**b**) The side-aspiration window at the tip of the Myriad device is shown with a fiber-optic attachment to maximize illumination at the bottom of the port

hypertension to prevent progressive hemorrhage. If the patient is not exhibiting clinical herniation syndromes, then hyperosmotic agents are withheld; temporary intracranial hypertension is advantageous during the initial cannulation procedure to provide backpressure against the port and assist with clot delivery into the port. For patients who are protecting their airway preoperatively, immediate post-procedure extubation is attempted.

BrainPath Evacuation of Intracerebral Hemorrhage
Operating Room Checklist

- Mayfield headholder skull pins
- Mayfield bed adapter
- Synaptive neuronavigation suite
  - Synaptive navigation reference frame
  - stereotactic pointer, non-sterile
  - stereotactic pointer, sterile
    (requires 4 sterile optical navigation spheres)
  - navigation reference frame sterile sleeve
- Storz endoscope tower
  - Storz exoscope camera and light source-sterile
- Mitaka pneumatic arm
  - clear plastic sterile drape
- NICO Myriad console
  - portable nitrogen tank
  - Myriad handpiece, needs to be primed
  - NICO BrainPath obturators
  - NICO BrainPath sheaths
  - NICO Shepherd's hook
- operating chair
  - pads for arm rests
  - sterile plastic sheaths for each arm rest
  - sterile gown for back of chair

- irrigating bipolar
- long black neuro bipolar
- electric high-speed drill
  - perforator drill bit
  - straight bit with footplate
  - insulated monopolar cautery
- suctions
  - rubber extensions
  - Frazier suctions size 10Fr and 12Fr
- Mizuho suction tips size 5 and 7, long and extra-long
- Leyla bar retractor system
- Greenberg retractor system
- Fishooks
- Gelfoam powder, Surgiflo with long applicator
- Surgicel
- cottonoids in 0.5x0.5 inch and 1x1 inch squares soaked in thrombin
- bone plating system
- small Duragen dural regeneration matrix
- Adherus dural sealant
- hydroxyapatite bone cement
- Vancomycin powder

**Fig. 15.6** Comprehensive checklist of equipment necessary for channel-based parafascicular evacuation of subcortical intracerebral hemorrhage. Equipment can be substituted as necessary and as resources are available for specific operative settings

## Patient and Head Positioning

Following radiographic target and trajectory planning, the patient's head is affixed to a three-point head fixation device to maintain stability and neuronavigation accuracy. The site of the craniotomy is planned preoperatively based on the port entry point and trajectory. This location is positioned at the highest point in the field. The head may remain in a neutral and slightly extended position for anterior corridors or turned for lateral or posterior corridors. The latter may require supporting the body with a bump or turning the body to a lateral position in order to maintain a neutral neck position. The incision is marked accordingly over the planned craniotomy. An incision in the eyebrow or forehead crease may accommodate an anterior approach, whereas a small vertical linear incision (~4–5 cm) over the parietal, temporal, or occipital bones would be suitable for lateral or posterior approaches. The patient's preoperative imaging is co-registered to his or her craniofacial features using the chosen stereotactic neuronavigation system. Incision is made, and the subperiosteal plane dissected. A small craniotomy the size of the skin opening is turned to accommodate the width of the port and still allow for adequate range of motion to align with the trajectory. The dura is opened sharply in a cruciate fashion just barely larger than the port; this contains the edematous brain tissue out of the field and maintains a seal around the port (Fig. 15.3). The exoscope is draped and brought into the field. A sulcus is selected for port entry, and the arachnoid sharply dissected. Adjacent vascular structures are mobilized and preserved as needed.

## Accessing the Lesion

The BrainPath obturator, sheath, and compatible neuronavigation probe are assembled and entered as a unit into the sulcus along the planned trajectory to the base of the target. Once the target is reached, the obturator and navigation probe are removed, and the sheath is docked in place with a retaining hook and retractor system (NICO Shepherd's Hook-Greenberg™, NICO Corporation, Indianapolis, IN; Greenberg® Retractor, Symmetry Surgical, Antioch, TN). This serves as the stable channel to the lesion for the remainder of the operation.

## Resection Techniques

Coagulated hematoma often extrudes spontaneously into the sheath channel. The hematoma is mechanically evacuated in a systematic fashion (NICO Myriad NOVUS®). The hematoma is gently guided into the sheath's channel and resected. Once healthy-appearing white matter is visualized, hemostasis is achieved in this location with bipolar electrocautery provided by long bayoneted forceps, flowable matrix with thrombin, or thrombin-soaked gelatin sponges. The retractor system is loosened, and the sheath is retracted by 1 cm increments for complete hematoma evacuation until it reaches the end of the cavity or cortical surface. Additionally, the sheath may be angulated in 10–15-degree increments if needed to access material that is out of site of the initial trajectory. The dura is reapproximated as able or closed with a dural substitute inlay. The craniotomy flap is replaced and secured to the skull with titanium miniplates and screws. The galea is reapproximated, and the skin closed with absorbable suture.

## Postoperative Care

All patients are admitted to the neurocritical care unit for close neurological monitoring. Patients with radiographic evidence of elevated intracranial pressure, cerebral edema, or obstructive hydrocephalus undergo placement of a ventriculostomy for external cerebrospinal fluid diversion and monitoring of intracranial pressures. The patients undergo immediate postoperative head CT to assess the resection cavity. The systolic blood pressure is maintained <180 mmHg. Prophylactic anticoagulation for the prevention of deep venous thrombosis is resumed 48 hours postoperatively if there is no evidence of recurrent hemorrhage. Levetiracetam is administered for 7 days or longer if the presentation is complicated by ongoing seizures. Alimentation by mouth or by a Dobhoff tube is resumed within 24 hours.

## Case Example

The patient is a 74-year-old Hispanic woman who presented to our institution. She had a history of type 2 diabetes mellitus and hypertension. Neuroimaging revealed a right spontaneous intraparenchymal hematoma centered in the basal ganglia measuring 4.8 × 3.0 × 4.0 cm (approximately 29 cc in volume) causing mass effect on the right lateral ventricle and 5 mm of right to left midline shift. CT angiography was negative for a vascular malformation or aneurysm. The presumed etiology was hypertension. On initial neurological examination, she was intubated, opening eyes to voice, briskly localizing with the right arm, withdrawing the right leg, and flaccid in the left extremities (GCS 9 T, ICH score 2). She underwent immediate MRI with DTI (Fig. 15.7). She was taken to the operating room emergently for a right frontal craniotomy through a forehead crease incision. The dura was opened, and the BrainPath port was inserted under image guidance to the base of the hematoma, which was resected with the use of a suction-aspiration device. The dura and skull defect were reconstructed. The patient ultimately made a reasonable postoperative recovery and was discharged to a subacute rehabilitation facility with residual left-sided hemiparesis.

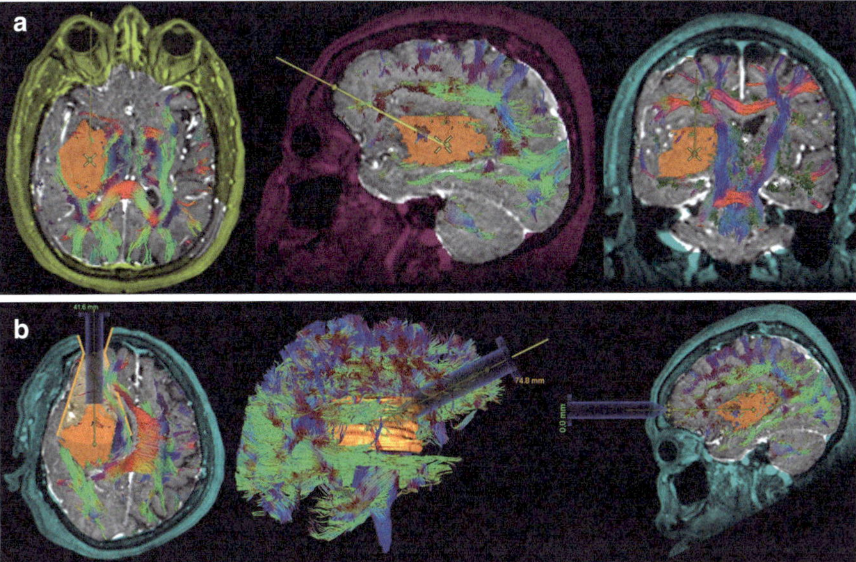

**Fig. 15.7** Magnetic resonance imaging with diffusion tensor sequences of a spontaneous right basal ganglia intraparenchymal hematoma in axial, sagittal, and coronal planes. Note the partial destruction and medial displacement of the corticospinal tracts in blue (coronal) and destruction and lateral displacement of the inferior longitudinal fasciculus in green (axial) (**a**)
Stereotactic guidance trajectory views of the planned approach to the intraparenchymal hematoma utilizing the Synaptive neuronavigation system. Note the 15-degree range of motion in all directions (left image), the 3D image of the trajectory and hematoma in relation to white matter tracts (middle image), and the sagittal trajectory view through the planned frontal craniotomy (right image) (**b**)

## Conclusion

Acute intracerebral hemorrhages located in deep subcortical white matter can be safely and efficiently accessed and evacuated with a trans-sulcal, parafascicular port-based technique. This technique, and the technology that enables its execution, aims to provide access and visibility to the lesion at hand while minimally disturbing intervening and adjacent brain matter. The techniques described here have been successfully employed at our institution, but can be modified to fit the neurosurgeon's particular context and resources.

## References


1. Gross BA, Jankowitz BT, Friedlander RM. Cerebral intraparenchymal hemorrhage: a review. JAMA. 2019;321(13):1295–303.
2. Ikram MA, Wieberdink RG, Koudstaal PJ. International epidemiology of intracerebral hemorrhage. Curr Atheroscler Rep. 2012;14(4):300–6.
3. Prasad K, Mendelow AD, Gregson B. Surgery for primary supratentorial intracerebral haemorrhage. Cochrane Database Syst Rev. 2008;(4):CD000200.
4. Hemphill JC III, Greenberg SM, Anderson CS, Becker K, Bendok BR, Cushman M, et al. Guidelines for the management of spontaneous intracerebral hemorrhage: a guideline for healthcare professionals from the American Heart Association/American Stroke Association. Stroke. 2015;46(7):2032–60.
5. Morgenstern LB, Frankowski RF, Shedden P, Pasteur W, Grotta JC. Surgical treatment for intracerebral hemorrhage (STICH): a single-center, randomized clinical trial. Neurology. 1998;51(5):1359–63.
6. Mendelow AD, Gregson BA, Fernandes HM, Murray GD, Teasdale GM, Hope DT, et al. Early surgery versus initial conservative treatment in patients with spontaneous supratentorial intracerebral haematomas in the International Surgical Trial in Intracerebral Haemorrhage (STICH): a randomised trial. Lancet. 2005;365(9457):387–97.
7. Gregson BA, Mitchell P, Mendelow AD. Surgical decision making in brain hemorrhage: new analysis of the STICH, STICH II, and STITCH(trauma) randomized trials. Stroke. 2019;50(5):1108–15.
8. Aronowski J, Zhao X. Molecular pathophysiology of cerebral hemorrhage: secondary brain injury. Stroke. 2011;42(6):1781–6.
9. Labib MA, Shah M, Kassam AB, Young R, Zucker L, Maioriello A, et al. The safety and feasibility of image-guided brainpath-mediated transsulcul hematoma evacuation: a multicenter study. Neurosurgery. 2017;80(4):515–24.
10. Bauer AM, Rasmussen PA, Bain MD. Initial single-center technical experience with the brain path system for acute intracerebral hemorrhage evacuation. Oper Neurosurg (Hagerstown, Md). 2017;13(1):69–76.
11. Phillips VL, Roy AK, Ratcliff J, Pradilla G. Minimally Invasive Parafascicular Surgery (MIPS) for spontaneous intracerebral hemorrhage compared to medical management: a case series comparison for a single institution. Stroke Res Treat. 2020;2020:1–10.
12. Mendelow AD, Gregson BA, Rowan EN, Murray GD, Gholkar A, Mitchell PM. Early surgery versus initial conservative treatment in patients with spontaneous supratentorial lobar intracerebral haematomas (STICH II): a randomised trial. Lancet (London, England). 2013;382(9890):397–408.

13. Vigneswaran K, Pradilla G. Chapter 27 – Tubular retractors for intraventricular tumors. In: Chaichana K, Quiñones-Hinojosa ABT-CO of MSA to IBT, editors. Comprehensive overview of modern surgical approaches to intrinsic brain tumors. Academic Press; 2019. p. 451–63. Available from: http://www.sciencedirect.com/science/article/pii/B9780128117835000276.
14. Hohne J, Brawanski A, Gassner HG, Schebesch K-M. Feasibility of the custom-made titanium cranioplasty CRANIOTOP((R)). Surg Neurol Int. 2013;4:88.
15. Jellison BJ, Field AS, Medow J, Lazar M, Salamat MS, Alexander AL. Diffusion tensor imaging of cerebral white matter: a pictorial review of physics, fiber tract anatomy, and tumor imaging patterns. AJNR Am J Neuroradiol. 2004;25(3):356–69.
16. Assaf Y, Pasternak O. Diffusion tensor imaging (DTI)-based white matter mapping in brain research: a review. J Mol Neurosci. 2008;34(1):51–61.
17. Roy A, Turan N, Pradilla G. Transcortical corridors. In: Evans J, Kenning T, Farrell C, Kshettry V, editors. Endoscopic and keyhole cranial base surgery. Springer: Cham; 2019. p. 173–83.
18. Nimsky C, Ganslandt O, Hastreiter P, Wang R, Benner T, Sorensen A, et al. Intraoperative diffusion-tensor MR imaging: shifting of white matter tracts during neurosurgical procedures – initial experience. Radiology. 2005;243(1):218–25.
19. Cartwright MM, Sekerak P, Mark J, Bailes J. Use of a novel navigable tubular retractor system in 1826 minimally invasive parafascicular surgery (MIPS) cases involving deep-seated brain tumors, hemorrhages and malformations. Interdiscip Neurosurg [Internet]. 2021;23:100919. Available from: http://www.sciencedirect.com/science/article/pii/S2214751920304801.

# Chapter 16
# Trans-sulcal, Channel-Based Parafascicular Surgery for Cavernous Angiomas and Other Vascular Lesions

Benjamin B. Whiting and Mark D. Bain

## Abbreviations

AVM    Arteriovenous malformation
DTI     Diffusion tensor imaging
fMRI   Functional magnetic resonance imaging
ICH    Intracerebral hemorrhage
MRI   Magnetic resonance imaging

Cavernous angiomas represent vascular lesions comprised of densely compacted capillaries without intervening cerebral tissue and surrounded by hemosiderin and gliosis [1]. While these have relatively low incidence in the general population (0.4–0.8%), they are the most common vascular malformation and can result in significant morbidity, most commonly via headaches, seizures, progressive neurological deficits, and intracranial hemorrhage [1]. Treatment options for cavernous angiomas include microsurgical resection, radiosurgery, and observation, each with their own associated risks. Often, open microsurgical intervention is deferred when these lesions are located in deep or eloquent brain tissue, even when these lesions are symptomatic. There is literature describing microsurgical approaches to these lesions with favorable neurological outcomes [2, 3]. However, these are technically difficult approaches that may not confer similar neurological results when applied to the general vascular neurosurgeon population. These deep and eloquently located lesions require significant dissection and retraction to obtain access. As such, there is a continuing effort in developing further approaches and techniques to minimize these approach-related issues. The use of a channel-based approach, entering

B. B. Whiting (✉) · M. D. Bain
Department of Neurosurgery, Cleveland Clinic Foundation, Cleveland, OH, USA
e-mail: whitinb@ccf.org; bainm@ccf.org

© Springer Nature Switzerland AG 2022
G. Zada et al. (eds.), *Subcortical Neurosurgery*,
https://doi.org/10.1007/978-3-030-95153-5_16

through a sulcus and traveling parallel to important fiber tracts, has shown particular promise in this regard.

The use of stereotaxis has been a mainstay of the treatment of deep-seated lesions, and vascular lesions are no exception. In 1960, Guiot and co-authors described the use of a stereotactic apparatus for the approach to two deeply located vascular malformations, both resulting in successful surgical treatment [4]. Riechert and Mundinger further advanced this technique in their description of the treatment of four patients with previously deemed inoperable arteriovenous angiomas via a stereotactic channel-based approach [5]. In their technique, the stereotactic apparatus was constructed, and the target point and coordinates were identified via angiography. Subsequent trephination was performed, and target needle was applied to the stereotactic frame. The dura was opened, and a small corticectomy was performed at the tip of the target needle. The needle was advanced to within 5 mm of the lesion. At this point, a channel was created by suctioning the layer of cerebral tissue surrounding the needle until the supplying blood vessel of the target was identified. The needle was subsequently removed, and the vascular lesion was treated along this channel. All four patients were treated successfully, and the authors described this as an indicated treatment option for subcortical lesions, particularly when these lesions are located in functionally important regions of the brain.

In the following years, stereotactic approach to deep-seated vascular lesions was evaluated using a number of different treatment methods, including anodal electrolysis, magnetic thrombosis, and direct electric current [6–8]. In 1977, Kandel and Peresedov described a technique using a conical device to allow access to deepseated aneurysms and AVMs for clipping through this cannula [8]. They began with angiography to identify feeding/origin vessels and select a target point. A burr hole was placed at a site chosen to avoid functionally important regions of the brain during insertion of the stereotactic device. After burr hole placement, the stereotactic device was affixed with the first of two attachments inserted within the cannula, and the combination was passed to the previously selected target point. Angiography was performed to confirm accurate placement at the target site. The first attachment was then replaced with a second attachment, a specially designed device with an aneurysm clip at the distal tip. The clip was deployed with controls on the proximal end of the device. After clip placement through the cannula, angiography was performed to confirm effective clip placement, and the patient was subsequently awakened to ensure normal function. Once deemed satisfactory, the patient was again anesthetized, and the cannula with attached device was removed from the brain. They published a series of eight patients (ten lesions) treated with this procedure/ device (four aneurysms and six AVMs). With this stereotactic approach, they experienced no mortalities with only a single case of hemiparesis lasting several days. In a similar stereotactic method, Sisti resected ten small, deeply located AVMs. Importantly, he utilized a trans-sulcal approach to these malformations as a means to "preserve the surrounding cortex" [9].

In 1982, Kelly utilized a similar stereotactic/stereoscopic angiography localization method when he first described the use of a uniquely designed self-retaining retractor passed parallel to the white matter fibers to approach and remove a deep-seated vascular malformation [10]. In subsequent publications, he was the first to describe a cylindrical retractor system that allowed access to deep-seated lesions [11, 12]. This device consisted of a hollow cylinder (either 2 or 3 cm in diameter) with dilators that fit inside with a wedged distal tip to allow ease of passing. They felt a cylindrical retractor resulted in less damage to surrounding brain tissue. While the majority of his experience was with tumors, his initial publication in 1986 described the treatment of nine vascular lesions (two cavernous angiomas, five thrombosed AVMs, and two active AVMs). Otsuki utilized a thin-walled cylindrical tube in conjunction with an endoscope to resect two cavernous angiomas [13]. Ross described a cylindrical retractor system for the resection of a diverse array of lesions, including cavernous angiomas [14]. He utilized a pial opening at the gyral crest and directly visualized lesions via a microscope aimed through the cylinder.

By the 2000s, publications regarding surgical approaches to deep lesions utilizing stereotaxis and cylindrical or tubular retractors were becoming more commonplace. In 2006, Ogura used a cylinder made of thin polyester as a conduit to deeply located lesions [15]. A transparent 0.1-mm-thick polyester film was cut into sheets and rolled around a holding needle. The needle was introduced into the brain transcortically to the target, and the holding needle was removed, allowing the polyester to naturally expand in the shape of a cylinder. Lesional resection was performed along this cylindrical path. The pressure exerted on the surrounding brain tissue by this cylinder was measured in two cases and was found to never exceed 10 mmHg (well below the pressures Rosenorn described as causing a considerable reduction in cerebral blood flow [30 mmHg] and ultimately resulting in cortical damage) [16]. The authors utilized this technique to remove 11 lesions, 1 of which was a cavernous angioma. Greenfield and colleagues used a spinal surgery tubular retractor system to access deep lesions, including one cavernous malformation [17]. Their technique consisted of a cortical entry site in non-eloquent location using an incision in the gyral crest. They described two main advantages of a tubular retraction system: (1) equal distribution of pressures to minimize injury and (2) splitting of deep white matter tracts, as opposed to transection. They also surmised the use of DTI and/or fMRI may aid in the surgical planning when these techniques are used. Fahim (2009) and Almenawer (2013) each used a similar technique with a spine tubular retraction system to resect, respectively, a choroidal AVM and two cavernomas [18, 19].

As channel-based approaches to deep-seated lesions increased in frequency, devices to aid these techniques became available on the market. One of these devices that has become particularly prominent is the BrainPath™ tubular retractor system (NICO Corp, Indianapolis, IN, USA). The BrainPath™ system includes a sheath and an obturator, the former being disposable and the latter reusable. The sheath is transparent and allows the obturator to fit within it. The head of the obturator is tapered to an atraumatic tip that extends beyond the distal edge of the sheath. To insert the device, a 3 cm craniotomy is turned with a small dural opening. The arachnoid is opened, and the sheath (with obturator inserted) is passed through the brain to the target point. When the appropriate depth has been reached, the obturator is removed, allowing a cylindrical channel within which the lesion can be addressed (either 11 or 13.5 mm in diameter). This requires the use of neuronavigation to plan an appropriate trajectory. As seen in techniques described previously, a trans-sulcal approach is ideal, as this reduces the amount of brain tissue manipulation. Additionally, when planning the trajectory, specific attention should be paid to avoiding disruption of important white matter tracts.

The BrainPath™ device has been used to treat a wide variety of deeply or eloquently located lesions (e.g., brain tumors, ICH, abscesses), and vascular lesions are no exception. One of the first published uses of this device for a vascular lesion was a case series by Ding and colleagues [20]. The authors discussed a channel-based, trans-sulcal resection of three cavernomas via BrainPath™. The first of three patients treated by this group was a young female who presented with ICH but was found to have a 4.5 cm cavernous malformation located in the anterior body of the corpus callosum with intraventricular extension. Using the BrainPath™ device via a right frontal approach, the lesion was initially debulked internally followed by circumferential dissection of the capsule after the lesion retracted inwardly. The patient was discharged 2 days after surgery without deficit, and post-operative MRI at 2 months demonstrated 8 mm residual. The second patient treated was another young female with a 7 mm cavernoma in the left inferior frontal lobe, posterior to Broca's area. Functional MRI demonstrated left dominant speech. As such, awake speech mapping was utilized during resection. The approach was via a left frontal craniotomy with trajectory obliquely through the left middle frontal gyrus. The cavernoma was resected en bloc, and the patient was discharged at her baseline exam. Post-operative MRI at 3 months showed complete resection of cavernoma. Lastly, the third patient presented with a 10 mm cavernoma within the left anterior body of the corpus callosum. A left frontal craniotomy was performed, and the lesion was resected en bloc. She was discharged without deficits, and post-operative MRI at 12 months demonstrated complete resection. Chen and colleagues described the use of the BrainPath™ system for the treatment of a ruptured periventricular aneurysm [21]. In the report, the patient was found to have a periventricular aneurysm located in the wall of the right lateral ventricular atrium. Feeding vessel was deemed to be the posterior choroidal artery. Endovascular treatment was attempted but was unable to be performed due to inability to safely access the distally located vessel and the significant amount of brain parenchyma supplied distal to the aneurysm. As such, the authors decided to move forward with channel-based treatment via BrainPath™. The sheath was advanced into the atrium of the right lateral ventricle. Hematoma was encountered and evacuated. The aneurysm was found to be fusiform and clipping was unable to be performed and electrocautery ligation of the aneurysm was performed. Scranton and colleagues further described the use of BrainPath™ for a trans-sulcal, parafascicular resection of two subcortical cavernomas [22]. The first case was a hemorrhagic cavernoma within the right thalamus with extension into the midbrain and cerebral peduncle. The second was a hemorrhagic cavernoma within the subcortical white matter, deep to the superior temporal and supramarginal gyri. Both cases utilized pre-operative DTI imaging for trajectory planning, and one utilized functional MRI. Witek and colleagues utilized a similar approach to resect a subcortical AVM adjacent to the right lateral ventricle [23]. Post-operative angiogram demonstrated complete resection of the AVM. While the authors state that AVMs amenable to this type of resection are likely rare, they demonstrated this system should be a consideration when planning treatment of small, deep, ruptured AVMs.

The use of trans-sulcal, channel-based techniques has been a long process of trial and error, with great strides in recent years. While the majority of this work has been in the treatment of tumors and intracerebral hemorrhage, there has been a consistent push toward more vascular applications, as demonstrated in this chapter. When considering the use of this technique for a vascular pathology, a number of factors must be considered. The sheath diameter is 13.5 mm which provides a suitable working space when tasked with treating a small- to moderate-sized lesion. However, this may not provide proper visualization and control for treating larger lesions, in particular large cavernous angiomas and arteriovenous malformations. Additionally, this window of visualization is less than ideal for treating lesions with high flow characteristics. As such, these types of lesions are not recommended for treatment with these channel-based approaches [23]. As with all trans-sulcal, parafascicular approaches, the surgeon must critically evaluate the trajectory of the channel to the lesion. If important white matter fibers are disrupted, the benefits of these less invasive techniques are negated. MRI with fiber tracking (i.e., DTI) and functional MRI can be useful in the pre-operative stages of planning. As expected, there is a learning curve with the application of these techniques, as greater experience allows greater comfortability with operating through a channel. If selecting a trans-sulcal, parafascicular channel-based approach for the treatment of a vascular lesion, the surgeon should have sufficient experience with using the devices and techniques.

Deep-seated and eloquently located vascular lesions remain some of the most challenging pathologies to treat, as the approach alone can subject the patient to significant morbidity and mortality. There has been significant effort in describing novel treatment options for these lesions that reduce these associated risks and provide patients with better outcomes. The application of trans-sulcal, channel-based parafascicular surgery for deep-seated cavernous angiomas and other vascular lesions has demonstrated to be a promising new option in carefully selected cases.

## References


1. Mouchtouris N, Chalouhi N, Chitale A, Starke MS, Tjoumakaris SI, Rosenwasser RH, et al. Management of cerebral cavernous malformations: from diagnosis to treatment. ScientificWorldJournal. 2015;2015:808314.
2. Chang EF, Gabriel RA, Potts MB, Berger MS, Lawton MT. Supratentorial cavernous malformations in eloquent and deep locations: surgical approaches and outcomes. Clinical article. J Neurosurg. 2011;114(3):814–27.
3. Steinberg GK, Chang SD, Gewirst RJ, Lopez JR. Microsurgical resection of brainstem, thalamic, and basal ganglia angiographically occult vascular malformations. Neurosurgery. 2000;46(2):260–70.

4. Guiot G, Rougerie J, Sachs M, Hertzog E, Molina P. Stereotactic localization of deep vascular intracerebral malformations. Sem Hop. 1960;36:1134–43.
5. Riechert T, Mundinger F. Combined stereotaxic operation for treatment of deep-seated angiomas and aneurysms. J Neurosurg. 1964;21:358–63.
6. Alksne JF. Stereotactic thrombosis of intracranial aneurysms. N Engl J Med. 1971;284(4):171–4.
7. Mullan S. Experiences with surgical thrombosis of intracranial berry aneurysms and carotid cavernous fistulas. J Neurosurg. 1974;41(6):657–70.
8. Kandel EI, Peresedov VV. Stereotactic clipping of arterial aneurysms and arteriovenous malformations. J Neurosurg. 1977;46(1):12–23.
9. Sisti MB, Soloman RA, Stein BM. Stereotactic craniotomy in the resection of small arteriovenous malformations. J Neurosurg. 1991;75(1):40–4.
10. Kelly PJ, Alker GJ Jr, Zoll JG. A microstereotactic approach to deep-seated arteriovenous malformations. Surg Neurol. 1982;17(4):260–2.
11. Kelly PJ. Computer-assisted stereotaxis: new approaches for the management of intracranial intra-axial tumors. Neurology. 1986;36(4):535–41.
12. Kelly PJ, Goerss SJ, Kall BA. The stereotaxic retractor in computer-assisted stereotaxic microsurgery. Technical Note. J Neurosurg. 1988;69(2):301–6.
13. Otsuki T, Jokura H, Yoshimoto T. Stereotactic guiding tube for open-system endoscopy: a new approach for the stereotactic endoscopic resection of intra-axial brain tumors. Neurosurgery. 1990;27(2):326–30.
14. Ross DA. A simple stereotactic retractor for use with the Leksell stereotactic system. Neurosurgery. 1993;32(3):475–6.
15. Ogura K, Tachibana E, Aoshima C, Sumitomo M. New microsurgical technique for intraparenchymal lesions of the brain: transcylinder approach. Acta Neurochir (Wien). 2006;148(7):779–85;discussion 785.
16. Rosenorn J, Diemer N. The risk of cerebral damage during graded brain retractor pressure in the rat. J Neurosurg. 1985;63(4):608–11.
17. Greenfield JP, Cobb WS, Tsouris AJ, Schwartz TH. Stereotactic minimally invasive tubular retractor system for deep brain lesions. Neurosurgery. 2008;63(4 Suppl 2):334–9; discussion 339–40.
18. Fahim DK, Relyea K, Nayar VV, Fox BD, Whitehead WE, Curry DJ, et al. Transtubular microendoscopic approach for resection of a choroidal arteriovenous malformation. J Neurosurg Pediatr. 2009;3(2):101–4.
19. Almenawer SA, Crevier L, Murty N, Kassam A, Reddy K. Minimal access to deep intracranial lesions using a serial dilatation technique: case-series and review of brain tubular retractor systems. Neurosurg Rev. 2013;36(2):321–9.
20. Ding D, Starke RM, Crowley RW, Liu KC. Endoport-assisted microsurgical resection of cerebral cavernous malformations. J Clin Neurosci. 2015;22(6):1025–9.
21. Chen CJ, Caruso J, Starke RM, Ding D, Buell T, Crowley RW, et al. Endoport-assisted microsurgical treatment of a ruptured periventricular aneurysm. Case Rep Neurol Med. 2016;2016:8654262.
22. Scranton RA, Fung SH, Britz GW. Transulcal parafascicular minimally invasive approach to deep and subcortical cavernomas: technical note. J Neurosurg. 2016;125(6):1360–6.
23. Witek AM, Moore NZ, Sebai MA, Bain MD. BrainPath-mediated resection of a ruptured subcortical arteriovenous malformation. Oper Neurosurg (Hagerstown). 2018;15(1):32–8.

# Chapter 17
# Surgical Resection of Intraventricular Tumors Using a Minimally Invasive Parafascicular (MIP) Approach with a Navigated Tubular Retractor System


Jonathan Weyhenmeyer, Robert A. Scranton, Charles Kulwin, and Mitesh V. Shah


## Traditional Approaches

The ventricular system is found deep within the brain, and the overlying neuro-anatomy and intricate vasculature can make surgical approaches challenging. The lateral ventricle encompasses a large area of the brain and can anatomically be divided into the frontal horn, body, atrium, occipital horn, and temporal horn. There are a variety of both primary and secondary pathologies that may appear in these areas (see Table 17.1). Additionally, the blood supply and venous drainage around and to various pathologies must also be considered during the approach. The venous drainage is especially important as violation may result in significant morbidity. The lateral ventricles contain the septal, caudate, and thalamostriate veins. The roof of the third ventricle contains the major outflow of the ventricle, basal ganglia, and thalamic veins, e.g., the internal cerebral veins, in the velum interpositum. Mass occupying pathologies in the lateral and third ventricles will distort the typical landmarks for ventricular surgery and may distort the locations of the major venous


J. Weyhenmeyer
Department of Neurosurgery, Indiana University School of Medicine, Indianapolis, IN, USA
e-mail: jweyhenm@iupui.edu

R. A. Scranton · M. V. Shah (✉)
Department of Neurosurgery, Indiana University School of Medicine, Indianapolis, USA
e-mail: mshah2@iu.edu

C. Kulwin
Goodman Campbell Brain and Spine, Carmel, IN, USA
e-mail: ckulwin@goodmancampbell.com



© Springer Nature Switzerland AG 2022
G. Zada et al. (eds.), *Subcortical Neurosurgery*,
https://doi.org/10.1007/978-3-030-95153-5_17

**Table 17.1** Tumors of the ventricles by location

| Lateral ventricle | Third ventricle |
| --- | --- |
| Neurocytoma | Colloid cyst |
| Subependymoma | Craniopharyngioma |
| Giant cell astrocytoma | Pineocytoma |
| Meningioma | Pineoblastoma |
| Choroid plexus papilloma | Germ cell tumors |

anatomy. As such, ventricular surgery requires careful study of the pre-operative MRI and, when indicated, vascular imaging including MR angiography, CT angiography, or digital subtraction angiography prior to the operation (Table 17.1).

Surgical approaches to the frontal horn include the frontal trans-basal, frontal transcortical, and anterior interhemispheric transcallosal. The frontal transcortical and anterior interhemispheric transcallosal approaches may be used for approaching the body as well. The frontal transcortical approach provides excellent visualization of large unilateral ventricular pathology, while the anterior interhemispheric transcallosal approach affords better visualization of the contralateral lateral ventricle. Several reports detail a higher post-operative seizure risk with a frontal transcortical approach as compared to the anterior interhemispheric transcallosal [5, 9, 15]; however, conflicting data does exist [13]. The frontal trans-basal approach has historically been used for pathology that emanates from the sellar or suprasellar cistern through the lamina terminalis. The operating angles for this approach require access to the third ventricle through the lamina terminalis. Given the tight working angles and eloquent surrounding anatomy, e.g., optic chiasm inferiorly, hypothalamus bilaterally, and close proximity to the cerebral vasculature, this approach is fraught with difficulty.

## *Anterior Interhemispheric Approach*

The most technically demanding approach to the frontal portion of the lateral ventricle is the anterior interhemispheric transcallosal approach. Through this approach, either ventricle may be accessed, tumors arising from the midline can be easily approached from either side, and if a lesion arises from the lateral wall, it is best visualized when a contralateral approach is used. For example, a mass arising from the lateral wall of the left lateral ventricle can be seen with a good working trajectory from a craniotomy performed on the right. While the approach may be implemented from either side, it is technically more challenging to perform on the left due to concern for draining veins from the dominant hemisphere.

First, a craniotomy is performed with exposure of the midline centered two thirds anterior to the coronal suture, one third posterior to the coronal suture. Bony removal must encompass exposure of the edge of the sagittal sinus in order to facilitate the interhemispheric trajectory. The dura is flapped toward midline with the base at the edge of the sagittal sinus. Retention sutures are placed to provide adequate retraction. Next, an interhemispheric dissection is performed taking care not to avulse any veins that may be attached to the superior sagittal sinus. In general, tributary veins to the anterior third of the sagittal sinus can be sacrificed without consequence; however, attempts should be made to save large tributaries. The interhemispheric dissection continues with small retractor blades until the bright white of the corpus callosum is seen. This dissection should occur in a plane parallel to a plane drawn from the coronal suture to the external auditory meatus (EAM) as this will point directly toward the foramen of Monro. The cingulate gyrus is often confused with the corpus callosum, which is seen as a bright white surface without the delicate vasculature typically seen on the cortical surface. The dissection may be aided with the use of an external ventricular drain or lumbar drain to relax the brain prior to dissection depending upon the pathology and presence of obstructive hydrocephalus. Attention is also paid to preserving the small arterioles arising from the pericallosal and callosomarginal artery. Identification of the pericallosal arteries overlying the corpus callosum is not required prior to the callosotomy provided the surgeon is comfortable that the corpus has been properly identified. Once the corpus callosum is reached, a 2–3 cm incision oriented in the sagittal plane is made to enter the ventricle. The incision should stay within the anterior third of the body. If the pericallosal arteries are identified, the incision should be placed between the arteries to avoid violation of their branching vessels. The laterality of the ventricle of entry is determined based on anatomic landmarks, e.g., choroid plexus, septal vein, and thalamostriate veins [14]. Care must be taken not to injure the fornix which can result in post-operative memory deficits. Techniques using both fixed and dynamic retraction have been described in the interhemispheric approach. Use of a fixed blade retraction system may lead to cortical and subcortical ischemia and/or contusion with extended time and excessive retraction force [1, 16]. Importantly, if too large of an incision is made in the corpus callosum, the surgeon runs the risk of performing a true callosotomy causing disconnection syndrome whereby the patient may present post-operatively with agnosia, ideational apraxia, alien hand, and/or alexia.

## *Transcortical Approach*

The transcortical route avoids some of the pitfalls of the transcallosal route but still comes with its own set of complications. The craniotomy for the transcortical approach is larger as the surgeon will require a wider medial-to-lateral working corridor. The craniotomy is centered approximately two thirds anterior to the coronal suture and runs 7–8 cm lateral to the sagittal suture. The sagittal sinus does not need to be exposed, and there is no requirement for coagulating venous tributaries. Once the dura is opened, the middle frontal gyrus is identified. A 2–3 cm corticectomy is made in the gyrus. Depending on the length for dissection, e.g., the degree of hydrocephalus present, a larger incision may be required due to the increased amount of tissue. Maintaining the planes of subcortical dissection in this approach is critical to ensure that the surgeon is able to reach the ventricle without significant complication. Some surgeons will place a ventricular catheter as guide for appropriately traversing to the ventricle. Another method involves the usage of surface anatomy. The anterior-posterior trajectory should be parallel to a plane drawn from the EAM to the coronal suture. The medial-lateral trajectory should proceed in line with a plane drawn from the ipsilateral middle frontal gyrus to the contralateral medial canthus [14]. Once the ventricle is entered, the surgeon should again orient based on the ventricular anatomy previously mentioned. Dynamic or fixed retraction can be used throughout the remainder of the procedure.

As discussed, it is unclear which approach represents a greater post-operative seizure risk. The transcortical route is an excellent choice for midline pathology such as colloid cysts given the trajectory; however, in more laterally based pathologies, it may be more difficult to visualize all the margins and vascular supply early in the operation. A challenging aspect of the transcortical route is the difficulty in limiting damage to the cortex and subcortical white matter pathways during resection or while instruments transit along the route. Unprotected repeated placement of instruments can lead to cortical injury. Traditionally a cotton patty or retractor blade may be placed along the path to assist in maintaining the operative corridor with the use of fixed retraction, dynamic retraction, or a combination of the two. The entry point and trajectory are often visualized using a hand-held navigation probe. The lack of continuous navigation can, at times, make a precise approach to the pathology difficult. Navigation instruments must be placed and removed during the phase of identifying the ventricle. Initial cortical opening can vary and can enlarge with blade retractors as necessary to access the depth of the lesion. Often the planned opening is enlarged more than anticipated by using the blade retractors.

## Tubular Retractor Systems

Many of these issues have been ameliorated with use of a navigated tubular retractor system such as the BrainPath (NICO Corporation, Indianapolis, Indiana). The closest historical corollary is Patrick Kelly's description of his use of a tubular retractor on a stereotactic arc for resection of deep-seated lesions [11]. The BrainPath device is a modern version where a small tubular retractor (inner diameter of 13.5 mm) system with inner cannula of varying lengths is combined with frameless stereotactic neuronavigation. A standard neuronavigational pointer can be inserted into the center of the cannula for continuous navigation while approaching a target destination. Additionally, a custom navigation array may be placed on the tubular retractor itself for use with a navigation guidance system (e.g., Synaptive guidance system). The advantage of this custom array is that it affords continuous navigation for the entirety of the procedure rather than just during the initial approach. This results in fewer instruments that are passed between the surgeon and assistant throughout the course of the operation creating a more efficient procedure, thereby decreasing surgeon fatigue and anesthetic time. The advantage of continuous navigation during the procedure becomes more obvious when approaching and resecting subcortical pathology as the visual anatomic clues available in ventricular surgery are lost.

Another decided advantage of a tubular retractor system for cranial neurosurgery is in the equal dispersion of the retraction force on the cortex and subcortical white matter [2]. This likely results in less trauma to these structures throughout the operation than with standard fixed retraction systems [4, 16]. Additionally, these tubular retractors are typically made of plastic, which is less likely to stick to the parenchyma as compared to a cotton patty.

At present, tubular retraction systems have been employed in a vast array of clinical scenarios for subcortical and intraventricular lesions. The most frequent usage of the system has been for the evacuation of spontaneous intracerebral hemorrhage, for which there are ongoing trials [12]. In addition, the tubular retractor has been utilized for subcortical high-grade gliomas, metastasis, vascular lesions, and intraventricular lesions such as colloid cysts and ependymal tumors [3, 6–8, 10].

## *Tubular Retractor Implementation*

Use of the modern tubular retractor begins with pre-operative planning to define a specific trajectory to the lesion that utilizes a sulcus and minimizes the need to traverse eloquent subcortical pathways. The sulcal approach minimizes the distance to the lesion traversed by the retractor. The craniotomy is usually 3–4 cm in diameter with the selected sulcus centrally located. Large veins that need to be dissected and preserved or avoided all together can often be found on the post-contrast MR imaging during the planning phase. The craniotomy is larger than the tubular retractor (about the size of a dime), but much smaller than an open approach, in order to permit for multiple degrees of freedom for rotating the retractor in the long axis in order to improve visualization, a maneuver often referred to as "wanding." Once the craniotomy is performed, stereotactic navigation is used to identify the entry point, and then a dural incision is made overlying the sulcus. Typically, this incision is small, approximately 1/2 inch by 1/2 inch, performed in the cruciate fashion, to permit entry of the retractor and trocar while preventing spinal fluid egress and brain shift. Care must be taken to not hyperventilate the patient or use hyperosmolar treatment to decrease the ICP when MIPS is used. This helps to avoid cortical sinking and injury to the veins that are tributaries to the midline. The minimal craniotomy and dural opening decrease brain shift, maintaining the accuracy of neural navigation. The tubular retractor and trocar are then assembled (Fig. 17.1a). The trocar extends 15 mm beyond the edge of the tubular retractor to facilitate parallel fascicular dissection during placement. The stereotactic navigation will provide feedback on the location of the tip of the retractor with the navigation guidance system; otherwise, a projection must be added. When the pre-selected intracranial target is reached, the tubular retractor must be advanced 15 mm before removing the trocar. We prefer to cannulate past the ependymal lining but just superficial to the lesion wall. The tubular retractor is then held in place, and a Shepherd's hook retractor

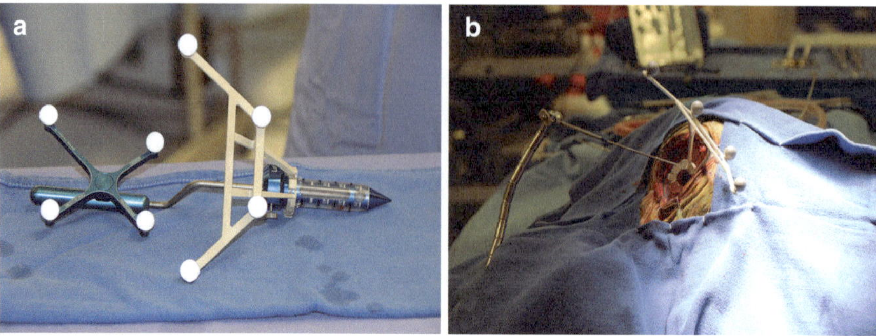

**Fig. 17.1** Retractor system and hands-free application. (**a**) Trocar and tubular retractor assembled with both Stealth and Synaptive navigation systems. (**b**) Implanted tubular retractor with Synaptive navigation and Shepherd's hook for hands-free stabilization

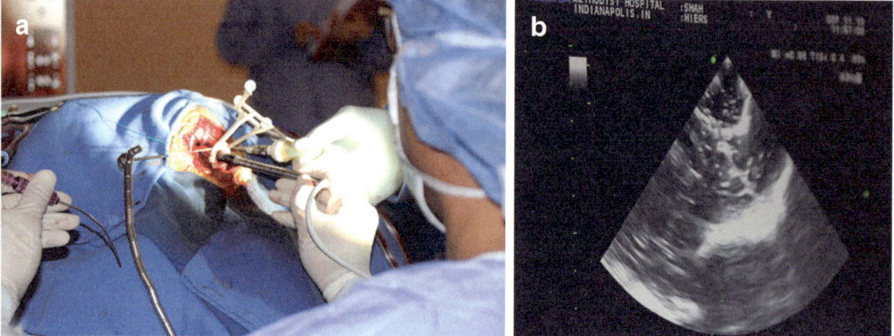

**Fig. 17.2** Intra-operative ultrasound. (**a**) Intra-operative ultrasound is used through the tubular retractor to appropriately visualize the tumor. (**b**) An intra-operative ultrasound image showing a heterogeneous tumor

system is assembled for stability (Fig. 17.1b). The loss of CSF from the ventricle may affect the accuracy of navigation. We utilize an intra-operative ultrasound probe which fits thru the retractor system to document successful cannulation next to lesion and as a guidance for confirming gross total removal (Fig. 17.2). We have also performed these cases in the IMRIS room, and we can safely get iMRI with tube left in the ventricle and the Shepherd's hook and navigation system removed from the wound. Following cannulation, the surgeon has the option of utilizing either an operating microscope or an exoscope. At our institution, we have predominantly utilized the Synaptive exoscope for most BrainPath cases. The advantages of the robotic digital microscope are the greater light, optical magnification, and greater depth of field than the standard microscopes. The robotic alignment down the axis of the navigated tube permits an efficient system to seamlessly remove deep-seated tumors. The robotic exoscopes now allows for stereoscopy. Olympus has developed a 3D exoscope, but it has manual arms and shorter working distance.

The key portion of the procedure is then performed. Continuous transgressions into the ventricle using bimanual techniques can be performed safely without both cortical and subcortical injury using a tubular system. Once the intracranial portion of the case is complete, the tubular retractor is detached from the Shepherd's hook and slowly removed from the brain under direct visualization. As the retractor is removed, careful attention is paid to the subcortical walls, and any bleeding, if encountered, is managed. This is typically not necessary with this system. Following removal of the retractor, the dura, craniotomy, and incision are closed in the usual fashion.

## Case Illustration 1

A 22-year-old male presented to the emergency room with complaints of fever, headaches, nausea, emesis, and blurry vision. He was initially worked up for sinusitis and meningitis. A head CT was obtained that demonstrated obstructive hydrocephalus and a cystic mass at the foramen of Monro consistent with a colloid cyst (Fig. 17.3a, b). Given his symptomatic obstructive hydrocephalus, he was offered resection utilizing transcortical approach using the BrainPath system.

The BrainPath and Stealth (Medtronic, Minneapolis, MN, USA) neuronavigation systems were appropriately registered, and an incision and craniotomy were planned such that they provided access to the right lateral ventricle and foramen of Monro via the chosen sulcus. After the craniotomy, a small 1/2 inch by 1/2 inch incision was made in the dura in a cruciate fashion. The arachnoid overlying the chosen sulcus was cut with an arachnoid knife. A 7.5 cm BrainPath tubular retractor was then paired with the trocar and placed in the sulcus. The navigation pointer was inserted into the center of the trocar and a 15 mm projection added to the pointer. The BrainPath trocar system was then passed into the right lateral ventricle under continuous navigation with careful attention to avoid entering the cyst at the foramen of Monro. After the trocar was removed and the BrainPath was fixed into place with the Shepherd's hook, the operating microscope was brought into the field. The cyst was readily visualized bulging out of the foramen of Monro. Anatomic cues, such as location of the septum pellucidum and the septal and thalamostriate veins, confirmed the laterality shown on the neuronavigation system. The cyst resection proceeded by decompressing the cyst, followed by piecemeal resection of the cyst capsule with careful attention to preserve the internal cerebral veins as well as the fornices. Following resection, the BrainPath was removed, and an EVD was left in the operative cavity. The patient was then sent to the ICU. A follow-up head CT was performed that showed adequate resection and decreased size of the lateral ventricles (Fig. 17.3c). The EVD was weaned over the coming days, and the patient was discharged to home. He did well post-operatively, returning to work within 1 month.

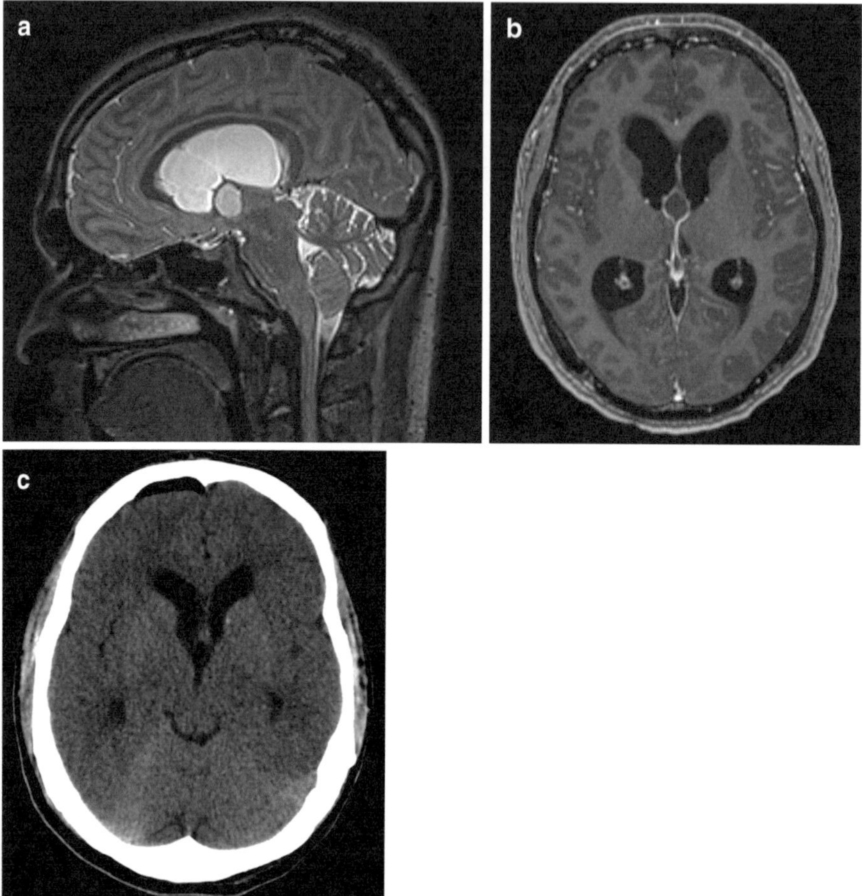

**Fig. 17.3** Pre- and post-operative images of a third ventricular colloid syst. (**a**) T2-weighted sagittal image with ventriculomegaly and clearly defined colloid cyst occupying the third ventricle. (**b**) T1 post-contrast image that shows the colloid cyst and venous anatomy with the internal cerebral veins coursing posteriorly around the cyst. (**c**) Post-operative CT showing ventricular decompression and resection of colloid cyst without significant intraventricular blood products

## Case Illustration 2

A 68-year-old female with a past medical history significant for breast cancer presented with headaches and nausea. A head CT and subsequent MRI were obtained that showed an intraventricular mass with hydrocephalus (Fig. 17.4a, b).

The patient was brought to the operating room and positioned supine. The Stealth (Medtronic) and Synaptive navigation systems were registered, and a right frontal approach with trans-sulcal access was planned to the ventricle. A 4 cm craniotomy was subsequently preformed, and the dura was opened in a cruciate fashion overlying the sulcus of interest. The right lateral ventricle was then accessed as previously

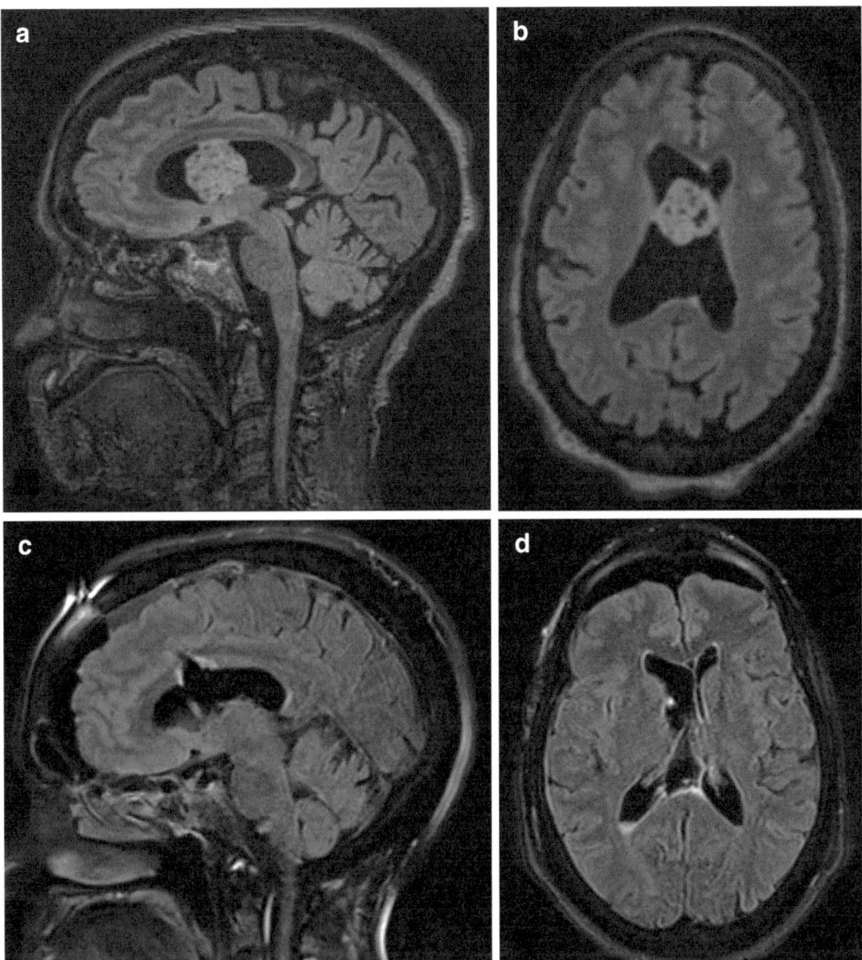

**Fig. 17.4** Pre- and post-operative images of an intraventricular subependymoma. (**a**, **b**) Pre-operative FLAIR MRI, sagittal, and axial slices displaying the intraventicular location and bowing of the septum pellucidum. (**c**) and (**d**). Post-operative FLAIR MRI, sagittal, and axial slices showing gross total resection of the lesion

described. Laterality was again conformed using anatomic cues and neuronavigation. The tumor was then visualized and resected using the NICO Myriad suction system, bipolar electrocautery, and microdissection techniques. After removal of the subependymoma, a septostomy was performed, connecting the two lateral ventricles. An EVD was left in place to monitor pressure post-operatively. She was sent to the ICU for close post-operative monitoring. Her post-operative MRI confirmed a gross total resection (Fig. 17.4c, d). She did well post-operatively but required discharge to inpatient rehabilitation for further balance and gait training prior to returning home.

## Case Illustration 3

A 49-year-old male presented after multiple episodes where he fell asleep while driving. A non-contrast head CT was obtained, and he was noted to have obstructive hydrocephalus secondary to an intraventricular mass. An MRI demonstrated a large sellar and suprasellar mass that extended through the third ventricle into the lateral ventricle with a cystic component in the lateral ventricle and notable obstructive hydrocephalus (Fig. 17.5a, b). Given the extent to which the tumor extended

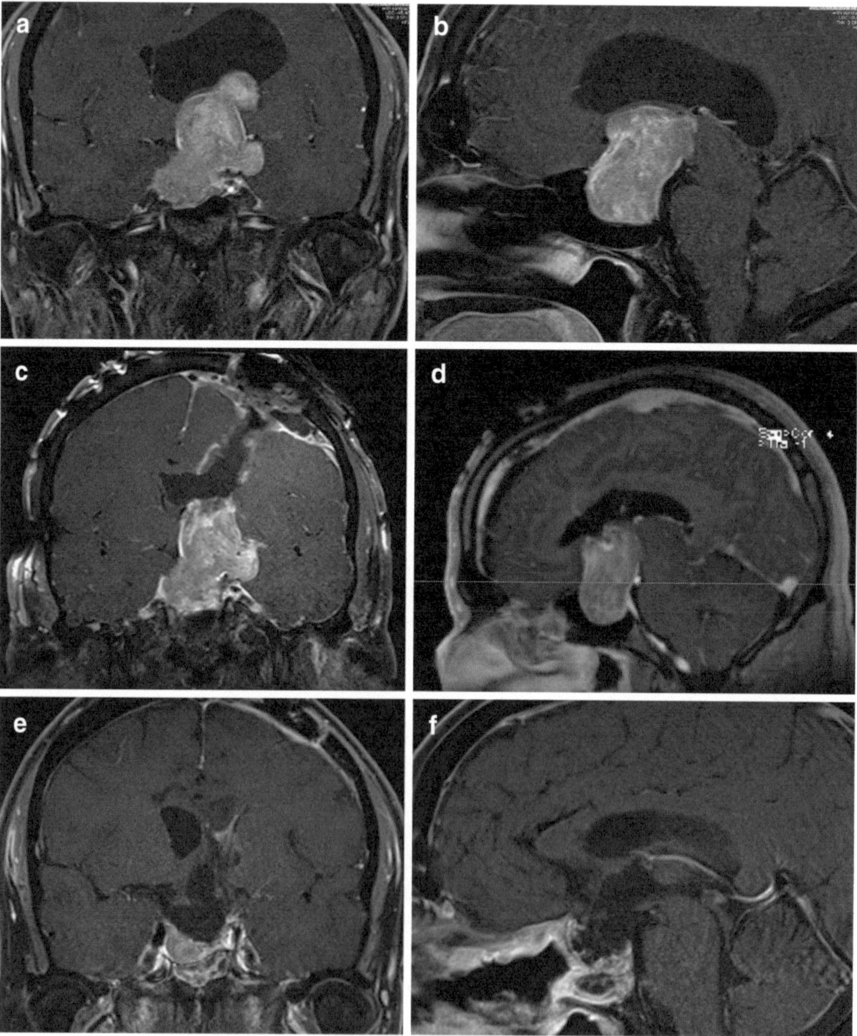

**Fig. 17.5** (**a, b**) Pre-operative T1-weighted post-contrast images of a pituitary adenoma extending into the third and lateral ventricles. (**c, d**) Intra-operative T1-weighted post-contrast images after resection of the lateral ventricular portion of the tumor via tubular retractor allowing for ventricular decompression. (**e, f**) Post-operative T1-weighted post-contrast images after transsphenoidal resection of remaining tumor. There is a small remnant along the right carotid artery

superiorly, we did not feel that this lesion could be appropriately addressed through a single transsphenoidal or transcranial approach. As such, the patient was offered a staged procedure whereby the lateral ventricular portion of the pituitary macroadenoma was removed with a trans-sulcal BrainPath approach first in order to address the hydrocephalus. The remainder of the tumor would then be removed through an endoscopic transsphenoidal approach.

An incision and craniotomy were planned that allowed for use of a sulcus to access the ventricle at a trajectory that would facilitate resection. The tubular retractor system was constructed, the arachnoid opened, and the sulcus cannulated as described previously. The tumor within the lateral ventricle was readily visible and resected with the assistance of an exoscope for visualization. Following resection, an intra-operative MRI was obtained (Fig. 17.5c, d) demonstrating significant debulking of the tumor and resolution of the ventricular obstruction. Three weeks later, the patient returned to the operating room for an endonasal transsphenoidal approach to complete the resection. Figure 17.5e, f shows the post-operative imaging at 6 months with a small amount of residual tumor in the right suprasellar region, adjacent to the cavernous sinus. There was no optic apparatus compression or hydrocephalus. The patient had no neurological deficits on exam, but has developed panhypopituitarism.

## Discussion

The trans-sulcal parafascicular approach with a tubular retractor affords a number of advantages when attempting to resect deep-seated lesions. The trans-sulcal approach helps to minimize cortical damage as compared to a standard open transcortical approach. Additionally, the trocar and tubular retractor help to disperse fibers radially rather than transect fascicles when traversing the subcortical white matter to the pathology of interest. The radial dispersion of forces also holds when the tubular retractor is fixed into place as the force on the brain parenchyma is applied in a radial fashion to all of the surrounding brain, rather than to a single side as is the case with a fixed straight retractor. In theory, this should result in less damage secondary to retraction as the force is spread out over a greater area. The tubular retractor also allows for easy "wanding" to assist in visualization in any plane. Finally, the 360-degree nature of the tube helps to protect the brain parenchyma when entering and exiting the operative field with instruments. In comparison to endoscopy, we have found that there is significantly less trauma to the ventricular ependymoma with the tubular retractor approach. The MIPS tube is significantly more robust than the endoscopic sheath and does not allow for shearing of the ependymal lining with varying degrees of forces. Coupled with the lack of a long lever arm, contrary to endoscopy, the surrounding tissues are readily protected. The other advantage of a tubular retractor system is that it permits a bimanual operation which greatly facilitates lesion resection in a timely manner.

It is important to emphasize that BrainPath is not the first tubular retractor engineered for minimally invasive cranially surgery. As noted previously, Patrick Kelly developed a tubular retractor system based on passing successively larger tubes to cannulate the parenchyma to the lesion of interest. More recently, Vycor has developed a ViewSite system that traverses the parenchyma via a corticectomy that is approximately the diameter of the retractor. From our perspective, there is an inherent advantage in utilizing a trans-sulcal as opposed to a transcortical approach in that the cortex is not violated. While vascular anatomy does run within the sulci, we have not found it difficult to avoid injury the superficial vascular structures with either the initial pial opening or during passing of the tubular retractor. From the time the sulcus entry point is identified to decannulation, it takes 1.5–2 minutes.

Implementation of any tubular retractor system for minimally invasive cranial surgery does come with a learning curve. It is necessary for the operator to become accustomed to operating within a tubular system as the visualization and angles required may at first seem challenging. Bayonetted instruments are required to allow for visualization while working in the operative field. While some surgeons utilize the BrainPath system with a traditional operating microscope, we have found improved visualization with an exoscope. The Synaptive exoscope increases the field of view for the surgeon and permits a comfortable viewing experience such that awkward positioning is not required.

In this chapter, we have presented three different cases of intraventricular tumors that were accessed and successfully resected with the BrainPath system. These cases encompassed a simple colloid cyst to a vastly overgrown pituitary macroadenoma with significant compression on surrounding neural structures. Resection of a colloid cyst with the BrainPath system should be considered similar to the more traditional interhemispheric approach in that both require operating in tight corridors and anatomic recognition to ensure that the surgeon is the proper ventricle. As such, the colloid cyst provides a good opportunity for a surgeon who is new to the BrainPath system. We consider both the subependymoma and pituitary macroadenoma to be more complex lesions to resect owing to their size and effect on ventricular morphology. If the decision is made to implement the BrainPath system, then it is preferred that the surgeon have some prior experience with the system before attempting to resect more complicated lesions located in the ventricles.

# References


1. Andrews RJ, Bringas JR. A review of brain retraction and recommendations for minimizing intraoperative brain injury. Neurosurgery. 1993;33:1052–63; discussion 1063–1054.
2. Assina R, Rubino S, Sarris CE, Gandhi CD, Prestigiacomo CJ. The history of brain retractors throughout the development of neurological surgery. Neurosurg Focus. 2014;36:E8.
3. Chen CJ, Caruso J, Starke RM, Ding D, Buell T, Crowley RW, et al. Endoport-assisted microsurgical treatment of a ruptured periventricular aneurysm. Case Rep Neurol Med. 2016;2016:8654262.

4. Cohen-Gadol AA. Minitubular transcortical microsurgical approach for gross total resection of third ventricular colloid cysts: technique and assessment. World Neurosurg. 2013;79(207):e207–10.
5. Desai KI, Nadkarni TD, Muzumdar DP, Goel AH. Surgical management of colloid cyst of the third ventricle–a study of 105 cases. Surg Neurol. 2002;57:295–302; discussion 302–294.
6. Ding D, Starke RM, Crowley RW, Liu KC. Endoport-assisted microsurgical resection of cerebral cavernous malformations. J Clin Neurosci. 2015;22:1025–9.
7. Eichberg DG, Buttrick SS, Sharaf JM, Snelling BM, Shah AH, Ivan ME, et al. Use of tubular retractor for rescction of colloid cysts: single surgeon experience and review of the literature. Oper Neurosurg (Hagerstown). 2019;16(5):571–9.
8. Eliyas JK, Glynn R, Kulwin CG, Rovin R, Young R, Alzate J, et al. Minimally invasive trans-sulcal resection of intraventricular and periventricular lesions through a tubular retractor system: multicentric experience and results. World Neurosurg. 2016;90:556–64.
9. Ellenbogen RG. Transcortical surgery for lateral ventricular tumors. Neurosurg Focus. 2001;10:E2.
10. Iyer R, Chaichana KL. Minimally invasive resection of deep-seated high-grade gliomas using tubular retractors and exoscopic visualization. J Neurol Surg A Cent Eur Neurosurg. 2018;79:330–6.
11. Kelly PJ, Goerss SJ, Kall BA. The stereotaxic retractor in computer-assisted stereotaxic microsurgery. Technical note. J Neurosurg. 1988;69:301–6.
12. Labib MA, Shah M, Kassam AB, Young R, Zucker L, Maioriello A, et al. The safety and feasibility of image-guided BrainPath-mediated transsulcul hematoma evacuation: a multicenter study. Neurosurgery. 2017;80:515–24.
13. Milligan BD, Meyer FB. Morbidity of transcallosal and transcortical approaches to lesions in and around the lateral and third ventricles: a single-institution experience. Neurosurgery. 2010;67:1483–96; discussion 1496.
14. Shucart W. Anterior transcollosal and transcortical approaches. In: Apuzzo M, editor. Surgery of the third ventricle. LWW; 1998.
15. Villani R, Tomei G. Approach to tumors of the third ventricle. In: Schmidek H, Roberts D, editors. Schmidek and Sweet's operative neurosurgical techniques: indications, methods, and results. 5th ed. Philadelphia: Saunders Elsevier; 2006. p. 772–85.
16. Zhong J, Dujovny M, Perlin AR, Perez-Arjona E, Park HK, Diaz FG. Brain retraction injury. Neurol Res. 2003;25:831–8.

# Chapter 18
# Future Directions

Gabriel Zada, Gustavo Pradilla, and J. D. Day

In this text, the editors have attempted to, for the first time, comprehensively present an informed approach pertaining to the structure, function, advanced neuro-imaging features, relevant pathology, access, instrumentation, and surgical techniques facilitating modern and safe surgery of the subcortical and intraventricular spaces of the human brain. The expertise and perspectives offered by leading neurological surgeons who have helped to shape this rapidly evolving niche of neurological surgery, and contributed to this reference, collectively provide a curated catalogue for students, trainees, and practicing surgeons who may be interested in current practices guiding treatment of complex subcortical pathology while always maintaining at the forefront of consideration the minimization of collateral damage and preservation of neurological function. It is without question that the particular topic covered by this compendium has been based considerably on recent advancements in neuro-imaging as well as optical and surgical instrumentation technology. Together, these capabilities have created a confluence of various working systems that neurological surgeons can now utilize with greater ease to accurately and more safely access deeper, more intricate, and potentially more eloquent neuroanatomical regions, definitively and safely treating a challenging subset of deeply located vascular and neoplastic lesions. The small field of neurological surgery is limited by its inability to routinely perform large, randomized controlled surgical trials to test the efficacy

G. Zada (✉)
Keck Hospital, Neurological Surgery, Los Angeles, CA, USA
e-mail: gzada@usc.edu

G. Pradilla
Neurological Surgery, Emory University School of Medicine, Atlanta, GA, USA
e-mail: gpradil@emory.edu

J. D. Day
Department of Neurosurgery, University of Arkansas for Medical Sciences,
Little Rock, AR, USA
e-mail: jdday@uams.edu

© Springer Nature Switzerland AG 2022
G. Zada et al. (eds.), *Subcortical Neurosurgery*,
https://doi.org/10.1007/978-3-030-95153-5_18

of each surgical approach or instrument. It is only with gradual evolution and step-wise advancements that surgeons share with one another, via references such as this, that neurosurgical practice can advance until supported by the required levels of evidence to definitively change practice. As an example, neurosurgeons may be on the verge of a new horizon with respect to the management of intracerebral hemorrhage, which is rapidly evolving and may indeed be supported by Level I evidence in the next several years. Advanced neuro-imaging such as diffusion tensor imaging has provided an ability to image and understand previously ignored subcortical fascicles. This has enhanced the ability to select best approaches to navigate around critical white matter tracts in a continuous effort to improve neurological outcomes while maximizing access to deeper subcortical regions. In conjunction with integrated neuro-navigation and ever-evolving miniaturized instrumentation and technology, surgical port retractors provide access to subcortical anatomical compartments with which a variety of tumors and vascular pathology can now be treated. Mapping out the future of this evolution is exciting and encouraging, and we will no doubt see the introduction of fully robotic systems that will provide additional miniaturization and potential for unparalleled tissue handling and maneuverability that is currently unachievable. Multi-port access to deep-seated lesions is another possibility that has not yet been fully harnessed by neurological surgeons, although has become a pillar of minimally invasive surgery in other anatomical compartments such as the thorax and abdomen. It is important to also consider that the entire landscape of management for tumor pathology is changing based on advancements in optical fluorescence and targeted and immune-based treatments. In the future, the role of the surgeon may evolve as tissue sampling and molecular characterization become even more paramount. It is an exciting time for neurological surgeons who perform complex cranial surgery in the subcortical space. The editors are honored to be a part of this journey and to collaborate with leaders in the field who have given these issues thorough consideration and will continue to help shape the future of subcortical neurosurgery for the benefit of generations of patients to come.

# Index